Principles of Specialty Nursing

Under the Auspices of the European Specialist Nurses Organisations (ESNO)

Series Editor
Ber Oomen, European Specialist Nurse Organisation, Arnhem, The Netherlands

The role of the specialist nurse in Europe is still not clearly defined. Despite the fact that there have been formal training programs – e.g. for nurse anaesthetists, operating room nurses, intensive care and mental health nurses – for years now, the practices, status, duration and content of training can vary greatly from country to country. Some other specialist roles, e.g. for Diabetes, Dialysis, Urology and Oncology, have successfully been established in Europe with the help of professional transnational collaborations.

Moreover, advances in medical technologies and more sophisticated treatment will not only require specialist nurses in order to ensure quality and safety of care, but will also call upon them to assume new roles in their professional field to compensate for physician shortages. Most of the available literature on specialty nursing practice currently comes from the USA, Canada, and Australia, and accordingly reflects evidence-based nursing in these countries.

Therefore, there is a need to establish European evidence-based practice on the basis of different clinical experiences. This series, which encompasses textbooks for each specialty, shapes evidence-based practice in Europe, while also integrating lessons learned from other continents. Moreover, it contributes to clarifying the status of the specialist nurse as an advanced practice nurse.

Each volume is dedicated to a specialty such as Mental health and Pyschiatry, firstly published, but also Oncology, Kidney Care, Prevention Control, Vaccination etc. and for most of them, textbooks are supported by ESNO member societies.

Ber Oomen • Silvana Gastaldi
Editors

Principles of Nursing Infection Prevention Control

Enhancing Preparedness:
Implementation Across Diverse Fields
(Volume 2)

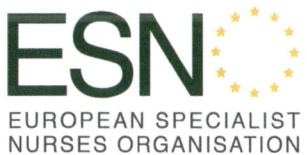

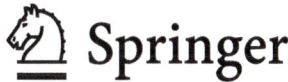

Editors
Ber Oomen
European Specialist Nurse
Organisation (ESNO)
Arnhem, The Netherlands

Silvana Gastaldi ⓘ
Independent Researcher
Mazzano, Italy

ISSN 2366-875X   ISSN 2366-8768   (electronic)
Principles of Specialty Nursing
ISBN 978-3-032-01445-0   ISBN 978-3-032-01446-7   (eBook)
https://doi.org/10.1007/978-3-032-01446-7

Foreword

As a Member of the European Parliament, advancing healthcare resilience across Europe is both a political priority and a personal mission, I very much welcome this second volume on Infection Prevention.

The challenges we face—pandemics, antimicrobial resistance, and increasing global health complexity—demand innovative, coordinated, and sustainable solutions. That's why I fully endorse this second volume on Nurses Roles in Infection Prevention, a book that unites expertise and forward-thinking strategies essential for safeguarding public health in a rapidly evolving world.

Preparedness is a necessity, not a luxury. The COVID-19 pandemic revealed vulnerabilities in our systems and emphasized the value of infection prevention, early response, and leadership at all levels. This book reflects those lessons and provides a guide for future readiness, spotlighting the essential roles of infection prevention and control (IPC), in the advanced nursing professional practice.

It also draws inspiration from Florence Nightingale, who laid the scientific foundations of modern nursing and public health through her focus on hygiene, data, and professionalism. Her vision of the nurse as an educated, responsible leader continues to resonate.

The contributions in *Infection Prevention* advance this legacy—recognizing nurses not only as caregivers but as leaders in combating infection and antimicrobial resistance. With sections on artificial intelligence, scientific rigor, and public health leadership, the book reinforces the need for education, certification, and autonomy for nurses.

As Europe aims to harmonize standards, reduce disparities, and confront global health threats, this book offers a practical, evidence-based roadmap. It highlights the essential role of nurses, who bring scientific expertise, leadership, and a deep commitment to care to the European patients and civil society.

I proudly endorse this work, which makes clear that preparedness is not just about the next crisis—it's about building a workforce capable and empowered to lead us through it.

MEP Andras Kulja, member of the European Parliament Committee on Public Health (SANT)

Preface

Infection prevention and control (IPC) is a critical element in safeguarding public health, where practitioners are at the frontline of patient care. As the world faces an ever-evolving landscape of infectious threats—from hospital-acquired infections to global pandemics—the need for comprehensive, evidence-based strategies in IPC has never been more urgent. *Principles of Nursing Infection Prevention Control* seeks to address these challenges by offering a detailed exploration of infection prevention within diverse contexts, combining historical insights with cutting-edge practices and global perspectives.

This two-volume work has been meticulously curated to serve as both a foundational text for those new to the field and a valuable resource for experienced professionals seeking to refine their practice. Volume 1 introduces readers to the global context of infection prevention, highlighting the essential role nurses play in maintaining patient safety, while also examining the historical and legislative frameworks that shape IPC today. Volume 2 delves into the practical applications of IPC across a variety of environments, emphasizing preparedness and adaptability in diverse healthcare settings.

By fostering an understanding of the fundamental principles of infection control and encouraging a multidisciplinary approach, this book aims to equip healthcare professionals with the tools needed to mitigate infection risks and promote patient safety across all levels of care. We hope this work serves as a catalyst for ongoing education, research, and innovation in this critical field.

Independent Researcher, Mazzano, Italy   Silvana Gastaldi
Arnhem, The Netherlands   Ber Oomen

Contents

Pandemic Preparedness and Infection Prevention and Control

1

Emilio Hornsey, Silvana Gastaldi ⓘ, and April Baller

Abstract

Pandemic preparedness is an evolving global priority requiring integrated strategies that encompass Infection Prevention and Control (IPC), public health, governance, and community engagement. This chapter explores the interconnections between IPC and pandemic preparedness, grounded in historical evidence and emerging paradigms. Lessons from SARS, H1N1, Ebola, and COVID-19 underscore the necessity of early detection, community trust, vaccine equity, and rapid innovation. Technological advances such as artificial intelligence, wastewater surveillance, and whole genome sequencing are revolutionizing disease forecasting and outbreak containment, yet they risk exacerbating inequities without deliberate policy interventions.

The WHO's Health Emergency Preparedness, Response and Resilience (HEPR) framework, the revised International Health Regulations (IHR 2005), and new global strategies on IPC set the stage for more coordinated, resilient responses. Nevertheless, contested areas—such as the expanding application of IPC outside healthcare settings, persistent global health inequities, and the fragility of health systems in humanitarian crises—demand renewed scrutiny.

E. Hornsey (✉)
UK Public Health Rapid Support Team, UK Health Security Agency/London School of
Hygiene & Tropical Medicine, London, UK
e-mail: Emilio.Hornsey@ukhsa.gov.uk

S. Gastaldi
Independent Researcher, Mazzano, Italy

A. Baller
WHO Health Emergencies Programme, Geneva, Switzerland

The chapter also highlights the crucial role of community health workers, adaptive healthcare infrastructure, and robust supply chain strategies in ensuring systemic resilience. Legal and nonbinding governance instruments—ranging from the WHO IPC framework to regional regulatory mechanisms—are discussed as foundations for coordinated action. An equity-centered, context-specific, and multidisciplinary approach emerges as essential for future pandemic preparedness, especially in the face of global challenges like climate change, geopolitical instability, and antimicrobial resistance.

Ultimately, IPC must be repositioned as both a core public health function and a driver of resilient, inclusive systems prepared to prevent and respond to pandemics across diverse settings.

Keywords

Pandemic preparedness · Infection prevention · Healthcare resilience · Climate change · Emerging diseases · Healthcare worker preparedness

1.1   Introduction

Pandemic preparedness is more than a political or technical requirement; it is a shared responsibility in an increasingly interconnected world. The COVID-19 pandemic brought this reality into sharp focus, exposing how un- or underprepared systems make societies vulnerable—from overflowing hospitals to widespread economic hardships. Infection Prevention and Control (IPC) is at the center of any response effort, providing a protective shield that can stop individual cases or small outbreaks from developing into large-scale epidemics.

While the global scale and implications of pandemics require specific considerations for preparedness, all pandemics start as smaller outbreaks or epidemics. So, immediate and locally implemented IPC interventions to avoid and minimize all outbreaks are key elements of pandemic preparedness.

The distinction between outbreaks, epidemics, and pandemics can be contested, and while there may be reasons for using a particular terminology, the WHO uses the declaration of a Public Health Emergency of International Concern (PHEIC[1]) to focus attention and mobilize resources.[2] The criteria used for this declaration include not just the number and rate of growth of infections but also the potential consequences of the outbreak.

---

[1] WHO Definition of PHEIC *"an extraordinary event which is determined to constitute a public health risk to other States through the international spread of disease and to potentially require a coordinated international response"*.

[2] Available at: https://www.who.int/news-room/questions-and-answers/item/emergencies-international-health-regulations-and-emergency-committees

1.1.1   Evolution of Pandemic Preparedness and IPC

Research by Laage-Thomsen and Frandsen has shown how pandemic preparedness plans developed in the early 2000s by countries like Denmark, Norway, and Sweden were significantly influenced by the World Health Organization's (WHO) growing emphasis on preparedness. These plans underwent crucial transformations following the H1N1 pandemic, which exposed weaknesses in health crisis management systems [1].

The International Health Regulations 2005 (IHR) [2] have been a cornerstone in aligning global pandemic responses. These regulations emphasize the necessity of robust surveillance systems, coordinated actions, and the protection of human rights during health emergencies. The IHR's universal scope ensures its relevance across diverse infectious threats, guiding nations in preventing the global spread of diseases while maintaining equity and transparency.

More recently based on lessons learnt from the COVID-19 pandemic, to strengthen pandemic preparedness and response, WHO launched the global architecture Health Emergency Preparedness, Prevention, Response and Resilience (HEPR) initiative, as well as advocating for the establishment of the Pandemic Agreement and Pandemic Fund [3]. There have also been amendments to IHR accordingly.

Similarly, the Global Strategy on Infection Prevention and Control [4], the Global Action Plan and monitoring framework 2024–2030 [5] (which have been endorsed by Member States through two resolutions), define strategic objectives to prevent healthcare-associated infections, through developing national IPC action plans for implementing national- and facility-level IPC programs, coordinating IPC with other health priorities, and monitoring implementation.

This chapter will showcase examples from previous pandemics to highlight lessons and evolutions in pandemic preparedness. It will also discuss areas for growth and advancement in pandemic preparedness as well as draw attention to contested and neglected needs with respect to IPC.

1.2   Historical Pandemics: Lessons Learnt and Implications

Experience can provide valuable lessons about pandemic response and preparedness. Each historical event has contributed unique insights to our understanding of effective IPC and public health and social measures (PHSM).

1.2.1   SARS (2002): The Power of Sharing Information

The SARS pandemic of 2002–2004 served as a crucial wake-up call for global health systems. Beginning in Asia, it rapidly spread across continents, disrupting lives and economies. The World Health Organization (WHO) led the efforts to share information between countries, demonstrating how transparency and collaboration can facilitate containment of an outbreak.

SARS underscored the importance of global surveillance networks like the Epidemic Intelligence from Open Sources (EIOS) initiative, which enables real-time sharing of epidemiological data. These systems help nations act quickly, limiting spread and minimizing harm. The outbreak also catalyzed the development of more robust response frameworks like the 2016 amendment of the IHR [2], which include commitments to transparent reporting and coordination for any new and evolving health threat.

1.2.2   H1N1 Influenza (2009): Vaccines as Game-Changers

The H1N1 pandemic demonstrated both the promise and challenges of vaccine development and distribution. The rapid development of an H1N1 vaccine was groundbreaking, but access inequities became apparent as high-income countries secured vaccines while others struggled.

This experience provided practical insights into how parallel investments in vaccine development, trials, licensing, and production could speed up availability of vaccines, which would later prove crucial during COVID-19 [6]. It also highlighted the importance of maintaining a well-funded, globally connected public health research ecosystem.

1.2.3   Ebola (2014–2016): The Value of Community Trust

The 2014–2016 Ebola outbreak in West Africa revealed the critical importance of community trust and engagement, in addition to IPC in pandemic response. While safe burial practices and quarantine measures were essential, their effectiveness hinged on community acceptance and trust in the healthcare system. In areas of Sierra Leone where community-based responses, rooted in social mobilization and community engagement, were utilized, transmission of EVD was halted more swiftly compared to other areas where the response was controlled centrally [7]. Research by Li, ZJ et al. has highlighted how a lack of preparedness within health and social care systems can lead to increased infection rates among healthcare providers, patients, and in the communities [8].

Health workers in Liberia and Sierra Leone successfully led education campaigns that helped communities understand the virus and necessary containment measures [9]. This experience demonstrated that pandemic response requires more than medical counter measures —it demands community engagement, resilience, and cultural sensitivity.

1.2.4   COVID-19 (2019–2024): Learning the Hard Way

The COVID-19 pandemic exposed significant vulnerabilities in healthcare systems, while simultaneously demonstrating humanity's capacity for rapid innovation.

Rapid development of therapeutics, vaccines, PPE, and disinfection tools are all examples of this; however, their impact was affected by the unequal access to resources across the world. COVID-19 highlighted that innovation requires interpretation and adaptation of guidance to meet the needs of all. For example, the promotion of natural ventilation in congregate settings.

During the COVID-19 pandemic, IPC expertise was sought more widely within the community (in addition to healthcare), to support congregate settings like schools, churches, prisons, and public transport (airplanes, cruises). There was a broader public recognition of what IPC entails, with the boundaries between IPC, PHSM, Health Protection and Hygiene becoming blurred in many contexts.

1.3   New Paradigms in Pandemic Preparedness

Pandemic preparedness in today's interconnected world requires innovative approaches that integrate technology, healthcare system resilience, and community engagement. We will discuss the impact of technological advancements, innovative approaches to surveillance, and different aspects of enhancing resilience.

1.3.1   Technological Integration in Preparedness

The integration of cutting-edge technology into pandemic preparedness represents a paradigm shift in how we approach the detection, management, and prevention of infectious diseases. Among the most transformative tools are artificial intelligence (AI) and big data analytics, which have revolutionized disease surveillance and outbreak prediction. These technologies enable health systems to move beyond reactive responses, empowering them to anticipate and mitigate risks before they escalate into global crises.

One of the most illustrative examples of technological advancements in disease surveillance is the World Health Organization's Epidemic Intelligence from Open Sources (EIOS) system. This platform leverages AI to automatically analyze a vast array of global health data, including news reports, social media updates, and official public health communications. By processing this information in real time, EIOS identifies potential outbreaks early, often before they are formally reported. This capacity for rapid detection not only accelerates public health responses, but also enhances global collaboration, by providing actionable intelligence to multiple stakeholders. For further details, the official WHO EIOS initiative can be explored at WHO EIOS.[3]

AI also now plays a role in predictive modeling, offering tools to forecast the trajectory of disease outbreaks. By integrating diverse data sources, such as environmental factors, population mobility, and epidemiological patterns, models provide governments and health organizations with actionable forecasts. For instance,

---

[3] Available at: https://www.who.int/initiatives/eios

during the COVID-19 pandemic, predictive modeling informed resource allocation and public health interventions, demonstrating its utility in real-world crisis management.

1.3.2 Pandemic Surveillance for IPC

IPC is, in some respects, a practical application of epidemiology, as IPC utilizes surveillance data among other forms of information to inform interventions, therefore advancements in capacity for surveillance and epidemiology provide IPC with data to guide action [10].

Wastewater surveillance has emerged as a valuable tool in pandemic preparedness, providing a noninvasive, cost-effective method for early detection of infectious disease outbreaks within communities [11]. By monitoring viral RNA and other biomarkers shed in human waste, public health authorities can track the prevalence and spread of pathogens such as SARS-CoV-2, sometimes before clinical cases are reported [12]. This approach enables timely public health interventions and resource allocation, particularly in areas with limited access to healthcare or diagnostic testing. It can also be targeted to specific sites like health facilities, making results even more relevant for IPC. As such, wastewater-based epidemiology serves as a critical component of integrated disease surveillance systems, enhancing situational awareness and response capabilities during public health emergencies [13].

Another critical technological advancement lies in Whole Genome Sequencing (WGS), which has become indispensable in tracking and understanding pathogens, even within healthcare facilities (healthcare-associated outbreaks). WGS allows for the precise identification of viral variants, tracking of transmission chains, and detection of emerging mutations associated with increased transmissibility, virulence, or immune escape. While WGS has been available for some time, the resources and lengthy time required for results has, until recently, meant that it could only be used for research or retrospective analysis of outbreaks. The speed with which WGS can now been conducted means that results can be used to inform interventions during responses [14]. Integrating WGS into routine surveillance frameworks enhances the capacity to monitor pathogen evolution and adapt response efforts dynamically, thereby strengthening preparedness and response. This technology became a cornerstone of the global response to COVID-19, allowing monitoring of viral mutations and the emergence of new variants. Such insights were instrumental in the development and adjustment of vaccines, as well as in guiding public health policies. Platforms like the Global Initiative on Sharing Avian Influenza Data (GISAID) exemplify the power of open data sharing, fostering global cooperation and transparency in genomic research. To explore GISAID's contributions, visit GISAID.org.[4]

---

[4] Available at: https://www.gisaid.org/

However positive these technological advancements are, they do not resolve the structural inequalities that hinder implementation. Hurdles such as disparities in digital infrastructure, data privacy concerns, and limited access in low-resource settings are some of many issues that continue to limit impact. Addressing these barriers requires strategic investments, international collaboration, and robust policy frameworks that prioritize equitable access and ethical use of technology.

Ultimately, the integration of AI, genomic sequencing, and digital tools into pandemic preparedness offers unprecedented opportunities to strengthen global health systems. By leveraging these innovations, public health responses can become more proactive, data-driven, and equitable, ensuring that we are better equipped to navigate the uncertainties of future pandemics.

1.3.3 Healthcare System Resilience: Examples of Supply Chains

Research by Shahid et al. has demonstrated that well-prepared general hospitals can significantly reduce the demand for specialized healthcare services during pandemics [9]. Their work emphasizes the fundamental importance of flexible infrastructure in healthcare settings, from primary care, where most of the health care is delivered, through to specialist services with integrated referral mechanisms. Modern healthcare facilities should be designed with adaptability in mind, incorporating modular spaces that can be quickly repurposed during surge events. This approach allows hospitals to rapidly scale their capacity while maintaining essential services [15].

The COVID-19 pandemic highlighted the critical nature of robust supply chain management in healthcare settings. Local manufacturing, developing reusable alternatives with decontamination protocols, combined with strategic stockpiling of critical supplies are vital approaches for maintaining healthcare resilience. This evolution in supply chain thinking represents a significant shift from the just-in-time inventory systems that proved vulnerable during recent health crises. This is especially pertinent in IPC, where many of the consumable supplies such as PPE and cleaning materials are low-margin, high-volume items, where economic pressures have led to highly centralized production.

1.3.4 Community Health Workers and Grassroots Implementation

Boyce and Katz's research on the role of community health workers (CHWs) in resource-constrained environments demonstrates how CHWs serve as essential bridges between formal healthcare systems and local communities [16]. CHWs play a multifaceted role in pandemic preparedness and response, operating at the crucial intersection of clinical care and community engagement.

The impact of CHWs stems from their deep understanding of local contexts and cultural nuances. Through building trust within their communities, they facilitate better acceptance and implementation of IPC measures. This trust-building process involves continuous engagement, culturally appropriate health education, and consistent presence in the community. Research has shown that communities with active CHW programs demonstrate significantly higher rates of adherence to public health measures during disease outbreaks.

Communication effectiveness represents another crucial aspect of CHW impact. Through their intimate knowledge of local dialects and languages, customs, and communication patterns, CHWs can translate complex medical concepts into accessible information for their communities. This capability proves especially valuable during rapidly evolving health crises, where quick dissemination of accurate information can save lives.

Furthermore, CHWs contribute significantly to early warning systems, through their constant presence in communities. Their ability to identify unusual health patterns or emerging concerns often provides the first indication of potential outbreaks. This early detection capability, combined with their established communication channels with formal health systems, creates an effective surveillance network that can trigger rapid response mechanisms when needed.

1.4   Integrating Law, Guidelines, and Governance for IPC in Pandemic Preparedness

1.4.1   Legal and Regulatory Frameworks

These provide the foundation for wider pandemic preparedness, defining the rights, responsibilities, and enforcement mechanisms for governments, institutions, and individuals. Globally, these include the previously mentioned IHR and the Pandemic Agreement. International Development Law Organization [17] has emphasized the critical role of comprehensive legal preparedness in addressing health threats and emergencies. These frameworks not only provide the structural guidelines for action, but also ensure that responses are coordinated, efficient, and equitable.

To strengthen these frameworks, governments and international bodies must prioritize the integration of adaptable legal measures into national and regional health policies, enabling more agile responses to emerging threats. A notable example is the Africa Centers for Disease Control and Prevention's (Africa CDC) Infection Prevention and Control (IPC) Legal Framework, which provides guidelines for member states to enhance IPC measures across the continent.[5]

1.4.2   Supporting Nonbinding Frameworks and Guidelines

Voluntary guidelines and technical recommendations help fill gaps, harmonize standards, and align evidence-based practice. The nonbinding WHO framework

---

[5] Available at: https://africacdc.org/news-item/africa-cdc-ipc-legal-framework/

and toolkit for IPC in outbreak preparedness, readiness, and response [18, 19] is one such resource, and complements legal and regulatory frameworks by offering an operational approach, tailored for national and healthcare facility level.

The WHO framework delineates three critical health emergency phases and the respective key activities that should be implemented:

1. *Preparedness phase (2 years to 6 months pre-outbreak)*: Establishing foundational IPC programs, coordination mechanisms, surge capacity, HAI systems and partnerships, stockpiling essential resources, and training personnel. These align with legal mandates to ensure readiness through enforceable protocols and budget allocations.
2. *Readiness phase (up to 6 months pre-outbreak)*: Adapting existing IPC protocols to specific threats, ensuring robust surveillance systems, and conducting simulation exercises. Legal frameworks support these actions by facilitating cross-border agreements and data sharing.
3. *Response phase (during the outbreak)*: Activating pre-developed IPC strategies, guidelines and protocols, optimizing human, financial and logistical resource allocation, and conducting intra/after-action reviews to refine ongoing responses. Legal provisions ensure swift implementation and compliance.

In addition to both binding and nonbinding legal frameworks and guidelines, effective governance and coordination mechanisms are vital to ensure both legal frameworks and implementation of operational guidelines are effectively aligned across different sectors and levels of government.

1.5 Contested and Critical Areas

1.5.1 Infection Prevention and Control in Communities

The WHO definition of IPC is as a "practical, evidence-based approach preventing patients and health workers from being harmed by avoidable infections"[6] and the USCDC describes the role of IPC to "prevent or stop the spread of infections in healthcare settings".[7] Recently, the term IPC has been used much more widely to describe community-based interventions that might otherwise or previously be described as health protection, hygiene or public health and social measures. The blurring of boundaries between IPC in health settings and hygiene measures in

---

[6] World Health Organization. Infection prevention and control [Internet]. Geneva: World Health Organization; [cited 2025 May 24]. Available from: https://www.who.int/health-topics/infection-prevention-and-control#tab=tab_1

[7] Centers for Disease Control and Prevention. About infection control [Internet]. Atlanta: Centers for Disease Control and Prevention; [cited 2025 May 24]. Available from: https://www.cdc.gov/infection-control/about/index.html

communities became more pronounced during the COVID 19 pandemic, when measures traditionally applied in health settings (such as masks) became common practice in the wider community. The name itself, 'infection prevention and control' does not recognize the setting, and the words taken literally could mean any community-based intervention. This lack of clarity among stakeholders has led, and may continue to lead to misunderstanding and misinterpretation in communication between agencies and individuals.

1.5.2   Inequity

By embedding equity into IPC strategies, public health systems can foster resilience, ensure inclusivity, and achieve better outcomes in controlling infectious diseases. These lessons from the COVID-19 pandemic provide a roadmap for building healthier, more equitable communities in the future.

An equitable approach to IPC will ensure that all populations benefit from protective measures, regardless of their socioeconomic status, geographic location, or other factors. Vaccine equity emerged as a critical challenge during the COVID-19 pandemic. Despite efforts, such as the COVAX initiative, low-income countries faced significant barriers to accessing vaccines. Many regions reported that less than half of their healthcare workers had been vaccinated during critical phases of the pandemic. A similar situation is now being experienced during the ongoing Mpox pandemic [20]. Likewise, PPE was bought by high-income countries at the expense of lower resource areas when supply chains were under pressure. There are long-standing issues of medical PPE not being designed specifically for health workers (who are 70% female) in the global south, as design and testing is based around males in the global north [21].

1.5.3   Humanitarian Crisis and Conflict

Conflict significantly undermines infection prevention and control (IPC) efforts by disrupting healthcare infrastructure, displacing populations, and limiting access to clean water, sanitation, and medical supplies. Health facilities may be damaged or destroyed, and health workers may face threats to their safety, leading to workforce shortages. Surveillance programs, that may provide early warning of a pandemic, become even more challenging. In these circumstances, basic IPC practices like hand hygiene, decontamination of medical devices, and isolation of infectious patients may become difficult or impossible to maintain, increasing the impact of disease outbreaks and the spread of antimicrobial resistance. The destabilizing effect of conflict on pandemic preparedness and IPC is an area of concern, as disrupted surveillance infrastructure and diversion of resources severely limit a country's ability to detect, respond to, and contain infectious disease outbreaks [22].

1.6   Conclusion

The evolution of infection prevention and control in the context of pandemic preparedness reflects our growing appreciation of the complexities between medical science, socioeconomic factors, and global cooperation within an increasingly interconnected and a rapidly evolving global landscape. Success requires integrating historical lessons with modern innovations while addressing political, financial, technical, and human elements of emergencies.

IPC needs to be integrated into resilient health systems, addressing current challenges such as antimicrobial resistance (AMR), alongside preparing for future health emergencies. Strong governance and leadership are central to this effort. At the national and subnational levels, dedicated IPC leadership ensures consistent oversight and coordination of measures. Interventions must also emphasize equity, inclusivity, and collaboration across sectors to address disparities in healthcare access and resources.

As health challenges continue, with prospects of increasing frequency, our ability to learn, adapt, and collaborate will determine our resilience against emerging and reemerging health threats.

Acknowledgments The UK Public Health Rapid Support Team is funded by UK Aid from the Department of Health and Social Care and is jointly run by the UK Health Security Agency and the London School of Hygiene & Tropical Medicine. The views expressed in this publication are those of the author(s) and not necessarily those of the Department of Health and Social Care.

References

1. Laage-Thomsen J, Frandsen SL. Pandemic preparedness systems and diverging COVID-19 responses within similar public health regimes: a comparative study of expert perceptions of pandemic response in Denmark, Norway, and Sweden. Global Health. 2022;18:3. https://doi.org/10.1186/s12992-022-00799-4.
2. World Health Organization, editor. International Health Regulations (2005). 3rd ed. World Health Organization; 2016. Available at https://iris.who.int/handle/10665/246107.
3. World Health Organization. Strengthening health emergency prevention, preparedness, response and resilience. Geneva: World Health Organization; 2023. Licence: CC BY-NC-SA 3.0 IGO.
4. World Health Organization. Global strategy on infection prevention and control. Geneva; 2023. Licence: CC BY-NC-SA 3.0 IGO.
5. World Health Organization. Global action plan and monitoring framework on infection prevention and control (IPC), 2024–2030: annexes. Geneva: World Health Organization; 2024. Available from: https://cdn.who.int/media/docs/default-source/integrated-health-services-(ihs)/ipc/ipc-global-action-plan/who_gampf_w_annexes.pdf?sfvrsn=aef723f7_3&ua=1.
6. Ankomah AA, Moa A, Chughtai AA. The long road of pandemic vaccine development to roll-out: a systematic review on the lessons learnt from the 2009 H1N1 influenza pandemic. Am J Infect Control. 2022;50(7):735–42. https://doi.org/10.1016/j.ajic.2022.01.026. Epub 2022 Feb 4. PMID: 35131349; PMCID: PMC8815192.
7. Bedson J, Jalloh MF, Pedi D, Bah S, Owen K, Oniba A, et al. Community engagement in outbreak response: lessons from the 2014–2016 Ebola outbreak in Sierra Leone. BMJ Glob Health. 2020;5(8):e002145. https://doi.org/10.1136/bmjgh-2019-002145.

8. Li ZJ, Tu WX, Wang XC, et al. A practical community-based response strategy to interrupt Ebola transmission in sierra Leone, 2014–2015. Infect Dis Poverty. 2016;5:74. https://doi.org/10.1186/s40249-016-0167-0.

9. Cénat JM, Broussard C, Darius WP, Onesi O, Auguste E, El Aouame AM, Ukwu G, Khodabocus SN, Labelle PR, Dalexis RD. Social mobilization, education, and prevention of the Ebola virus disease: a scoping review. Prev Med. 2023;166:107328. https://doi.org/10.1016/j.ypmed.2022.107328. Epub 2022 Nov 8.

10. Kim JO, St. John KH, Coffin SE. Epidemiology and infection prevention and control. In: Pediatric infectious diseases; 2008. p. 385–91. https://doi.org/10.1016/B978-0-323-02041-1.50046-8. Epub 2020 Jun 22. PMCID: PMC7310929.

11. Wise J. Poliovirus is detected in sewage from north and east London. BMJ. 2022;377:o1546. https://doi.org/10.1136/bmj.o1546.

12. Trigo-Tasende N, Vallejo JA, Rumbo-Feal S, et al. Wastewater early warning system for SARS-CoV-2 outbreaks and variants in a Coruña, Spain. Environ Sci Pollut Res. 2023;30:79315–34. https://doi.org/10.1007/s11356-023-27877-3.

13. Grassly NC, et al. Global wastewater surveillance for pathogens with pandemic potential: opportunities and challenges. Lancet Microbe. 2025;6(1):100939.

14. World Health Organization. Whole genome sequencing as a tool to strength en foodborne disease surveillance and response. Module 2. Whole genome sequencing in foodborne disease outbreak investigations. Geneva: World Health Organization; 2023. Licence: CC BY-NC-SA 3.0 IGO.

15. Łukasik M, Porębska A. Responsiveness and adaptability of healthcare facilities in emergency scenarios: COVID-19 experience. Int J Environ Res Public Health. 2022;19(2):675. https://doi.org/10.3390/ijerph19020675. PMID: 35055493; PMCID: PMC8775513.

16. Shahid A, Zahra T, Mahwish R, Zaidi SMAA. Preparedness of public hospitals for the coronavirus (COVID-19) pandemic in Lahore District, Pakistan. Cureus. 2022;14(2):e22477. https://doi.org/10.7759/cureus.22477. PMID: 35371716; PMCID: PMC8943522.

17. Boyce MR, Katz R. Community health workers and pandemic preparedness: current and prospective roles. Front Public Health. 2019;26(7):62. https://doi.org/10.3389/fpubh.2019.00062. PMID: 30972316; PMCID: PMC6443984.

18. International Development Law Organization (IDLO). Preventing pandemics through the rule of law: strengthening countries' legal preparedness for public health emergencies. Rome: IDLO; 2023.

19. World Health Organization. Framework and toolkit for infection prevention and control in outbreak preparedness, readiness and response at the health care facility level. Geneva: World Health Organization; 2022. Licence: CC BY-NC-SA 3.0 IGO.

20. Adepoju P. African mpox surges show lack of vaccine access. Lancet. 2024;404(10447):18. https://doi.org/10.1016/S0140-6736(24)01393-X. PMID: 38972316.

21. Thompson R, et al. Fit for women? Safe and decent PPE for women health and care workers Women in Global Health; 2021. Available from: https://womeningh.org/wp-content/uploads/2022/11/WGH-Fit-for-Women-report-2021.pdf.

22. Lowe H, Woodd S, Lange IL, Janjanin S, Barnet J, Graham W. Challenges and opportunities for infection prevention and control in hospitals in conflict-affected settings: a qualitative study. Confl Health. 2021;15(1):94. https://doi.org/10.1186/s13031-021-00428-8. Erratum in: Confl Health. 2022;16(1):2. https://doi.org/10.1186/s13031-022-00433-5. PMID: 34930364; PMCID: PMC8686079.

Compassionate Care and Infection Prevention: A Holistic Guide to Safeguarding Health and Well-Being

2

Julie Storr ⓘ

During the COVID-19 pandemic, we have left too many people alone unnecessarily, deprived of human contact other than healthcare workers, and with many people in care spending their last moments alone. Clinical isolation should never mean human isolation. The harms of this human disconnection can be immense, in some cases greater than the harms of the infection.

ESNO (2022)

Abstract

The ethical concerns and unintended consequences associated with the precautionary measures espoused by IPC guidance has come to the fore in recent years. The COVID-19 pandemic intensified the tension between IPC measures and the need for their compassionate implementation. Evidence on the impact of compassion on improved patient outcomes, suggests that empathy-driven care enhances treatment effectiveness, fosters a supportive environment, and strengthens primary healthcare systems. The visitor restrictions imposed across health care settings resulted in prolonged isolation, emotional distress, and ethical dilemmas for patients, families, and healthcare providers. Recent discourse suggests a need to move away from a pure focus on the biomedical model towards a more person-centred approach to IPC, emphasizing the need to balance safety with psychosocial well-being, including the need for humane IPC policies and their implementation. Seven practice, policy, and research considerations are presented to address these issues and novel frameworks such as the Ethical

J. Storr (✉)
S3 Global Health (KS Healthcare Consulting), Glasgow, Scotland, UK

13

Infection Prevention and Control Decision-Making Framework that aim to guide practitioners in making balanced, ethical decisions across various healthcare settings.

Keywords

Compassion · Person-centredness · Fundamental care · Decision-making · Ethics

2.1   Introduction

Upon prompting a large language model with a question on the extent of the published literature addressing nursing and compassion, the generated text highlights that a great deal of material exists on the theoretical foundations, the existence of models of compassionate care, its impact on patient outcomes, the challenges and barriers and the value of compassion embedded in nursing curricula [1]. When undertaking the same task but replacing the word nursing with IPC the result suggests that although there is growing interest in this intersection, publications are not as extensive as in the general nursing compassion literature. This starting point acts as a bellwether for the chapter which will drill into these matters looking at the available evidence to explore what is meant by compassionate care in the context of IPC but framed within the wider context of person-centredness, since compassion is but one element of person-centredness. The quotation at the start of this chapter from the European Specialist Nurses Association [2] outlines in a powerful and a profound way a key focus of the topic under the spotlight in which an example from the COVID-19 pandemic will be used to highlight critical points around compassion and IPC and the important role that nurses play in implementing IPC given their ubiquity within the health care workforce.

2.2   Learning from the Past

IPC came to prominence in the latter half of the twentieth century with its focus on stopping potential pathogens from spreading in hospitals. The traditional weapons in the IPC armoury have been described as those mainly informed by biological sciences, epidemiology, and surveillance. Historically IPC was implemented mainly through education—teach it and they will do it [3]. Training was focused on ensuring policies were translated into practice and its impact was measured through audit and in some cases informed by legal frameworks. Incorporating the social sciences within IPC was not high on the agenda. Storr [4] emphasised the importance of applying IPC from a holistic, rights-based perspective that addressed dignity of the patient and was based on ethical principles. She raised the issue of the unintended consequences of some IPC guidelines, referencing a paper by Braut and Holt [5] on MRSA challenges, highlighting cases where colonised patients with dementia were isolated for long periods and in some cases denied access to their family physician, with consultations taking place in a parking lot. These authors highlighted the balancing act between implementing guidelines to ensure patient and health worker safety while at the same time being aware of the ethical dilemmas such implementation can raise and asked the question "Oh God, what are we doing". Parallels were drawn to previous infectious diseases and lessons learned (or not), for example, from the stigma surrounding the treatment of those with HIV and AIDS.

2.3   The Evolving Role of Compassion in Achieving Safe, Quality Care

Compassion has been described as having three essential elements that are not necessarily sequential; awareness of the suffering of others (cognitive appraisal); the ability to empathise or demonstrate an empathic response with the suffering of others; and importantly empathic resonance coupled with action to relieve and prevent suffering [6, 7]. This third element takes compassion one step beyond empathy in that it also requires action to alleviate suffering. Klein-Bingham et al. [7] summarise the essence of the matter, drawing on the seminal work of Kruk by stating that "ethical, respectful and compassionate care, and the fundamentals of systems thinking, and quality improvement should be additional core competencies [for health professionals]" [8]. Kleine-Bingham et al. go on to highlight that when patients perceive their health care provider as being compassionate, health outcomes improve and cite the work of Trzeciak and Mazzarelli [9], and the World Health Organization [10]. In their book, Trzeciak et al. have brought to the world's attention the growing evidence that demonstrates how compassionate care can have a tangible impact on patient outcome including on specific illnesses such as migraine, and also how it can enhance immune responses and reduce depression.

A more recent publication [11] on compassion and primary healthcare (PHC) has kept the issue in the global spotlight and reinforces its critical role in the delivery of quality care. Informed by frontline realities, the report details examples of how compassion helps to improve PHC by creating a supportive environment for both patients and staff. One of the key messages of the report is the critical role of leaders and the importance of effective leadership, including role modelling, in driving a culture where compassion thrives. In a recent narrative review, Ahmed et al. [12] drill further into these matters, exploring the existing literature on compassion and leadership and their combined impact on patient safety and healthcare quality. Their findings indicate that both compassion and transformational leadership play a crucial role in fostering a positive organisational culture within healthcare settings. Specifically, leaders who demonstrate compassion are more effective in encouraging healthcare professionals to prioritise patient safety and quality and act as role models in inspiring their teams to deliver safer, patient-centred care. In a similar vein, Pattison et al. [13] explore what they describe as relational leadership styles, which embrace compassionate, collective, and transformational leadership, and its relationship with fundamental care. The fundamentals of care theoretical framework [14] explains, guides, and predicts nursing interactions with patients, carers, and their families at the point of care. Fundamental care has been described as a central tenet of care, which "involves actions on the part of the nurse that respect and focus on a person's essential needs to ensure their physical and psychosocial well-being" [15]. Indeed awareness of the importance of the psychosocial aspects of the patient experience have been described as making a significant contribution to the value and understanding of compassion in recent years [6].

2.4   IPC and Compassion—Lessons from a Modern Pandemic

In their literature review on the epidemiology of compassion, Addis and colleagues [6] describe the causal pathways leading from suffering to a compassionate response as non-linear and complex. In 2020 these complexities came to the fore in relation to the provision and implementation of IPC guidance within a compassionate milieu. During the COVID-19 pandemic IPC measures, including strict visitor restrictions in healthcare and aged care settings, were implemented to protect public health. While initially accepted as necessary, these measures had profound emotional and ethical consequences to everyone involved—both healthcare professionals and patients and their loved ones. Measures often involved separating loved ones for extended periods. Some healthcare institutions exercised discretion, but inconsistencies in decision-making led to prolonged isolation for many and in some cases people suffered and died without loved ones near.

Attempts were made to highlight the need for balancing safety with compassionate care, emphasising that IPC should enable, not prevent, human connection and that IPC decisions should balance both physical safety and psychosocial well-being [16]. In an open letter published in the Nursing Times, five considerations were presented to help stimulate action and empower and support those on the receiving end of restrictions and those being told to enforce them in a non-negotiable manner. These can be summarised as follows: IPC should enable not prevent safe entry for family and close friends into long-term care facilities, even during lockdowns. IPC decision-making must balance safety and compassionate care, avoiding unnecessary restrictions, and recognising the caregiving role of families alongside paid caregivers [17].

Acknowledgement of the need to rebalance the concept of safety with the need for compassion saw a number of organisations step forward. The ESNO issued its position statement that was touched on earlier in the chapter. Entitled "clinical isolation should never mean human isolation" [2] the position statement included a three-pronged call to action to all healthcare organisations: first that all stakeholders recognise and mitigate the impact that clinical isolation has on the physical, psychological, and social well-being of persons; second that IPC measures informed by the best available evidence, balanced with the holistic needs of patients and relatives are implemented humanely and from a perspective of person-centredness (in particular during end-of-life and maternity stages), and limited to the immediate crisis only, and finally support for those wishing the right to "speak out" to promote compassion, connectivity, and encourage those in responsible position to initiated education with a preference in interdisciplinary context and above all in collaboration with patient organisations and institutional representatives.

Before moving on you are now invited to pause for a moment and to consider your own IPC guidance and, in particular, the extent to which it addresses the importance of communication with patients in a way that embraces compassion. To what extent does it highlight the need to address the impact that precautionary measures might have on the psychosocial well-being of the recipient of those precautions and their loved ones?

2.5   Person-Centredness and the Quest to Humanise IPC

The Health Foundation [18] identified a framework for person-centred care in which they highlight how such care involves healthcare professionals working collaboratively with service users. They explain how person-centred care supports people to more effectively manage and make informed decisions about their own health and healthcare. Within such a framework people are treated with dignity, compassion, and respect and care is coordinated, personalised, and enabling. Building on this, Storr et al. [19] reflect on whether IPC, rooted in a biomedical model centred around germ theory, dominated the entire health system during the 2020 pandemic and appeared to shape hospital visitor policies. Furthermore, that the biomedical narrative dominated the pandemic response and likely eclipsed other ways of thinking about what is right and just. Acolin and colleagues [20] have also suggested that this biomedical model shaped the COVID-19 response, and they called for a paradigm shift to overcome some of the person-centred failures this resulted in. In interviews with relatives restricted from visiting their loved ones, Loft et al. [21] explain how relatives saw the restrictions as a necessary evil. As Storr et al. [19] emphasise, if IPC is to be humanised, there is a need to challenge this "necessary evil" mantra, and strive for person-centred and safe solutions to the challenges posed by infection. All health workers, including nurses, have a role to play in this; however, for person-centred IPC to be fully realised, action is needed at both the practice and policy level as well as the need to undertake further research in this neglected area. Storr et al. present seven considerations in this regard (Box 2.1).

> **Box 2.1: Seven Practice, Policy, and Research Considerations [19]**
> 1. International and national IPC guidance and implementation resources must address principles of person-centredness. Values such as critical thinking and responding to unexpected and sub-optimal conditions alongside following guidelines and algorithms by rote should be emphasized.
> 2. Nurses and IPC leaders must be included in ethical decision-making processes in future pandemics, at all levels.

(continued)

Box 2.1 (continued)

3. Where not in place, collaboration between IPC and nurse training institutions must exist to strengthen aspects of compassion-informed decision-making and ethical competence.

4. Policy briefs should be available and must focus on person-centred mitigations associated with the non-transmission related consequences of each element of the IPC hierarchy of controls.

5. A research agenda that aims to reach a model of embodied compassion in IPC decision-making throughout the health system, using the COVID-19 experience as an example, should exist.

6. Research should ensure that perspectives from low-, middle- and high-income settings are considered and that the factors influencing the ability to implement person-centred approaches be considered.

7. International and national IPC guidance and any IPC guidance that includes restrictions should be accompanied by implementation tools to support front line staff including unambiguous definitions re local discretion and an emphasis on healthcare professionals and patients /loved ones working together in decision-making.

That multiple factors affect decision-making in healthcare cannot be over stated. At the practice level for example, the capacity and capability to practice compassion informed decision-making will be influenced by the following (not exhaustive): the available evidence-based guidance (and their specificity or ambiguity); health worker competence; perceptions of risk; fear and uncertainty and the influence of prevailing information and mis-information. Structurally, decisions will also be influenced by available resources that enable or prevent safe practices. And decisions will also be influenced by the culture and leadership within an organisation. There is much to learn from historical efforts to strengthen compassion within nursing. In the English NHS, following a national strategy centered on compassion, a review highlighted professional anger, distress and resistance from nurses who perceived the strategy to be a top-down initiative that failed to take account of structural constraints on nurses' ability to put compassionate care into practice [22].

2.6   Integrating IPC Logic and Relational Ethical Logic

McMillan and colleagues [23] posed the question "can IPC logic and relational ethical logic be integrated to inform decision-making and policy in relation to the issues raised by visitor restrictions?" A recent publication by the American and Canadian professional societies for IPC practitioners suggests the answer is a resounding "yes". The Ethical Infection Prevention and Control (EIPAC) Decision-Making Framework [24] highlights how to identify and apply relevant, ethical decision-making principles to the practice of IPC in a stepwise manner. It aims to support frontline practitioners in their IPC-related decision-making both in acute and long-term care and *it* provides a set of scenarios to illustrate how the framework can be applied in a range of settings.

In addition to these scenarios, practical resources to support practitioners to implement compassion-informed IPC practices have been developed. In the context of long-term care, IPC experts worked with civil society groups in Scotland to co-develop a website that acted as a repository of freely available and accessible resources for anyone undertaking or supporting safe and compassionate human interaction in care homes, under the strapline "safe practices with compassion" [25]. A central pillar of the resources was a set of visual scenarios that brought this to life, uniquely from the perspective of carers/relatives, and these were launched on a unique website (www.enablesafecare.org). At each step, the relevant IPC measures and their rationale were described with the aim of empowering people to act with both compassion and safety. Storr et al. emphasised that the resources could be adapted and encouraged their widespread use to help redress the imbalance between IPC and compassion.

2.7   Conclusion

Although there has been great progress in recent years, the pandemic demonstrated that IPC guidance and its implementation continued to overlook to some extent the psychosocial effects of both the infection and the IPC precautions necessary to keep people safe on those with infections and their loved ones. The need within IPC to balance the technical, scientific side of the specialty with the compassion necessary to humanise the application of IPC precautions requires ongoing leadership and role modelling not least to advocate for a health service that embeds compassion within policies and strategies, including training approaches, and their implementation. WHO [11] outlines the importance of raising awareness of the value of compassion in healthcare. The report suggests that making compassion tangible and visible through concrete actions can create a positive cascade effect, generating new norms of interaction. It goes on to state that a key aspect of this awareness is recognising that every individual interacting within the system holds immense power through the compassion they relay. As Ahmed and colleagues [12] highlight, compassion is a behaviour that is not only inherited but can also be learnt.

References

1. Open AI. ChatGPT (GPT-4) [Large language model]. https://openai.com. Accessed 13 Feb 2025.
2. ESNO. Clinical isolation should never mean human isolation. Position Statement Infection Prevention and Compassion. 2022. http://esno.org/assets/files/Position_Statement_IPC_and_Compassion_2022.pdf. Accessed 18 Feb 2025.

3. Storr J, Wigglesworth N, Kilpatrick C. Integrating human factors with infection prevention and control: thought paper. Health Foundation 2013. https://www.health.org.uk/reports-and-analysis/reports/integrating-human-factors-with-infection-prevention-and-control. Accessed 18 Feb 2025.

4. Storr J. Just infection prevention and control. In: Elliott P, Storr J, Jeanes A, editors. Infection prevention and control: perceptions and perspectives. Boca Raton: Taylor and Francis; 2016.

5. Braut GS, Holt J. Meticillin-resistant Staphylococcus aureus infection—the infectious stigma of our time? J Hosp Infect. 2011;77(2):148–52.

6. Addiss DG, Richards A, Adiabu S, et al. Epidemiology of compassion: a literature review. Front Psychol. 2022;13:992705. Published 2022 Nov 17.

7. Kleine-Bingham M, Mensah Abrampah N, Ako-Egbe L, Syed SB. Communicating with compassion—service user perspectives. In: Elliott P, Storr J, Jeanes A, editors. Infection prevention and control—social science perspectives. CRC Press; 2023.

8. Kruk ME, Gage AD, Arsenault C, et al. High-quality health systems in the sustainable development goals era: time for a revolution. Lancet Glob Health. 2018;6(11):e1196–252.

9. Trzeciak S, Mazzarelli A. Compassionomics – the revolutionary scientific evidence that caring makes a difference. Pensacola: The Studer Group, LLC; 2019.

10. WHO. Scoping report: compassion and quality of care. Geneva: World Health Organization; 2018.

11. WHO. Compassion and primary health care. Geneva: World Health Organization; 2024. https://iris.who.int/bitstream/handle/10665/380286/9789240105249-eng.pdf?sequence=1. Accessed 18 Feb 2025

12. Ahmed Z, Ellahham S, Soomro M, Shams S, Latif K. Exploring the impact of compassion and leadership on patient safety and quality in healthcare systems: a narrative review. BMJ Open Qual. 2024;13(Suppl 2):e002651. Published 7 May 2024.

13. Pattison N, Corser R. Compassionate, collective or transformational nursing leadership to ensure fundamentals of care are achieved: a new challenge or non-sequitur? J Adv Nurs. 2023;79(3):942–50.

14. Kitson AL. The fundamentals of care framework as a point-of-care nursing theory. Nurs Res. 2018;67(2):99–107.

15. Mudd A, Feo R, Conroy T, Kitson A. Where and how does fundamental care fit within seminal nursing theories: a narrative review and synthesis of key nursing concepts. J Clin Nurs. 2020;29(19–20):3652–66.

16. Storr J, Kilpatrick C, Vassallo A. Safe infection prevention and control practices with compassion—a positive legacy of COVID-19. Am J Infect Control. 2021;49(3):407–8.

17. Storr J. Open letter: infection prevention and control should never be at the expense of compassionate care. Nurs Times 16 Oct 2020. https://www.nursingtimes.net/opinion/open-letter-infection-prevention-and-control-should-never-be-at-the-expense-of-compassionate-care-16-10-2020/. Accessed 18 Feb 2025.

18. Health Foundation. Person-centred care made simple: what everyone should know about person-centred care. London: Health Foundation; 2014. https://www.health.org.uk/publications/person-centred-care-made-simple

19. Storr J, Kilpatrick C, Seale H. The relevance of nursing to the achievement of person-centred infection prevention and control. J Res Nurs. Published online 10 Dec 2024.

20. Acolin J, Fishman P. Beyond the biomedical, towards the agentic: a paradigm shift for population health science. Soc Sci Med. 2023;326:115950.

21. Loft MI, Guldager R, Poulsen I. Caring from a distance: how a COVID-19 visitor ban affects relatives when a loved one is admitted to a neurological or neurosurgical ward. J Res Nurs. 2022;27(6):532–42.

22. O'Driscoll M, Allan H, Liu L, Corbett K, Serrant L. Compassion in practice—evaluating the awareness, involvement and perceived impact of a national nursing and midwifery strategy amongst healthcare professionals in NHS trusts in England. J Clin Nurs. 2018;27(5–6):e1097–109.
23. McMillan K, Wright DK, McPherson CJ, Ma K, Bitzas V. Visitor restrictions, palliative care, and epistemic agency: a qualitative study of nurses' relational practice during the coronavirus pandemic. Glob Qual Nurs Res. 2021:8.
24. APIC/IPAC. Association for Professionals in Infection Control and Epidemiology (APIC). APIC/IPAC-Canada Ethical Infection Prevention and Control (EIPAC) decision-making framework. 2024. https://apic.org/apic-ipac-canada-ethical-infection-prevention-and-control-eipac-decision-making-framework/. Accessed 18 Feb 2025.
25. Storr J, Kilpatrick C, Hall S, Chraiti M-N. Applying workflow analysis techniques in care homes in the context of IPC and COVID-19. Antimicrob Resist Infect Control. 2021;10(1):P103.

Emerging Infections and Global Health

3

David Valente Peres and Isabel Neves

Abstract

Emerging and re-emerging infectious diseases are epiphenomena of human existence and our interactions with each other and with nature. The growth of societies creates opportunities for infectious agents to emerge in new ecological niches. This is not new, except that our increasingly aggressive action on the environment induces increasingly extreme reactions from nature. Science will find medicines, vaccines and diagnostics that save lives. But to prevent new diseases we have to think collectively about how to live in harmony with nature, even though it can always surprise us.

This chapter characterizes the scale of this problem and what can be done to prevent and control it.

D. V. Peres (✉)
Infection and Antimicrobial Resistance Control Department, Matosinhos Local Health Unit, Matosinhos, Portugal

Portuguese National Infection Control Association (ANCI), Lisbon, Portugal

I. Neves
Infection and Antimicrobial Resistance Control Department, Matosinhos Local Health Unit, Matosinhos, Portugal

Portuguese National Infection Control Association (ANCI), Lisbon, Portugal

Infectious Diseases Department, Matosinhos Local Health Unit, Matosinhos, Portugal

Keywords

Emerging infectious diseases · Global health · One health · Communicable diseases

3.1 Concepts and Historical Perspective

3.1.1 Historical Perspective

From ancient times to the present day, humanity has experienced infectious diseases, which have impacted both the development of society and medicine. Sakai and Morimoto [1] reviewed several historical and current infectious diseases in a paper that helps us understand this evolution and the concept of emergence and re-emergence (Table 3.1).

Table 3.1 Five periods in the history of medicine

History of medicine and medical education	Infectious diseases	Diagnosis and treatment
Western classic medicine (ancient-fifteenth century) **Ancient medical documents** (Hippocrates, Galen) **Scholastic education** (*lectio, disputatio*)	**Plague of Athens** (BC429–) **Antonine Plague** (165–) **Plague of Justinian** (541–) **Black Death** (1347–)	Diagnosis and prognosis by signs (uroscopy, pulse-reading) Hygienic therapy (regimen, herbals, venesection)
Traditional Western medicine (sixteenth-eighteenth century) **Anatomical research** **Lecture-based education** (*theoria, practica,* anatomy/surgery, botany/pharmaceutics) **Clinical observations**	**Syphilis (1494–)** **Malaria** **Smallpox** (Vaccination, 1798)	
Early modern medicine (nineteenth century) **Basic medicine** (anatomy, physiology, pathology, pharmacology, hygiene) **Clinical medicine** (internal medicine, surgery, etc.) **Cell theory (1838–1839)**	**Cholera** (pandemic, 1817–) **Dysentery**	Diagnosis by autopsy after death Innovation of surgery (anesthesia, disinfection) Discovery of pathogenic bacteria
Late modem medicine (1900–1980s) **Basic research** (bacteriology, biochemistry, cell Biology) **Antibiotics** (penicillin, 1941)	**Influenza** (Spanish flu, 1918–1920) **Tuberculosis**	Antibiotics Discovery of viruses
Exact medicine (1990s–) **Basic research** (molecular biology immunology) **Clinical and translational research**	**Antimicrobial resistance** **AIDS** (1981–) **COVID-19 (2019–)**	Diagnosis by medical imaging in vivo Scientific verification Partnership with patients Clinical cooperation

After the advent of antibiotics, it was thought that we would no longer suffer from epidemics or pandemics. But the experience with the human immunodeficiency virus (HIV)/ acquired immunodeficiency syndrome (AIDS), the return of cholera to the Americas in 1991, the plague outbreak in India in 1994, the resurgence of Ebola in Zaire in 1995, the emergence of severe acute respiratory syndrome (SARS) in 2003 and COVID-19 in 2019, created awareness of vulnerability to epidemics and the impact of associated morbidity and mortality. The term "emerging and re-emerging diseases" arose to explain that the world had entered an era with increasing risk of epidemics.

3.1.2 Concept

What are emerging and re-emerging diseases?

- **Emerging infectious diseases** are newly identified and previously unknown infections that cause local or international public health problems. Examples: HIV/AIDS (1981), Nipah virus (1999), SARS (2002), MERS (2012), COVID-19 (2019).
- **Re-emerging infectious diseases** are diseases that reappear after a significant decline, rapidly increasing in incidence or geographic extent (e.g., West Nile in the United States of America—USA and Russia in 1999) or in resistant forms (e.g., methicillin-resistant *Staphylococcus aureus*—MRSA).

But Morens and Fauci [2] expand this concept even more, specifically with two other definitions:

- **Deliberately emerging infectious diseases**—those that are associated with intent to harm, including mass bioterrorism.
- **Accidentally emerging infectious diseases**—those created by humans that are released unintentionally, e.g., epizootic vaccinia and transmissible vaccine-derived polioviruses.

In Image 3.1 we can see the global extent of newly emerging, re-emerging, and "deliberately emerging" infectious disease in the last four decades.

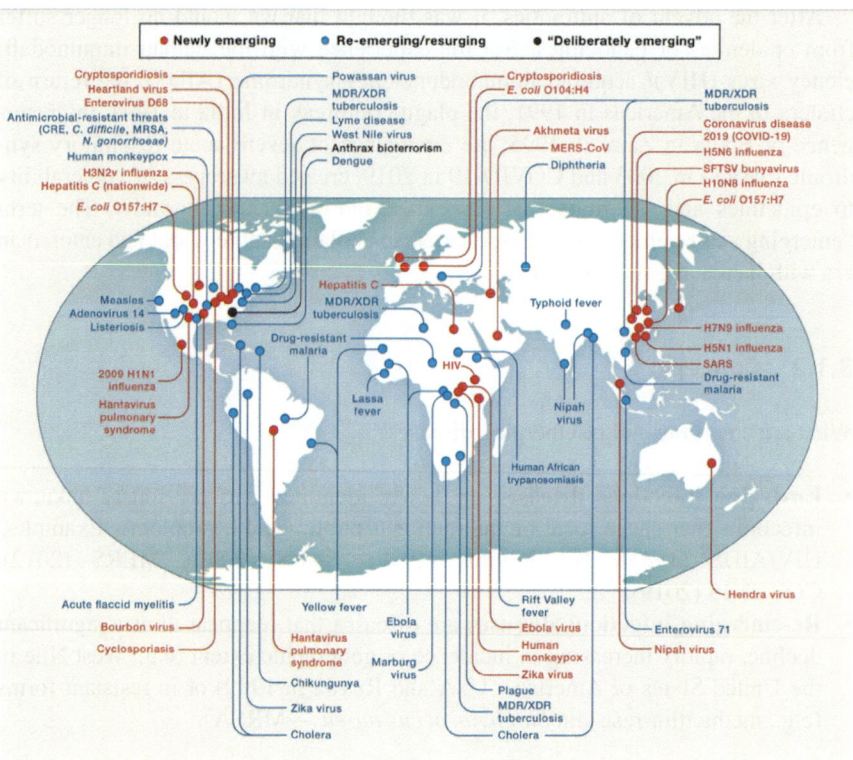

Image 3.1 The global extent of newly emerging, re-emerging, and 'deliberately emerging' infectious disease from 1981 to the 2020. (Source: Morens and Fauci [2])

3.2   Predisposing Factors

Common infections and related immune responses or inflammatory processes contribute to the multifactorial aetiology of morbid conditions that, together, make a substantial contribution to overall mortality. Infectious causation is suspected for many others because of strong evidence of association [3]. As Morens and Fauci [2] mention "the triad of causation of emerging and other diseases, as conceptualized for over a century, represents interactions between infectious agents, their hosts, and the environment. This conceptualization acknowledges the reality that, while infectious diseases themselves are necessarily 'caused' by microbial agents, emergences that produce epidemics and pandemics are also significantly determined by co-factors related to the host and to host-environmental interactions". Image 3.2 associates this triad of causation to the predisposing factors that contribute to disease (re) emergence and persistence [2].

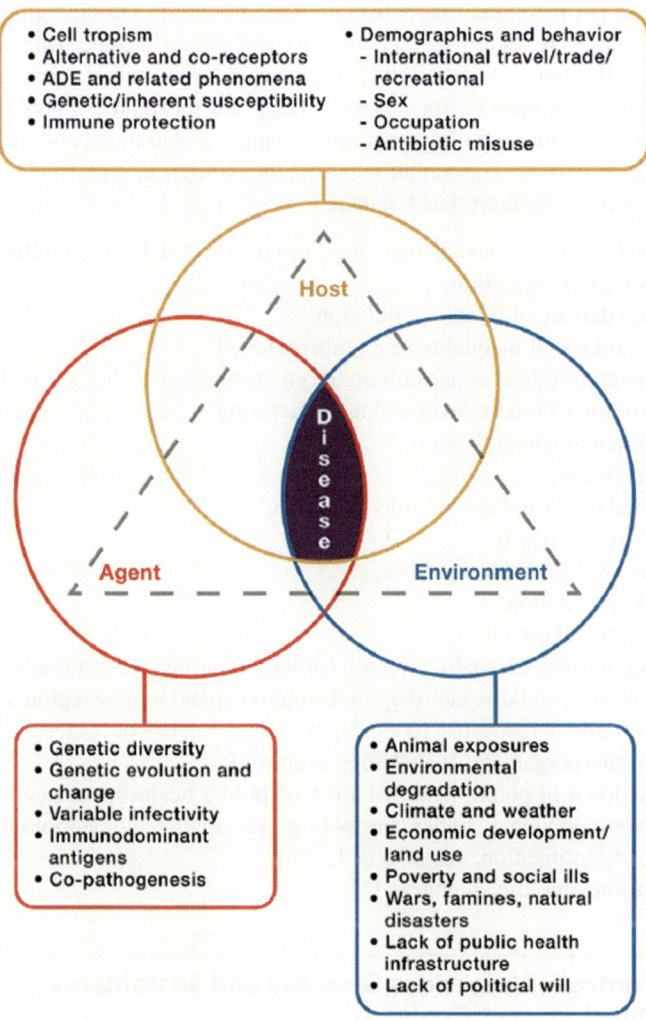

Image 3.2 Infectious Agents, Hosts, and the Environment: Determinants of Disease Emergence and Persistence Diseases, including emerging diseases, result from interactions between infectious agents, hosts, and the environment. (Source: Morens and Fauci [2])

McArthur [4] mentions that between 1940 and 2004, 335 emerging infectious diseases events were identified. The majority (60.3%) originated from wild animal reservoirs with approximately 1 in 5 transmitted from animal reservoir hosts to humans by disease vectors, for example, ticks and mosquitoes. This information reinforces the significance of demographic change, global travel and trade, and climate change as drivers. This author lists, too, the biological, social and environmental drivers, which are interrelated, namely:

- Microbial adaptation and change (e.g., genetic drift and shift in influenza A);
- Susceptibility to infection;
- Increased density of human population;
- Poverty and social inequality (e.g., tuberculosis);
- Stress from farm land expansion on the environment;
- Globalization of food market and manufacturing;
- Environmental contamination;
- Climate change;
- Additional opportunities for emerging infections:
  - Population growth;
  - Spread in healthcare facilities;
  - Aging population;
  - International travel;
  - Changing and expanding vector habitats (warmer temperatures may allow mosquitoes, and diseases they transmit, to expand to new regions);
  - Antimicrobial resistance (contributes to reemergence of bacteria, viruses, and other microorganisms that change overtime);
  - Breakdown in public health; failure of public health measures for diseases that were previously under control (e.g.: vaccination, epidemiological control of cases/notification, vector population);
  - Intentional biological attacks [4].

3.3 Control of Infectious Diseases and Sustainable Development Goals

In a review of Graham and Sullivan [5] they mention that "the approach to new pandemic threats has generally been reactive, and specific medical interventions have not been available in time to make a substantial impact on the immediate outbreak". However, "technical advances have provided tools that have made a more proactive approach feasible and a critical determinant for achieving the **Sustainable Development Goals** (SDGs) established by the United Nations (UN) in 2015" [5].

In this context these authors correlate the goals for the control of infectious diseases with the SDG's (Table 3.2).

Table 3.2 Interface between SDGs and the risk of emerging infectious diseases

Goals for the control of infectious disease	Relevant SDG(s)
Reduce human contact with pathogens found in conditions of poor sanitation (rodent- and vector-borne diseases), alternative food sources (bushmeat hunting), untreated water (parasites and bacteria) and altered-pathogen reservoirs resulting from climate change or deforestation.	1 - No poverty; 2 - Zero hunger; 6 - Clean water and sanitation; 13 - Climate action; 14 - Life below water; 15 - Life on land
Reduce pathogen exposure and disease severity via better understanding of how infectious diseases are transmitted, lowering resistance to seeking care and knowing the value of medical interventions such as vaccination.	3 - Good health and well-being; 4 - Quality education
Reduce the spread of sexually transmitted viruses, such as HIV and HPV, for which young women have the highest risk of acquisition.	5 - Gender equality
Reduce exposure to mosquitoes and other transmission vectors by improving and maintaining general infrastructure and living conditions (reduce standing water, protect indoor spaces with screens); build capacity for surveillance and early diagnosis in low- and middle-income countries and maintain public health systems and access to medical care to contain outbreaks and prevent pandemics.	7 - Affordable and clean energy; 9 - Industry and infrastructure; 10 - Reduced inequalities; 11 - Sustainable cities; 12 - Responsible consumption and production; 16 - Peace, justice and strong institutions; 17 - Partnership for the goals
Reduce pathogen transmission from high-risk occupations related to the hunting or selling of wild animals in mixed-species marketplaces and diminish the prevalence of commercial sex work and crowded living conditions that provide avenues for the transmission of some viruses.	8 - Decent work and economic growth

Adapted from: Graham and Sullivan [5]

3.4   Zoonotic and Vector-Borne Diseases

According to the World Health Organization (WHO), a **ZOONOSIS** is an infectious disease that has jumped from a non-human animal to humans [6]. Some important facts about zoonosis:

- Zoonotic pathogens may be bacterial, viral or parasitic, or may involve unconventional agents and can spread to humans through direct contact or through food, water or the environment.
- They represent a major public health problem around the world due to our close relationship with animals in agriculture, as companions and in the natural environment.
- Zoonoses can cause disruptions in the production and trade of animal products for food and other uses.

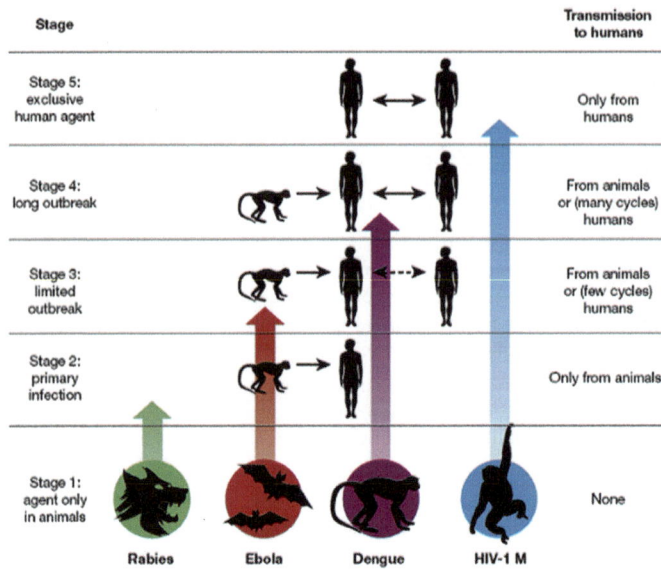

Image 3.3 Illustration of five stages through which pathogens of animals evolve to cause diseases confined to humans. (Source: Wolfe at al. [7])

- They comprise a large percentage of all newly identified infectious diseases, as well as many existing ones. Some diseases (such as HIV) begin as a zoonosis but later mutate into human-only strains.
- Some zoonoses can cause recurring disease outbreaks, such as Ebola virus disease and salmonellosis.
- Others, such as the novel coronavirus that causes COVID-19, have the potential to cause global pandemics [6].

In Image 3.3 it can be seen the five stages in which an animal exclusive disease can evolve to a human-exclusive disease. In order for this to happen, there are several risk factors, namely:

- Markets selling the meat (or by-products) of wild animals are particularly high risk due to the large number of new or undocumented pathogens known to exist in some wild animal populations.
- Agricultural workers, in areas with a high use of antibiotics for farm animals, may be at increased risk of pathogens resistant to current antimicrobial drugs.

- People living adjacent to wilderness areas (or in semi-urban areas) with higher numbers of wild animals are at risk of disease from animals such as rats, foxes or raccoons.
- Urbanization and the destruction of natural habitats increase the risk of zoonotic diseases by increasing contact between humans and wild animals [6].

As Peterson et al. [8] mention "enhanced surveillance of infections in travellers, migrants, persons working with animals and persons living in regions with a high risk of vector-borne disease outbreaks is crucial to identify outbreaks at an early stage. A valuable source of information regarding emerging infectious diseases are the weekly communicable disease threat reports and risk assessments provided by the ECDC [9] that can be used when triaging patients".

Other important concept is **VECTORS**. They are living organisms that can transmit infectious pathogens between humans, or from animals to humans. Many of these vectors are bloodsucking insects, which ingest disease-producing microorganisms during a blood meal from an infected host (human or animal) and later transmit it into a new host, after the pathogen has replicated. Often, once a vector becomes infectious, they are capable of transmitting the pathogen for the rest of their life during each subsequent bite/blood meal [10].

According to the WHO, **VECTOR-BORNE DISEASES** are "human illnesses caused by parasites, viruses and bacteria that are transmitted by vectors. Every year there are more than 700,000 deaths from these diseases. The burden is highest in tropical and subtropical areas, and they disproportionately affect the poorest populations. Since 2014, major outbreaks of dengue, malaria, chikungunya, yellow fever and zika have afflicted populations, claimed lives, and overwhelmed health systems in many countries. Other diseases such as chikungunya, leishmaniasis and lymphatic filariasis cause chronic suffering, life-long morbidity, disability and occasional stigmatization." [10].

In response to this problem, the WHO's "Global Response to Vector Control 2017–2030" was implemented, with the following pillars of action:

- Strengthen inter- and intra-sectoral action and collaboration;
- Engage and mobilize communities;
- Enhance vector surveillance, and monitoring and evaluation of interventions;
- Scale up and integrate tools and approaches [11].

In Europe, there is the VectorNet, a network for medical and veterinary entomology, which is a project of ECDC and the European Food Safety Authority (EFSA) that aims to contribute to improving preparedness and response for vector-borne diseases, following a "One-Health" approach. In its website, "Vector Maps" provide information on the European distribution of several mosquitoes, ticks, sandfly and biting midge species, which can be vectors of pathogens affecting human or animal health [12].

3.5   Bioterrorism and Accidents

Bioterrorism can be defined as using microorganisms or infected samples to cause terror and panic in populations. In a historical review, Barras and Greub [13] summarize the main events, such as the following examples:

- In 1993, the Japanese Doomsday cult Aum Shinrikyo sprayed anthrax spores from the top of a cooling tower in Tokyo in a failed attempt to start an epidemic;
- In 1995, the same group used a similar chemical weapon in an attack on the Tokyo subway system that caused 13 deaths and many injuries;
- In 2001, an attacker with unknown motives caused terror and chaos in the USA by sending letters containing anthrax to the offices of two senators and several members of the media, resulting in five deaths.

The authors conclude that "more broadly, although the problem of bioterrorism is undoubtedly important, it should not cause us to overreact and obfuscate the reality of real and important preventable infections" [13].

There is, too, the possibility of biological threats of accidental etiology, such as the example of an accident in 2014, involving live anthrax bacteria at the North-American Centers for Disease Control and Prevention (CDC), that potentially exposed dozens of workers to the pathogen. This accident triggered measures to improve laboratory quality and safety [14]. Bloom and Cadarette have the opinion that "as long as stores of dangerous pathogens, such as anthrax and smallpox, are maintained (for research purposes), the potential for a damaging accident or intentional attack will remain" [15].

3.6   Antimicrobial Resistance

Antimicrobial Resistance (AMR) is the ability of bacteria, fungi or parasites to become resistant to the action of one or more antimicrobials. People don't become resistant to antimicrobials, but microorganisms do. Some facts about this global problem:

- AMR is responsible for more than 35,000 deaths each year in the European Union and the latest data show significant upward trends in the number of infections and deaths attributable to almost all combinations of antibiotic resistance in bacteria, especially in healthcare settings.
- Around 70% of cases of infections caused by resistant bacteria are healthcare-associated infections.
- A continued rise in resistance would result in ten million deaths worldwide by 2050, reducing global gross domestic product by 2% to 3.5% and costing the global economy up to $100 trillion [16].
- One of the challenges associated with this problem continues to be the lack of literacy among the population: according to data from the 2022 Eurobarometer

survey of the European population, around 8% of antibiotics were taken without a prescription and only half of those surveyed knew that antibiotics are not effective against viruses [17].

3.6.1   What Will the Future Look Like?

If urgent action is not taken, serious health, social and economic consequences are expected:

- Simple infections may become difficult or impossible to treat;
- Surgical procedures, organ transplants and cancer treatments will be moot, as patients rely on the availability of effective antimicrobials to prevent and treat infections;
- Healthcare facilities will be overcrowded with patients with infections, putting pressure on resources and increasing the demand for specialist care;
- Prolonged hospital stays, increased healthcare costs and decreased productivity due to illness or premature death will lead to an increased economic impact on individuals, families and societies.

Paradoxically, the pipeline of new antimicrobials is scarce, given that their research and production are not profitable (e.g., an antihypertensive or antidiabetic drug is taken for life, while an antimicrobial is used occasionally and for a short period). So, antimicrobial resistance poses a threat to global stability and security.

3.6.2   How Does Resistance Spread?

Resistant microorganisms are found in humans, animals, plants and the environment (in water, sewage, soil and air), and spread can occur from all of these means (Image 3.4). Sources can be:

- Healthcare: contact between patients, professionals and visitors, contaminated surfaces or devices;
- Inappropriate use of antibiotics: in humans and animals (production, domestic);
- Food contamination;
- Tourism and imports;
- Environmental contamination: wastewater and effluents;
- Environmental contamination: Animal production, use of manure for fertilization.

The challenges of AMR cannot be understood or addressed separately from the triple planetary crisis: climate change, loss of biodiversity and pollution and waste, because they are all associated with unsustainable consumption and production patterns [19].

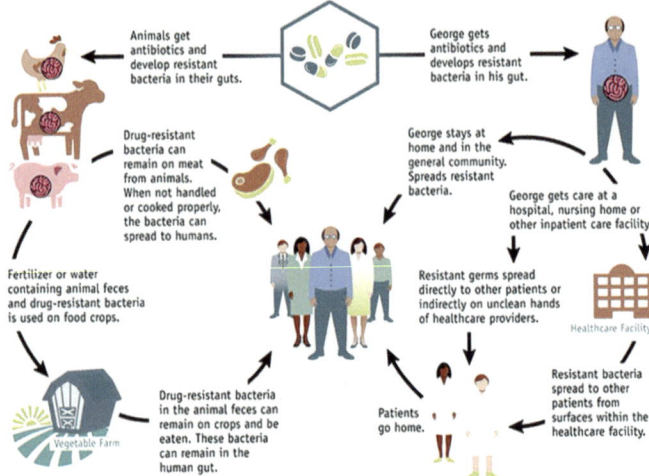

Image 3.4 How antimicrobial resistance can spread. (Source: CDC [18])

3.6.3   Strategies to Manage the Problem

Alert to this crisis, in 2015 the World Health Assembly adopted the "Global Action Plan on Antimicrobial Resistance", which outlines five objectives:

1. to improve awareness and understanding of AMR through effective communication, education and training;
2. to strengthen the knowledge and evidence base through surveillance and research;
3. to reduce the incidence of infection through effective sanitation, hygiene and infection prevention measures;
4. to optimize the use of antimicrobial medicines in human and animal health;
5. to develop the economic case for sustainable investment that takes account of the needs of all countries and to increase investment in new medicines, diagnostic tools, vaccines and other interventions [20].

In June 2017, the European Commission adopted the "One Health Action Plan against AMR". The main objectives of this plan are based on three main pillars: to make the EU a best practice region; to boost research, development and innovation; and to put the issue on the global agenda [21].

Table 3.3 WHO Bacterial Priority Pathogens List, 2024 update

Priority	Pathogen and resistance
PRIORITY 1: CRITICAL	*Acinetobacter baumannii* carbapenem-resistant *Enterobacterales* 3rd generation cephalosporin-resistant *Enterobacterales* carbapenem-resistant
PRIORITY 2: HIGH	*Salmonella Typhi* fluoroquinolone-resistant *Shigella* spp. fluoroquinolone-resistant *Enterococcus faecium* vancomycin-resistant *Pseudomonas aeruginosa* carbapenem-resistant Non-typhoidal *Salmonella* fluoroquinolone-resistant *Neisseria gonorrhoeae* 3rd generation cephalosporin, and/or fluoroquinolone-resistant *Staphylococcus aureus* methicillin-resistant (MRSA)
PRIORITY 3: MEDIUM	Group A *Streptococci* macrolide-resistant *Streptococcus pneumoniae* macrolide-resistant *Haemophilus influenzae* ampicillin-resistant Group B *Streptococci* penicillin-resistant
(included after an independent analysis)	*Mycobacterium tuberculosis*, rifampicin-resistant

Adapted from WHO [23]

In 2019, the WHO declared AMR as one of the top ten global public health threats facing humanity. Tackling AMR in the human health sector needs global efforts focused on several key areas: robust infection prevention and control measures, ensuring equitable access to diagnostics and treatment, adequate surveillance to detect emerging trends in AMR and substantial investment in research and development for the creation of new medicines, diagnostics and prevention tools [22]. In 2024, the WHO updated its "Bacterial Priority Pathogen List", a prioritization of antibiotic-resistant bacterial pathogens to address the evolving challenges of antibiotic resistance. The list categorizes these pathogens into critical, high and medium priority groups to inform research and development and public health interventions (Table 3.3) [23].

3.6.4   The "One Health" Approach

"One Health" is an integrated and unifying approach that aims to sustainably balance and optimize the health of people, animals and ecosystems, recognizing that the health of humans, domestic and wild animals, and ecosystems are intimately linked and interdependent. This approach mobilizes multiple sectors, disciplines and communities at various levels of society to work to promote global health and combat AMR, contributing to sustainable development [17].

In the implementation of "One Health" strategies,

- Limiting the emergence and spread of resistant pathogens is essential to preserve the ability to treat diseases in humans, animals and plants, reduce food safety risks, protect the environment and sustain progress;
- The global response to AMR relies on collaboration between sectors that have traditionally fallen into separate policy spheres;
- The dimensions of AMR require action at local, national and global levels;
- Country implementation is key to a successful response, as it is in countries that the work of addressing the many challenges of AMR takes place;
- A legal and regulatory framework that addresses the factors impacting AMR is needed;
- While countries may have different processes for developing their One Health plan, a robust multi-sectoral coordination system was highlighted as essential;
- Ensure continued political engagement, including budget and technical capacity across sectors;
- Countries need to explore innovative incentives and financial schemes, and make the investment case to secure sustainable financing;
- Environmental monitoring and surveillance and greater prioritization of research are also essential to provide more data and evidence and better understand the complex dynamics of AMR (this will ensure informed decision-making to prioritize interventions).

Therefore, strengthening national, regional and global surveillance systems, engaging the private sector and industry, implementing data-driven practices and reporting are essential [17].

3.7 Social and Economic Consequences

When dealing with an epidemic or pandemic, several social and economic consequences should be considered, namely:

- Direct costs for the health system, inherent to the treatment and reduced response capacity;
- Direct and indirect costs (suffering and disability) for patients and their families and, indirectly, for society due to lost productivity;
- Social and economic disruption due to the implementation of public health measures (isolation and social distancing);
- Decrease in commercial exchanges due to perceived risk of transmission. For example: the ban imposed by the European Union on the export of beef, which lasted 10 years after the outbreak of the Variant of Creutzfeldt-Jakob Disease (CJDv) in the United Kingdom.
- Mobility limitations of individuals, with tourism activity affected, with economic consequences for places where this activity is essential. Ex: Dengue in Brazil.

In this topic, United Nations did a snapshot of the socioeconomic impact of the COVID-19 pandemic in June 2020, describing the following challenges: [24].

(a) Poverty increase (estimated 40–60 million people pushed into extreme poverty because of the economic shocks from COVID-19);
(b) COVID-19 impact on women (unpaid care work has increased and quarantining has caused a spike in domestic violence levels);
(c) Students out of school (nearly 1.2 billion learners were affected by school closure);
(d) Lack of adequate social protection (55% of the world's population are not covered by social insurance or social assistance);
(e) Slum dwellers (over 90% of COVID-19 cases happened in urban areas);
    – With over one billion people living in informal settlements and slum-like conditions, COVID-19 exacerbated the vulnerability of these population groups.
(f) Income and jobs lost (about 1.6 billion informal workers lost 60% of their income);
(g) Increase in food insecurity (it was estimated that, by the end of 2020, about 265 million people in low and middle-income countries would be at risk of acute food insecurity).
(h) Dramatic fall in tourism (considered one of the hardest hits by the COVID-19 outbreak, with potential loss of 850 million to 1.1 billion international tourists and estimated 100 and 120 million jobs at risk).

In this report, it was described that the United Nations has mobilized the full capacity of the UN system, to support national authorities in developing public health preparedness and response plans to the COVID-19 and this support was delivered through the UN global framework for the immediate socio-economic response to COVID-19. The socio-economic response complemented the UN health response, led by WHO [24].

3.8 Preparedness and Response to Communicable Disease Threats

In this topic, an important document is the International Health Regulations (IHR) that provides the international legal framework for the prevention and response to the international spread of diseases. The IHR are an instrument of international law, adopted pursuant to Article 21 of the WHO Constitution, and are legally binding on 196 States Parties (including all the 194 Member States of WHO).

The IHR (2005), successor to the International Health Regulations of 1951, was designed to maximize collective efforts to manage public health events while minimizing disruption to travel and trade [25].

By the analysis of Table 3.4 it can be said that IHR is all-risk approach (biological, chemical, radionuclear) in which all countries must be able to detect, assess, notify and declare an occurrence, regardless of its etiology (natural, accidental or

Table 3.4 Five reasons why the IHR is important

Reason	Comments
Health threats have no borders.	The IHR strengthen countries capabilities to control diseases that cross borders at ports, airports and ground crossings.
Travel and trade are made safer.	The IHR promote trade and tourism in countries and prevent economic damage.
Global health security is enhanced.	The IHR establish an early warning system not only for disasters but also for anything that threatens human health and livelihoods.
Daily threats are kept under control.	The IHR guide countries to detect, access and respond to threats and inform other countries quickly.
All sectors benefit.	The IHR prepare all sectors for potential emergencies through coordination and information sharing.

intentional). This occurrence—classified as a **"Public Health Emergency of International Concern"**—should obey to certain characteristics, namely:

- Serious impact on Public Health;
- Unusual or unexpected;
- Significant risk for international spread;
- Significant risk to international trade and traffic [25].

In 2024 new amendments to the IHR were made, namely:

- introducing a definition of a pandemic emergency to trigger more effective international collaboration in response to events that are at risk of becoming, or have become, a pandemic.
- a commitment to solidarity and equity on strengthening access to medical products and financing.
- establishment of the States Parties Committee to facilitate the effective implementation of the amended Regulations [26].

In the preparedness for these threats at national level, Bloom and Cadarette [15] warn that "insufficient coordination among stakeholder organizations leads to inefficiency and missed opportunities. Many responses are available and required to proactively reduce the risk posed by infectious disease threats and prepare for inevitable outbreaks". In Table 3.5, these authors describe the needed responses.

In the document "Health emergencies in Europe: Making sure every country is ready", WHO states that "universal health coverage and health emergency capacity, or emergency preparedness, are two sides of the same coin in a people-centred health system. When countries strengthen their emergency preparedness and response capacities, they also strengthen their health system's ability to provide universal health coverage." To do so, they recommend that countries have "Health

Emergencies Programmes" in which a "health emergency management cycle" defines its rhythm [27]. This cycle is composed of four phases:

1. Prevention and control of infectious diseases (through vaccination, for example);
2. Preparedness (develop, test and evaluate their national plans and strengthen their capacities);
3. Response (response, life-saving health interventions and pre-positioned essential health packages);
4. Recovery (learn from experience and build back better).

In this area, WHO implemented the "R&D Blueprint", which is a "global strategy and preparedness plan that allows the rapid activation of research and development activities during epidemics. Its aim is to fast-track the availability of effective tests, vaccines and medicines that can be used to save lives and avert large scale crises." [28] In its document "An R&D Blueprint for Action to Prevent Epidemics – Update 2017" it describes its *modus operandi*, divided in "preparedness" and "response plan". The first one is structured with three approaches, namely:

Table 3.5 Responses to be considered to manage infectious disease threats at national level

Responses
• Health systems strengthening
• Improved (sustainable) urban infrastructure
• Improved public health infrastructure, including clean water and sanitation
• Increased routine immunization
• Mass vaccination following detection of outbreak-prone diseases (e.g., yellow fever)
• Surveillance of infectious disease in human and animal populations, including rates of resistance
– Building local (laboratory and epidemiological) capacity to diagnose and report cases of infectious disease
– Leveraging opportunities for informal surveillance (e.g., Google Flu Trends (no longer operating publicly), ProMED)
• Surveillance of possible terrorist organizations and activities
• Monitoring of biocontainment procedures and capabilities in microbiology laboratories
• Regular monitoring of preparedness for outbreaks and biosecurity incidents at national and supranational levels (e.g., joint external evaluations)
• Regulation of access to antimicrobials for both humans and livestock
• Investment in R&D of biomedical countermeasures
– Vaccines
– Antimicrobials
– Diagnostics
– Monoclonal antibodies and other novel treatments
– Platform technologies
• Supply chain strengthening and improved systems for rapid distribution of countermeasures in the event of an emergency
• Coordination of efforts

Source: Bloom and Cadarette [15] (licensed under CC-BY 4.0)

1. Improving Coordination & Fostering an Enabling Environment;
2. Accelerating Research and Development (R&D) Processes;
3. Developing New Norms & Standards Tailored to the Epidemic Context [29].

WHO defines, too, a list of which diseases pose the greatest public health risk due to their epidemic potential and/or whether there is no or insufficient counter-measures. At present, the priority diseases are:

- COVID-19;
- Crimean-Congo haemorrhagic fever;
- Ebola and Marburg virus diseases;
- Lassa fever;
- Middle East respiratory syndrome coronavirus (MERS-CoV) and SARS;
- Nipah and henipaviral diseases;
- Rift Valley fever;
- Zika;
- "Disease X".

"Disease X" represents the knowledge that a serious international epidemic could be caused by a pathogen currently unknown to cause human disease [30].

In this context, we can give the example of the COVID-19 pandemic:

- Just a few weeks after declaring COVID-19 as a public health emergency of international concern, the WHO published a coordinated global research road-map, identifying knowledge gaps that the world urgently needed scientists to fill to find solutions to address the COVID-19 pandemic.
- Fourteen months later, research into most of the knowledge gaps began, pro-gressed and has provided answers to several knowledge gaps identified in the roadmap.
- Most notably, research and development has delivered safe and effective COVID-19 vaccines at unprecedented speed [31].

At local level, Weber et al. [32] mentions that "assessing and managing the threat of an emerging infectious disease requires an understanding of the biology of the pathogen, its epidemiology, the clinical manifestations of infection, the methods of diagnosis, and therapies (if available). In addition, there are a number of issues more specific to infection control" [28]. They structure these factors in Table 3.6.

The same authors state that every healthcare facility should have a highly com-municable disease management plan, in which the following items should be addressed [30].

Table 3.6 Factors to be considered when assessing and managing the threat of an emerging infectious disease in healthcare facilities

Pathogen
Taxonomy (provides clues regarding transmission routes, environmental stability, germicide susceptibility)
Hosts
Epidemiology
Locations of endemicity (i.e., locations in the world where sources or reservoirs reside)
Incubation period
Transmission routes
Infectivity (i.e., communicability)
Duration of infectivity
Clinical
Symptoms
Signs
Risk factors for acquisition of infection
Morbidity
Mortality
Risk factors for morbidity and mortality
Diagnostic methods (sensitivity, specificity, biosafety)
Therapy (availability, efficacy, safety)
Infection control
Environmental survival
Germicide susceptibility
Isolation recommendations
Recommended personal protective equipment
Pre-exposure prophylaxis (availability, efficacy, safety)
Postexposure prophylaxis (availability, efficacy, safety)
Recommended biosafety level in the laboratory
Recommended waste disposal (liquids and solids)

Source: Weber et al. [32]

3.8.1 Organizational Aspects

- Build a Contingency Plan for Public Health Emergencies;
- Incorporate the Contingency Plan into the Disaster Plan;
- Base the plan on the transmission routes of the pathogen;
- Include a Command Structure in the Plan:
- Carry out simulations periodically;
- Include scenarios with a single suspected patient, or groups of patients;
- Ensure communication with Health Authorities.

3.8.2 Screening and Signage (when appropriate)

- Place signs at every entrance to the hospital and clinics that should include: epidemiologic clues to possible disease exposure (i.e., travel locations), signs and symptoms of infection, and who to notify in the presence of these.

- Include information about the signs and symptoms of the disease in all contacts with the patient and who to contact prior to arrival at the health care facility.
- Screen patients at the time of contact with healthcare.
- Include screening information and alerts (when screening is required) in the electronic medical record.
- Use appropriate sign on the door of isolation of all suspected patients.
- Emphasize respiratory hygiene, for diseases transmitted via droplet or airborne routes.
- Emphasize the importance of hand hygiene.
- Messages should be in several languages.

3.8.3   Triage

- Train frontline healthcare professionals (HCP) in appropriate use of personal protective equipment (PPE).
- Guarantee availability of adequate PPE.
- Have a designated location to place suspected patient(s), ideally a private room, access to a sink and toilet, with (central or portable) ventilation system adequate to airborne route (i.e., negative pressure, out-exhausted air, 6 to 12 air exchanges per hour).
- Have an internal communication protocol to alert key HCP (e.g., disaster manager, infection control professional) when in the presence of a suspected.
- Avoid unnecessary blood tests (or other procedures) that may place HCP at risk.
- Have a well-defined protocol for transporting a suspect patient within the healthcare unit, as well as, to other institutions.
- Emphasize respiratory etiquette, for diseases transmitted by droplets or particles.
- Emphasize the importance of hand hygiene.
- Key messages should be in several languages.

3.8.4   Inpatient Care

- Have a protocol for the inpatient location that will provide care to a patient with a highly communicative disease.
- In the inpatient care unit designate areas that are high risk (i.e., potentially contaminated) and low risk (i.e., areas that are not contaminated).
- Have a well-trained healthcare care team. For highly communicable diseases ideally provide three-step training:
  - basic individual training on PPE donning and doffing (that should include how to manage contamination of the environment and breach of the PPE);
  - team training using mannequins;
  - team training in the designated containment unit.

- Have a written list for training with donning and doffing steps (CDC and ECDC have guidance in this area [33–35]).
- Screen and exclude HCP unable to wear the proper PPE.
- Consider excluding from the healthcare team personnel at high risk for disease acquisition or more severe illness, such as persons with non-intact skin, pregnancy and immunocompromised persons.
- Consider excluding trainees from providing care.
- Guarantee adequate PPE supply.
- If needed, have dedicated point of care laboratory equipment.
- Safely dispose solid and liquid waste.
- Restrict visitors (if indicated) and maintain a log of all visitors.
- Maintain a log of all HCP providing care.
- Develop a plan for managing HCP with unprotected exposure to the infectious agent (e.g., needlestick).
- Assure that care team members receive proper rest (this will avoid adverse events related to human failure).

In this major paper, Weber et al. highlight the importance of the existence, in every healthcare facilities, of "policies and plans in place for early identification of patients with a highly communicable disease, immediate isolation, and proper management to prevent transmission to HCP, other patients, and visitors" [32].

3.9 Conclusion

The emergence of communicable diseases in the human population is one of the consequences of globalization and economic development, as it brings zoonotic reservoirs closer to humans.

According to the "One Health" concept, controlling these threats must integrate a multisectoral approach that, simultaneously, is dependent on achieving the 17 UN Sustainable Development Goals.

During a "Public Health Emergency of International Concern", all components of the health sector will be under tension. Advance planning, capacity building and training are of utmost importance in dealing with the threat.

At local level, all health units must have contingency plans that allow early identification of suspects; implementation of containment measures; communication to reference entities and adequate management to avoid nosocomial transmission.

Prof. Alexandra Levitt, an expert on emerging diseases and other public health threats, gives us three advices when dealing with communicable disease threats namely: "be prepared for the unexpected" (when it comes to infectious microorganisms); "we are all in it together" (with the phenomena of globalization, wherever we live, we are all at risk) and the importance of participating in a strong public health system, in the pursuit of prevention of disease spread among the community [36].

References

1. Sakai T, Morimoto Y. The history of infectious diseases and medicine. Pathogens. 2022;11(10):1147. https://doi.org/10.3390/pathogens11101147.
2. Morens DM, Fauci AS. Emerging pandemic diseases: how we got to COVID-19. Cell. 2020;182(5):1077–92. https://doi.org/10.1016/j.cell.2020.08.021.
3. Mercer AJ. Updating the epidemiological transition model. Epidemiol Infect. 2018;146(6):680–7. https://doi.org/10.1017/S0950268818000572.
4. McArthur DB. Emerging infectious diseases. Nurs Clin North Am. 2019;54(2):297–311. https://doi.org/10.1016/j.cnur.2019.02.006.
5. Graham BS, Sullivan NJ. Emerging viral diseases from a vaccinology perspective: preparing for the next pandemic. Nat Immunol. 2018;19(1):20–8. https://doi.org/10.1038/s41590-017-0007-9.
6. WHO. Zoonoses [internet]. Geneva: World Health Organization. Available at: https://www.who.int/news-room/fact-sheets/detail/zoonoses.
7. Wolfe ND, Dunavan CP, Diamond J. Origins of major human infectious diseases. Nature. 2007;447(7142):279–83. https://doi.org/10.1038/nature05775.
8. Petersen E, Petrosillo N, Koopmans M, ESCMID Emerging Infections Task Force Expert Panel. Emerging infections-an increasingly important topic: review by the emerging infections task force. Clin Microbiol Infect. 2018;24(4):369–75. https://doi.org/10.1016/j.cmi.2017.10.035.
9. ECDC. Publications and data [internet]. Geneva: World Health Organization. Available at: https://www.ecdc.europa.eu/en/publications-data.
10. WHO. Vector-borne diseases [internet]. Geneva: World Health Organization. Available at: https://www.who.int/news-room/fact-sheets/detail/vector-borne-diseases.
11. WHO. Global vector control response 2017–2030. Geneva: World Health Organization; 2017.
12. ECDC. European network for medical and veterinary entomology (VectorNet) [internet]. Stockholm: European Centre for Disease Prevention and Control; 2023. Available at: https://www.ecdc.europa.eu/en/about-us/partnerships-and-networks/disease-and-laboratory-networks/vector-net
13. Barras V, Greub G. History of biological warfare and bioterrorism. Clin Microbiol Infect. 2014;20(6):497–502. https://doi.org/10.1111/1469-0691.12706.
14. CDC. CDC director releases after-action report on recent anthrax incident; highlights steps to improve laboratory quality and safety [internet]. Atlanta: Centers for Disease Control and Prevention; 2014. Available at: https://archive.cdc.gov/www_cdc_gov/media/releases/2014/p0711-lab-safety.html.
15. Bloom DE, Cadarette D. Infectious disease threats in the twenty-first century: strengthening the global response. Front Immunol. 2019;10:549. https://doi.org/10.3389/fimmu.2019.00549.
16. EC. EU Action on Antimicrobial Resistance [internet]. Brussels: European Comission. Available at: https://health.ec.europa.eu/antimicrobial-resistance/eu-action-antimicrobial-resistance_en.
17. EU. Report Special Eurobarometer 522 – Antimicrobial resistance. Brussels: European Union. February – March 2022. https://doi.org/10.2875/16102.
18. CDC. Antimicrobial Resistance Facts [internet]. Atlanta: Centers for Disease Control and Prevention: 9 September 2024. Available at: https://www.cdc.gov/narms/resistance/index.html.
19. United Nations Environment Programme. Bracing for superbugs: strengthening environmental action in the one health response to antimicrobial resistance. Geneva: United Nations; 2023.
20. WHO. Global action plan on antimicrobial resistance. Geneva: World Health Organization; 2015.
21. EC. A European one health action plan against antimicrobial resistance (AMR). Brussels: Directorate-General for Health and Food Safety – European Comission; 2017.
22. EClinicalMedicine. Antimicrobial resistance: a top ten global public health threat. EClinicalMedicine. 2021;41:101221. https://doi.org/10.1016/j.eclinm.2021.101221.

23. WHO. WHO Bacterial Priority Pathogens List, 2024: bacterial pathogens of public health importance to guide research, development and strategies to prevent and control antimicrobial resistance. Geneva: World Health Organization; 2024.
24. UN. Brief #2: putting the UN framework for socio-economic response to COVID-19 into action: insights. New York: United Nations; 2020.
25. WHO. International health regulations—2005. 3rd ed. Geneva: World Health Organization; 2016.
26. WHO. World health assembly agreement reached on wide-ranging, decisive package of amendments to improve the international health regulations [internet]. Geneva: World Health Organization; 2024. Available at: https://www.who.int/news/item/01-06-2024-world-health-assembly-agreement-reached-on-wide-ranging%2D%2Ddecisive-package-of-amendments-to-improve-the-international-health-regulations%2D%2Dand-sets-date-for-finalizing-negotiations-on-a-proposed-pandemic-agreement.
27. WHO. Health emergencies in Europe: making sure every country is ready. Geneva: Regional Office for Europe of the World Health Organization; 2019.
28. WHO. R&D Blueprint [internet]. Geneva: World Health Organization. Available at: https://www.who.int/teams/blueprint.
29. WHO. An R&D blueprint for action to prevent epidemics – update 2017 – accelerating R&D and saving lives. Geneva: World Health Organization. p. 2017.
30. WHO. Prioritizing diseases for research and development in emergency contexts [internet]. Geneva: World Health Organization; 2025. Available at: https://www.who.int/activities/prioritizing-diseases-for-research-and-development-in-emergency-contexts
31. WHO. COVID-19 research and innovation achievements. Geneva: World Health Organization; 2021.
32. Weber DJ, Rutala WA, Fischer WA, Kanamori H, Sickbert-Bennett EE. Emerging infectious diseases: focus on infection control issues for novel coronaviruses (severe acute respiratory syndrome-CoV and middle east respiratory syndrome-CoV), hemorrhagic fever viruses (Lassa and Ebola), and highly pathogenic avian influenza viruses, A(H5N1) and A(H7N9). Am J Infect Control. 2016;44(5 Suppl):e91–e100. https://doi.org/10.1016/j.ajic.2015.11.018.
33. CDC. Personal protective equipment (PPE): protect the worker with PPE [internet]. Atlanta: Centers for Disease Control and Prevention, National Institute for occupational Safety and Health, 2022. Available at: https://www.cdc.gov/niosh/learning/safetyculturehc/module-3/7.html.
34. ECDC. Safe use of personal protective equipment in the treatment of infectious diseases of high consequence. Stockholm: European Centre for Disease Prevention and Control; 2014.
35. ECDC. Guidance for wearing and removing personal protective equipment in healthcare settings for the care of patients with suspected or confirmed COVID-19. Stockholm: European Centre for Disease Prevention and Control; 2020.
36. Levitt AM. Deadly outbreaks. 2nd ed. New York: Skyhorse Publishing; 2015.

The Role of Antiseptics in Wound Healing, Wound Disinfection, and Biofilm Management with a Focus on Povidone-Iodine (PVP-I)

4

Luc Gryson, Tine Gryson, and Tom Gryson

Abstract

Wound healing is a multifaceted biological process influenced by microbial dynamics, biofilms, and the choice of antiseptics. Chronic wounds often harbour biofilms—structured microbial communities that resist antimicrobial treatments and hinder healing. Among the widely available antiseptics, Povidone-Iodine (PVP-I) demonstrates exceptional efficacy in wound sanitation due to its broad-spectrum antimicrobial activity, its ability to disrupt biofilms, low resistance-inducing effect, and minimal cytotoxicity. PVP-I acts by penetrating biofilm matrices, eradicating embedded microorganisms, and reducing microbial load, thereby accelerating healing in acute, chronic, and surgical wounds. It is versatile and is available in various formulations such as solutions, ointments, and dressings, tailored to clinical needs.

Comparative studies highlight PVP-I's superior biofilm-disrupting properties and antimicrobial efficacy over alternatives like chlorhexidine, silver-based agents, and polyhexamethylene biguanide. Practical application involves integration with complementary therapies, including debridement and negative

L. Gryson (✉)
Centre for Continuous Education, WOUND-Ex, Poperinge, Belgium

ZOWE School for Nursing, Bruges, Belgium
e-mail: luc@cnpv.be

T. Gryson
Centre for Continuous Education, WOUND-Ex, Poperinge, Belgium

University of Ghent, Ghent, Belgium

Centre Hospitalier de Luxembourg (CHL), Luxembourg, Luxembourg

T. Gryson
Centre for Continuous Education, WOUND-Ex, Poperinge, Belgium

© The Author(s), under exclusive license to Springer Nature Switzerland AG 2025
B. Oomen, S. Gastaldi (eds.), *Principles of Nursing Infection Prevention Control*,
Principles of Specialty Nursing, https://doi.org/10.1007/978-3-032-01446-7_4

pressure wound therapy, to optimize treatment outcomes. Proposed algorithms emphasize structured care strategies, addressing infection control, biofilm management, and wound monitoring. Future developments in antiseptic therapies may leverage nanotechnology and personalized treatments based on wound microbiology and patient characteristics.

PVP-I remains a cornerstone in modern wound care due to its safety, effectiveness, and versatility, offering healthcare providers a reliable tool to manage infections, promote healing, and improve patient outcomes, particularly in biofilm-associated chronic wounds.

Keywords

Wound healing · Biofilms · Povidone-Iodine (PVP-I) · Antiseptics · Chronic wounds · Antimicrobial efficacy · Infection control · Biofilm disruption

4.1   Introduction

Wound healing is a complex biological process that is influenced by a variety of factors, including microbial dynamics, the presence of biofilms, and the choice of antiseptics used in treatment. Achieving optimal wound healing requires adequate treatment to prevent infections, promote tissue regeneration, and restore normal tissue function. The use of antiseptics plays a crucial role in wound disinfection and in the promotion of a conducive environment for healing.

Chronic wounds often contain biofilms, impeding healing and contributing to persistent infections [1]. Consequently, microbial biofilms pose a significant challenge in the treatment of chronic wounds. Biofilms are structured communities of microorganisms encapsulated in a self-produced extracellular matrix, which makes them more resistant to various antimicrobials and the host's immune response. Understanding the microbial dynamics of these biofilms is essential for effective treatment. Studies indicate that biofilms slow wound healing, emphasizing the necessity of well-designed antiseptic protocols [2, 3].

The practical application of antiseptics such as PVP-I in wound treatment extends beyond disinfection. Research demonstrates the unique ability of PVP-I to disrupt biofilm structures commonly present in chronic wounds [4, 5]. The efficacy of PVP-I, combined with its relatively low toxicity, make it a first-line tool in wound infection prevention and control, promoting healing in biofilm-infected wounds.

4.2   Microbial Dynamics and Biofilms in Wounds

4.2.1   Understanding Wound Microbiology

Wound microbiology is an important element in wound treatment because the presence and activity of microorganisms can significantly influence the healing process. Wounds provide a favourable environment for microbial colonization due to nutrient and fluid availability and a compromised immune response. Microbial dynamics in wounds are influenced by the interaction between aerobic, facultative anaerobic, obligate anaerobic bacteria and the host immune response. The microorganisms work together in synergy, increasing their collective resilience to antimicrobial treatments. Understanding the nature of the present microorganisms, their mutual interplay and interaction with the tissue is essential for effective care and the development of appropriate wound management strategies.

Wound biofilms are invisible to the eye, consist of diverse pathogens, often thriving in the nutrient-rich, oxygen-poor and mildly basic environment of chronic wounds [6]. The resistance to treatment of biofilm infected wounds demonstrates the need for an effective strategy to disrupt these inherently complex microbial communities [1, 7].

4.2.2   Common Pathogens in Wound Infections

Wound infections are usually caused by a variety of pathogens, including bacteria, fungi, and, in some cases, viruses. Chronic wounds are primarily infested by Gram-positive bacteria, Gram-negative bacteria, and anaerobic species [8].

The ESKAPE pathogens (*Enterococcus faecium, Staphylococcus aureus, Klebsiella pneumoniae, Acinetobacter baumannii, Pseudomonas aeruginosa,* and Enterobacter species) are the most common bacterial species causing wound infections [9, 10]. These require particular attention due to their role in multidrug resistance and persistence of biofilms.

4.2.3   Biofilms and Chronic Wounds

Chronic wounds are characterized by prolonged inflammation and persistent local infection, generally caused by the presence of biofilms. Biofilms are structured communities of microorganisms encapsulated in a self-produced extracellular matrix that attaches to the surface of wounds. Biofilms act as physical barriers for antimicrobials, reducing the efficacy of many antiseptics, and protect the microorganisms embedded in them from the host's immune system [11]. Biofilms aid bacterial survival by increasing resistance to antimicrobial treatment [12]. As biofilms develop, microorganisms within them are in constant communication, a process known as quorum sensing [13]. Biofilms contribute to long-term inflammation, impaired healing, and an increased risk of persistent infection [3, 14]. Biofilms do create a hypoxic and basic environment and consume the essential nutrients present in the wounds. The interactions between the various pathogens present in biofilms negatively affect wound healing [15]. The microorganisms embedded in biofilms are highly resistant to antibiotics, posing a major challenge in the care for chronic wounds [14]. The application of antiseptics is fundamental in controlling the microbial load, especially in the context of biofilm-infected wounds [16]. Biofilm formation involves several phases [14].

1. **Initial reversible attachment**: Microorganisms attach to the wound surface through weak, reversible interactions.
2. **Irreversible attachment**: Microorganisms produce extracellular polymeric substances (EPS) which anchor them firmly to the surface.
3. **Maturation**: The biofilm grows and forms complex, three-dimensional structures with channels for the exchange of nutrients and waste products.
4. **Dispersion**: Cells originating from the biofilm spread to colonize new areas.

Biofilms exhibit various resistance mechanisms to standard wound treatments [17]:

- **Physical barrier**: The EPS matrix acts as a physical barrier and prevents penetration of antibiotics and antiseptics.
- **Altered microbial metabolism**: Microorganisms in biofilms often enter a slow-growing or dormant state, making them less susceptible to antibiotics that target actively dividing cells.
- **Genetic exchange**: The proximity of cells in biofilms facilitates the exchange of genetic material, including antibiotic resistance genes.
- **Phenotypic diversity**: Biofilms contain a diverse population of cells with varying levels of resistance, ensuring the survival of some cells even under antimicrobial pressure.

4.3   Antiseptics

4.3.1   Introduction

Effective wound management promotes healing and prevents complications, such as infections. Antiseptics play an important role in controlling wound contamination, reducing bacterial load, and disrupting biofilm formation. They are used topically to reduce the microbial load on the wound surface, lowering the risk of infection and promoting a favourable environment for healing. Among the various antiseptics, povidone iodine has demonstrated significant efficacy due to its broad-spectrum antimicrobial activity, biofilm-disrupting properties, relatively low cytotoxicity, and ease of use. Studies underscore the importance of selecting antiseptics that target planktonic bacteria and biofilms while minimizing cytotoxicity to host tissues [4, 5].

4.3.2   Use of Antiseptics in Wound Treatment

4.3.2.1 Historical Context

The use of antiseptics dates to ancient civilizations, where natural substances such as honey and vinegar were applied for their antimicrobial properties. The modern era of antiseptics began in the nineteenth century with the introduction of carbolic acid by Joseph Lister, which revolutionized surgical practice by significantly reducing postoperative infections. Since then, the development and use of antiseptics has evolved, with a variety of products currently being available that target a broad spectrum of pathogens. [18].

4.3.2.2 Use of Antiseptics

Antiseptics are important in the prevention and treatment of infections in both acute and chronic wounds. The adequate use of antiseptics set the stage for optimal wound healing by reducing the microbial load on the wound surface and by disrupting the structural integrity of biofilms that impede healing [16]. Microbial resistance, cytotoxicity, and tolerability influence the choice of a product. Unlike antibiotics, antiseptics show a limited tendency to induce microbial resistance due to their multiple target sites. However, inappropriate use, such as suboptimal concentrations or incomplete application, can contribute to microbial adaptation.

4.3.2.3 Antiseptics from Clinical Practice [19]

- **Chlorhexidine (CHX):** [20]
    - Benefits: Has a broad-spectrum and long-lasting residual effect, is effective against a wide range of bacteria, and is often used.
    - Limitations: Reduced efficacy in the presence of organic matter; it has a certain cytotoxicity and a risk of anaphylactic reactions and cross-resistance.
- **Povidone-Iodine (PVP-I):**
    - Advantages: It has broad-spectrum activity, no known resistance, minimal toxicity, and is available in a variety of forms. PVP-I is safe when used correctly and has few long-term side effects. PVP-I knows an exceptionally low occurrence of allergy and contact dermatitis, found in only 0.4% of the documented cases [21].
    - Limitations: Exposure to large amounts of iodine can lead to hyper- or hypothyroidism [22].
- **Silver-based products:** [23]
    - Benefits: It is used in various wound dressings due to its long-lasting antimicrobial activity. It is effective against many antibiotic-resistant bacteria.
    - Limitations: Potential cytotoxicity, more expensive and risk of resistance development [24].
- **Poly hexamethylene biguanide (PHMB):**
    - Benefits: It is a broad-spectrum antiseptic, with an antiparasitic activity. It exhibits few toxicity problems that are often associated with other antimicrobials [25].

– Limitations: it has a slower action than PVP-I and requires an exposure time of minimum 15 minutes to achieve complete bactericidal efficacy [20] (Table 4.1).

4.3.2.4 Antiseptic Efficacy Studies

To evaluate the antimicrobial efficacy of antiseptics, both laboratory-based and clinical studies are used.

In vitro studies allow precise control over experimental conditions, allowing for detailed analysis of antiseptic activity against specific pathogens [4]. These studies use biofilm models to evaluate the effectiveness of antiseptics against biofilm-forming bacteria and provide insight into their potential clinical performance [27, 28].

In vivo studies are based on clinical trials. They assess the efficacy of antiseptics in real-world wound situations and results are subject to the variability of patient and wound-specific factors. These studies are especially useful in determining the practical effectiveness of antiseptics in promoting wound healing [5, 29].

4.3.2.5 Factors Affecting the Effectiveness of Antiseptics

Several factors influence the efficacy of antiseptics [32]

- **Concentration and contact time**: Higher concentrations and longer contact times generally enhance antimicrobial activity.
- **Wound environment**: The presence of organic matter, such as blood and exudate, can reduce the efficacy of antiseptics.
- **Microbial load and presence of biofilm**: High microbial load and biofilm formation can hinder antiseptic penetration and activity.
- **Patient factors**: Individual patient factors, including immune status and comorbidities, can influence the efficacy of antiseptic treatment.

4.3.3 PVP-I Compared to Other Antiseptics

The performance of PVP-I compared to other antiseptics, such as poly hexamethylene biguanide, chlorhexidine, and silver-based agents:

Table 4.1 Characteristics and efficacy of common antiseptics in wound care

Antiseptic	Spectrum of activity	Disruption of the biofilm	Cytotoxicity	Main applications
PVP-I	Gram-positive and gram-negative bacteria, fungi, yeasts, viruses	High	Low	Acute and chronic wounds, infected wounds, biofilms
CHX	Gram-positive and gram-negative bacteria, fungi	Moderate	Moderate	Surgical wounds
PHMB	Gram-positive and gram-negative bacteria, fungi	Moderate	Low	Infected wounds, biofilms

Table designed by the author [4, 20, 26]

- **Polyhexanide**: Studies highlight that PVP-I has superior anti-biofilm activity compared to polyhexanide [4].
- **Silver**: While silver dressings are effective against planktonic bacteria, PVP-I has a broader spectrum of activity and lower risk of microbial resistance. Additionally, PVP-I is more cost-effective [33].
- **Chlorhexidine**: PVP-I has better antimicrobial activity compared to chlorhexidine, making it more effective in controlling resistant bacteria. Chlorhexidine has a longer effect but has a narrower spectrum and shows cross-resistance [34] (Table 4.2).

Among the available antiseptics, PVP-I stands out for the following: [4, 35]

- Broad-spectrum efficacy: Effective against bacteria, fungi, viruses, and protozoa, including antibiotic-resistant strains.
- Low resistance development: In contrast to antibiotics, the risk of resistance development against PVP-I is minimal.
- Versatility: Applicable in various forms such as solutions, ointments, and dressings, making it suitable for different types of wounds.
- Minimal toxicity: Generally, well tolerated with low cytotoxicity to human cells.
- Minimal allergic reactions when used properly.

4.4 Focus on Povidone-Iodine

4.4.1 Role of Povidone Iodine and Microbial Dynamics

Studies highlight the biofilm-disrupting properties of PVP-I, underscoring its ability to break down the extracellular biofilm matrix and eradicating embedded microorganisms [4, 5]. PVP-I also exhibits rapid antimicrobial activity and significant reductions in microbial load with minimal exposure time [34].

Table 4.2 Comparative efficacy of antiseptics in targeting biofilms

Antiseptic	Pathogens targeted	Disruption of the biofilm	Application Time
PVP-I	Gram-positive and gram-negative bacteria, fungi, viruses	High	< 5 min
CHX	Gram-positive bacteria	Moderate	10 min
Silver ions	Broad range of bacteria, fungi, and viruses	Moderate	> 30 min
PHMB	Gram-positive and gram-negative bacteria, fungi	Moderate	30 min

Table designed by the author [4, 5, 30, 34]

4.4.2 Operation of PVP-I

Povidone-iodine is an iodophor known for its broad-spectrum antimicrobial activity, and anti-inflammatory effect. This anti-inflammatory effect is believed to leverage multiple mechanisms. PVP-I is a complex of iodine with polyvinylpyrrolidone (PVP), which acts as a carrier and stabilizer, allowing the slow release of free iodine. Povidone-iodine exhibits bactericide activity by targeting essential bacterial cellular mechanisms and structures. It binds to microbial proteins, thereby disrupting enzymatic activity crucial for bacterial survival, and interacts with microbial cell membranes, causing structural damage. The free iodine released by PVP-I is able to penetrate the microbial cell wall. It oxidizes nucleotides, fatty acids, and amino acids in bacterial cell membranes and denatures and deactivates cytosolic enzymes involved in its respiratory chain. By affecting DNA/RNA synthesis, thereby hindering microbial replication, and the destruction of proteins essential to bacterial functioning, cell death is induced [38].

Cytotoxicity studies show that iodine exerts its bactericidal effects before it affects individual human cells.

Povidone-iodine is one of the few topical antimicrobials that is effective against a wide range of microorganisms, including bacteria, viruses, fungi and spores, protozoa, and amoebic cysts [21]. Classic antimicrobial tests have shown that povidone-iodine can quickly kill bacterial strains responsible for nosocomial infections, such as methicillin-resistant Staphylococcus aureus (MRSA), vancomycin-resistant Entercocci (VRE), and other antibiotic-resistant strains, within 20–30 s of exposure. Alternatives such as chlorhexidine require longer exposure times, and encounter more bacterial resistance [4, 29].

4.4.3 Specific Efficacy Against Biofilms and Resistant Strains

PVP-I is effective against biofilms due to its ability to penetrate their matrix and kill microbial cells. Studies show that PVP-I not only effectively destroys existing biofilms but also impedes the formation of biofilms, underscoring its role in wound infection prevention [4, 5].

The sustained effectiveness of povidone-iodine in wound healing, in the presence of biofilms, has been demonstrated [4, 29]. PVP-I inhibits the growth of *S. epidermidis* and *S. aureus* and is able to prevent the formation of staphylococcal biofilms at low concentrations [36]. In addition, povidone-iodine demonstrated efficacy against biofilms consisting of MRSA and *Candida albicans*, even at highly diluted concentrations. The capacity to remove biofilms exceeded that of other agents such as PHMB, octenidine, chlorhexidine, mupirocin, and fusidic acid [37].

4.4.4   Clinical Applications in Different Types of Wounds

PVP-I is versatile, its broad-spectrum activity and absence of resistance make it useful in the care for acute, chronic, and surgical wounds. The rapid antimicrobial action helps reduce the risk of infection and promotes faster healing. In chronic wounds, such as diabetic foot ulcers and venous leg ulcers, PVP-I helps control biofilm-associated infections and reduces microbial load, supporting the healing process. PVP-I is also often used in preoperative skin preparation and postoperative wound care to prevent postoperative wound infections [33, 35, 38].

4.4.5   Cytotoxicity and Tissue Compatibility

1. **Cytotoxic effects:**

   - Although PVP-I exhibits some cytotoxic effects in vitro, its benefits in controlling infections and promoting healing outweigh its potential harms in clinical settings. The use of stabilizers has further minimized the risks of cytotoxicity [33, 35].
   - PVP-I may exhibit, (dose-dependent), cytotoxicity, potentially delaying healing if used excessively. This emphasizes the importance of adhering to recommended concentrations to balance antimicrobial efficacy with cellular viability [39].

2. **Patient-specific considerations:**

   - Variability in tissue response requires an individualized approach (e.g. diabetic patients) [7].

4.4.6   Application

4.4.6.1 Presentations

PVP-I is available in multiple forms, including solutions, ointments, gels, and impregnated dressings, each tailored for different wound care needs. The choice of a specific formulation depends on wound characteristics and treatment goals:

1. **Solutions:**

   - Used for irrigation, cleaning and disinfection of acute and chronic wounds.
   - Delivered via sprays or direct application to the wound bed.
   - Active even with short exposure times (<5 min).

2. **Ointments and gels:**

- Ideal for wounds at risk of drying out or that need a barrier against environmental contamination.
- Ointments provide a sustained antimicrobial effect while maintaining a moist wound environment.
- Ideal in the treatment of chronic wounds with a biofilm present [18, 40].

3. **Impregnated bandages:**

- Release PVP-I gradually, while maintaining long-term antimicrobial activity.
- Particularly effective in treating critically colonized or biofilm-laden wounds [7, 40].
- Impregnated dressings provide prolonged contact-time but may not be suitable for wounds with heavy exudate.

4. **Additional applications:**

- Combining PVP-I with debridement or negative pressure wound therapy (NPWT) improves efficacy [7].

Improper use can lead to suboptimal results, such as insufficient reduction of microbial load or excessive drying of the wound bed.

4.4.6.2 Method of Use

Differences in use between healthcare providers may negatively affect outcomes. Standardized protocols for application improve the product's overall effectiveness. The choice between solution, ointment or dressing depends on the type of wound and the clinical goals [40].

4.4.6.3 Frequency of Use

Frequent application is recommended to maintain antimicrobial efficacy [1, 7].

4.4.6.4 Patient Safety

Contraindications, such as hypersensitivity to the product or dysfunction of the thyroid gland, should be observed.

4.4.7 Considerations

The cost-effectiveness makes PVP-I easily and widely accessible. Training of healthcare providers to properly utilize antiseptics remains important [7]. The colour properties of PVP-I can affect patient compliance, highlighting the need for patient education.

While PVP-I can be an important tool in wound care, its use requires careful consideration of the benefits and individual risks and contra-indications in patient-centred care strategies.

4.5   Practical Applications of PVP-I in Wound Treatment

The practical application of povidone-iodine in wound management lies at the intersection of antimicrobial efficacy, biofilm disruption, and patient safety. PVP-I is a widely used antiseptic in wound care, effective against a broad spectrum of pathogens, including bacteria, fungi, viruses, and protozoa. The application of PVP-I in wound management involves solutions, ointments, and dressings, each tailored to specific clinical scenarios. PVP-I significantly reduces microbial load, prevents the formation of biofilms, and promotes the healing of chronic wounds. [35, 5] Successful treatment of diabetic foot ulcers and pressure ulcers with PVP-I-based products has been demonstrated. [35, 41] PVP-I is also used in postoperative wound care to prevent surgical site infections (SSIs). Its broad-spectrum activity is particularly beneficial in the treatment of polymicrobial infections [33].

The efficiency of PVP-I in wound care is influenced by several factors, including the concentration of the antiseptic, the duration of exposure, and the inherent properties of the wound. Studies have provided valuable insights into the optimal conditions for PVP-I application, highlighting the importance of short exposure times and proper formulation to maximize antimicrobial efficacy while minimizing cytotoxic effects [5, 35]. In vitro and ex vivo models validate the biofilm-disrupting properties of PVP-I, even in the presence of multidrug-resistant pathogens. PVP-I exhibits low cytotoxicity when used appropriately [4, 5, 21].

4.5.1   Consensus Guidelines for Biofilm Management in Chronic Wounds

Biofilms pose a major challenge in the treatment of chronic wounds due to their resistance to conventional treatments. Consensus guidelines [40, 7, 3] recommend a multifaceted approach to biofilm management, including debridement with regular removal of necrotic tissue and biofilm, as well as the use of broad-spectrum antiseptics to disrupt biofilm structure and reduce microbial load. Consensus guidelines promote the application of dressings impregnated with antiseptics, to maintain a persistent antimicrobial effect, and a regular assessment of the wound evolution and microbial load to allow for treatment adjustment if necessary.

4.5.2   Integration of PVP-I with Complementary Therapies

1. **Debridement:**
   - Mechanical or enzymatic debridement removes necrotic tissue and biofilms, thereby improving PVP-I penetration and accelerating healing [42].
2. **Negative pressure wound therapy (NPWT):**
   - Applying PVP-I solutions in combination with NPWT improves wound bed cleanliness and promotes granulation tissue formation [43, 11].

3. **Antibiotic stewardship:**
   - The use of PVP-I may reduce reliance on systemic antibiotics and may thereby address concerns about antimicrobial resistance by antibiotic overuse [31].

4.5.3 An Algorithm for the Treatment of Chronic, Non-healing Wounds Due to Local Infection and/or Biofilm

4.5.3.1 Chronic Wound Challenges

Chronic, non-healing wounds pose significant clinical challenges due to their multifactorial nature, often with persistent local infection, biofilm formation, and impaired host response.

The need for a structured approach stems from:

- **The complexity of biofilm-associated wounds:** Biofilms are highly resistant to antimicrobial agents and host defences. Targeted interventions to disrupt biofilm structures and early intervention with antiseptics prevent the formation of biofilm [1, 3, 40].
- **Limitations of current practices:** Empirical wound care often lacks precision and uniformity, leading to longer healing times and higher healthcare costs. Combined mechanical, chemical, and antimicrobial interventions are shown to be more effective [1, 7].
- **The role of PVP-I in biofilm management:** PVP-I has demonstrated superior anti-biofilm activity, making it a cornerstone of the proposed algorithm [40].

4.5.3.2 Components of the Algorithm

The use of antiseptics in wound care involves several key steps to ensure efficacy and safety, by addressing critical aspects of wound management: [40]

1. **Assessment and Diagnosis**
   - Assess wound size, depth, exudate levels, and the integrity of surrounding skin to establish a baseline. The use of a wound analysis model such as TIME can be helpful.
   - **Microbial analysis:** Perform swabs and/or biopsies if necessary to identify pathogens and confirm the presence of biofilm. Fluorescence imaging can be of value to detect biofilm regions [44].
   - **Risk stratification:** Classify wounds based on the severity of the infection, and the likelihood of biofilm formation. Identify comorbidities and consider patient factors such as diabetes, venous insufficiency, and lifestyle.

2. **Preparation and Cleaning**
   - **Debridement:** Use sharp, ultrasonic, enzymatic, or autolytic debridement to remove necrotic tissue and biofilm residues. This allows effective antiseptic penetration and reduces the microbial load [1, 3].
   - **Antiseptic irrigation:** Preferably use PVP-I soap solution for wound irrigation. The broad-spectrum antimicrobial activity combined with the detergent action of the soap component effectively removes plankton bacteria and residual biofilms [40]. Rinse and clean the wound thoroughly to remove dirt and exudate, then irrigate with a physiological saline solution.
   - **Pain management:** Administer local anaesthetics or systemic analgesics when needed to improve patient comfort and compliance during debridement.

3. **Biofilm Disruption and Infection Control**
   - **Anti-biofilm agents:** Apply the antiseptic evenly and directly to the wound bed. PVP-I is able to disrupt extracellular polymeric substances and penetrate biofilm matrixes. Ensure even coverage and ensure sufficient contact time, at least 1 minute in the case of PVP-I, to enable it to exert its effect.
   - **Dressing selection:** Maintain antiseptic action between dressing changes by applying PVP-I dressings or gels over the entire wound bed.

   1. Choose an appropriate dressing to provide sustained antimicrobial action (e.g., PVP-I impregnated mesh) while maintaining a moist environment conducive to healing.
   2. Cover with a suitable secondary dressing.
   3. Fix with tape or a suitable bandage.

   - **Frequency of application:** Repeat this care at least every 24 h.
   - **Systemic antibiotics:** Use systemic antibiotics judiciously and only when clinical signs of systemic infection, such as cellulitis or sepsis, are apparent. This prevents the unnecessary development of antibiotic resistance.

4. **Healing Optimization**
   - **Moisture balance:** Ensure an optimal moist wound environment with the help of appropriate dressings.
   - **Inflammation control:** Address excessive inflammation with systemic anti-inflammatory medications and maintain a balanced microbiological wound environment conducive to healing [3].
   - **Nutritional support:** Evaluate and address potentially underlying nutritional deficiencies that may hinder wound healing.
   - **Complementary therapies:** Consider advanced interventions such as negative pressure therapy (NPWT) or hyperbaric oxygen therapy.

5. **Monitoring and Re-evaluation**
   - **Regular assessments:** Conduct periodic assessments to evaluate the progress of the wound. Assess the wound for infection or recurrence of biofilm based on the wound exudate present and adjust treatment strategies accordingly. Check for potential side effects of the antiseptic agent [1].
   - **Use of digital technologies:** Leverage imaging tools and electronic health records to track healing trends and optimize care plans.
   - **Early intervention for recurrence:** Address reinfection or biofilm formation immediately [1].

4.5.4 Implementation in Clinical Practice

The proposed algorithm provides a flexible framework that can be adapted to different healthcare settings. Some main points of attention in the implementation of a wound treatment algorithm are proper training of care personnel and education addressing key concepts (e.g. biofilms) and tools (e.g. antiseptics, wound dressings) in wound management, while also providing the right resources such as antiseptics and advanced dressings and involving patients in their treatment.

This algorithm provides a structured, evidence-based approach to treat chronic, non-healing wounds complicated by local infection and/or biofilms, with the aim to improve wound healing.

4.6 Conclusion

Antiseptics play a vital role in the prevention of infections and in promoting healing in both acute and chronic wounds. They help maintain an optimal wound environment, reduce microbial load, and are an essential tool in the treatment of biofilm-associated infections. The use of antiseptics is important to minimize the risk of complications and improve patient outcomes.

The treatment of chronic wounds complicated by biofilms requires a multifaceted approach that includes the use of effective antiseptics. By understanding the microbial dynamics within biofilms and the practical application of antiseptics, healthcare providers can positively influence the course of wound evolution. Povidone-iodine remains an important tool in wound management due to its broad-spectrum antimicrobial activity, biofilm-disrupting properties, and minimal toxicity. Its ability to penetrate biofilms and effectively target antibiotic-resistant strains makes it a valuable tool in wound management. The large variety of PVP-I application modalities allows for it to be used in various types of wounds, including acute, chronic, surgical wounds and various wound care scenarios. It provides clinicians with a reliable and effective antiseptic option. By combining PVP-I with other treatment methods, effectiveness can be improved.

Important here are combination therapies that leverage the synergistic effects of multiple antimicrobials or interventions. The application of nanotechnology is being investigated to further improve the release and effectiveness of antiseptics.

A better understanding of the mechanisms of biofilm formation and the development of targeted strategies to eradicate biofilms is preeminent. It is expected that personalized treatments based on individual patient characteristics and patient specific wound microbiology will improve wound care outcomes.

References

1. Schultz G, Bjarnsholt T, James GA, Leaper DJ, McBain AJ, Malone M, Stoodley P, Swanson T, Tachi M, Wolcott RD. Global wound biofilm expert panel. Consensus guidelines for the identification and treatment of biofilms in chronic nonhealing wounds. Wound Repair Regen. 2017;25(5):744–57. https://doi.org/10.1111/wrr.12590. Epub 2017 Dec 12
2. Gajula B, Munnamgi S, Basu S. How bacterial biofilms affect chronic wound healing: a narrative review. Int J Sur Global Health. 2020;3(2020):e16. https://doi.org/10.1097/GH9.0000000000000016.
3. Metcalf D, Parsons D, Bowler P. Wound biofilm and therapeutic strategies; 2016. https://doi.org/10.5772/63238.
4. Gryson L, I. MSF, et al. Anti-biofilm activity of povidone-iodine and polyhexamethylene biguanide: evidence from in vitro tests. Curr Microbiol. 2023;80(5):161. https://doi.org/10.1007/s00284-023-03257-5. PMID: 37004626; PMCID: PMC10067645
5. Johani K, Malone M, Jensen SO, Dickson HG, Gosbell IB, Hu H, Yang Q, Schultz G, Vickery K. Evaluation of short exposure times of antimicrobial wound solutions against microbial biofilms: from in vitro to in vivo. J Antimicrob Chemother. 2018;73(2):494–502. https://doi.org/10.1093/jac/dkx391. PMID: 29165561; PMCID: PMC5890786.
6. Anju VT, Busi S, Imchen M, Kumavath R, Mohan MS, Salim SA, Subhaswaraj P, Dyavaiah M. Polymicrobial infections and biofilms: clinical significance and eradication strategies. Antibiotics (Basel). 2022;11(12):1731. https://doi.org/10.3390/antibiotics11121731. PMID: 36551388; PMCID: PMC9774821.
7. Snyder RJ, Bohn G, Hanft J, Harkless L, Kim P, Lavery L, Schultz G, Wolcott R. Wound biofilm: current perspectives and strategies on biofilm disruption and treatments. Wounds. 2017;29(6):S1–S17.
8. Bowler PG, Duerden BI, Armstrong DG. Wound microbiology and associated approaches to wound management. Clin Microbiol Rev. 2001;14(2):244–69. https://doi.org/10.1128/CMR.14.2.244-269.2001. PMID: 11292638; PMCID: PMC88973.
9. Puca V, Marulli RZ, Grande R, Vitale I, Niro A, Molinaro G, Prezioso S, Muraro R, Di Giovanni P. Microbial species isolated from infected wounds and antimicrobial resistance analysis: data emerging from a three-years retrospective study. Antibiotics (Basel). 2021;10(10):1162. https://doi.org/10.3390/antibiotics10101162. PMID: 34680743; PMCID: PMC8532735.
10. Pendleton JN, Gorman SP, Gilmore BF. Clinical relevance of the ESKAPE pathogens. Expert Rev Anti-Infect Ther. 2013;11(3):297–308. https://doi.org/10.1586/eri.13.12.
11. Phillips PL, Yang Q, Schultz GS. The effect of negative pressure wound therapy with periodic instillation using antimicrobial solutions on Pseudomonas aeruginosa biofilm on porcine skin explants. Int Wound J. 2013;10:48–55. https://doi.org/10.1111/iwj.12180.
12. Hurlow J, Couch K, Laforet K, Bolton L, Metcalf D, Bowler P. Clinical biofilms: a challenging frontier in wound care. Adv Wound Care (New Rochelle). 2015;4(5):295–301. https://doi.org/10.1089/wound.2014.0567. PMID: 26005595; PMCID: PMC4432968.
13. Rhoads DD, Wolcott RD, Percival SL. Biofilms in wounds: management strategies. J Wound Care. 2008;17(11):502–8. https://doi.org/10.12968/jowc.2008.17.11.31479.

14. Mirghani R, Saba T, Khaliq H, Mitchell J, Do L, Chambi L, Diaz K, Kennedy T, Alkassab K, Huynh T, Elmi M, Martinez J, Sawan S, Rijal G. Biofilms: formation, drug resistance and alternatives to conventional approaches. AIMS Microbiol. 2022;8(3):239–77. https://doi.org/10.3934/microbiol.2022019. PMID: 36317001; PMCID: PMC9576500.

15. Durand BARN, Pouget C, Magnan C, Molle V, Lavigne JP, Dunyach-Remy C. Bacterial interactions in the context of chronic wound biofilm: a review. Microorganisms. 2022;10(8):1500. https://doi.org/10.3390/microorganisms10081500. PMID: 35893558; PMCID: PMC9332326.

16. Diban F, Di Lodovico S, Di Fermo P, D'Ercole S, D'Arcangelo S, Di Giulio M, Cellini L. Biofilms in chronic wound infections: innovative antimicrobial approaches using the in vitro Lubbock chronic wound biofilm model. Int J Mol Sci. 2023;24(2):1004. https://doi.org/10.3390/ijms24021004. PMID: 36674518; PMCID: PMC9862456.

17. Shree P, Kant Singh C, Kaur Sodhi K, Niranjane Surya J, Kumar Singh D. Biofilms: Understanding the structure and contribution towards bacterial resistance in antibiotics. Med Microecol 2023;16:100084, ISSN 2590-0978. https://doi.org/10.1016/j.medmic.2023.100084. https://www.sciencedirect.com/science/article/pii/S2590097823000095.

18. Toledo-Pereyra LH. Joseph Lister's surgical revolution. J Invest Surg. 2010;23(5):241–3. https://doi.org/10.3109/08941939.2010.520574.

19. McDonnell G, Russell AD. Antiseptics and disinfectants: activity, action, and resistance. Clin Microbiol Rev. 1999;12(1):147–79. https://doi.org/10.1128/CMR.12.1.147. Erratum in: Clin Microbiol Rev 2001 Jan;14(1):227. PMID: 9880479; PMCID: PMC88911.

20. Nair HKR, et al. International consensus document: use of wound antiseptics in practice. Wounds International; 2023. Available online at www.woundsinternational.com

21. Lachapelle J-M. A comparison of the irritant and allergenic properties of antiseptics. Eur J Dermatol. 2014;24(1):3–9. https://doi.org/10.1684/ejd.2013.2198.

22. Burchés-Feliciano MJ, Argente-Pla M, García-Malpartida K, Rubio-Almanza M, Merino-Torres JF. Hyperthyroidism induced by topical iodine. Endocrinol Nutr. 2015;62(9):465–6. https://doi.org/10.1016/j.endonu.2015.05.012. English, Spanish. Epub 2015 Aug 12

23. Burd A, Kwok CH, Hung SC, Chan HS, Gu H, Lam WK, Huang L. A comparative study of the cytotoxicity of silver-based dressings in monolayer cell, tissue explant, and animal models. Wound Repair Regen. 2007;15(1):94–104. https://doi.org/10.1111/j.1524-475X.2006.00190.x.

24. Salisbury AM, Chen R, Mullin M, Foulkes L, Percival SL. In vitro evaluation of resistance development to silver sulfadiazine and subsequent cross-resistance to antibiotics. Surg Technol Int 2022 ;40:55–60. doi: https://doi.org/10.52198/22.STI.40.WH1541.

25. Worsley A, Vassileva K, Tsui J, Song W, Good L. Polyhexamethylene Biguanide:Polyurethane Blend Nanofibrous Membranes for Wound Infection Control. Polymers (Basel). 2019;11(5):915. https://doi.org/10.3390/polym11050915. PMID: 31121845; PMCID: PMC6572704.

26. Babalska ZŁ, Korbecka-Paczkowska M, Karpiński TM. Wound antiseptics and European guidelines for antiseptic application in wound treatment. Pharmaceuticals (Basel). 2021;14(12):1253. https://doi.org/10.3390/ph14121253. PMID: 34959654; PMCID: PMC8708894.

27. Oates A, Lindsay S, Mistry H, et al. Modelling antisepsis using defined populations of facultative and anaerobic wound pathogens grown in a basally perfused biofilm model. Biofouling. 2018;34 https://doi.org/10.1080/08927014.2018.1466115.

28. Touzel RE, Sutton JM, Wand ME. Establishment of a multi-species biofilm model to evaluate chlorhexidine efficacy. J Hosp Infect. 2016;92(2):154–60. https://doi.org/10.1016/j.jhin.2015.09.013. Epub 2015 Oct 23

29. Al-Kaisy AA, Salih SA. Role of the antioxidant effect of vitamin e with vitamin C and topical povidone-iodine ointment in the treatment of burns. Ann Burns Fire Disasters. 2005;18(1):19–30. PMID: 21990974; PMCID: PMC3187962

30. International consensus. Appropriate use of silver dressings in wounds. An expert working group consensus. London: Wounds International. 2012. Available to download from: www.woundsinternational.com.

31. Barreto R, Barrois B, Lambert J, Malhotra-Kumar S, Santos-Fernandes S, Monstrey S. Addressing the challenges in antisepsis: focus on povidone iodine. Int J Antimicrob Agents. 2020;56(3):106064. https://doi.org/10.1016/j.ijantimicag.2020.106064. ISSN 0924-8579. https://www.sciencedirect.com/science/article/pii/S092485792030234X

32. Atiyeh BS, Dibo SA, Hayek SN. Wound cleansing, topical antiseptics and wound healing. Int Wound J. 2009;6(6):420–30. https://doi.org/10.1111/j.1742-481X.2009.00639.x. PMID: 20051094; PMCID: PMC7951490.

33. Monstrey SJ, Govaers K, Lejuste P, Lepelletier D, Ribeiro de Oliveira P. Evaluation of the role of povidone iodine in the prevention of surgical site infections. Surg Open Sci. 2023;13:9–17. https://doi.org/10.1016/j.sopen.2023.03.005. PMID: 37034245; PMCID: PMC10074992

34. Block C, Robenshtok E, Simhon A, et al. Evaluation of chlorhexidine and povidone iodine activity against methicillin-resistant Staphylococcus aureus and vancomycin-resistant enterococcus faecalis using a surface test. J Hosp Infect. 2000;46(2):147–52. https://doi.org/10.1053/jhin.2000.0805.

35. Bigliardi PL, Alsagoff SAL, El-Kafrawi HY, Pyon JK, Wa CTC, Villa MA. Povidone iodine in wound healing: a review of current concepts and practices. Int J Surg. 2017;44:260–8. https://doi.org/10.1016/j.ijsu.2017.06.073. Epub 2017 Jun 23

36. Oduwole K, Glynn A, Molony D, Murray D, Rowe S, Holland L, McCormack D, O'Gara J. Anti-biofilm activity of sub-inhibitory povidone-iodine concentrations against staphylococcus epidermidis and staphylococcus aureus. J Orthopaed Res Off Pub Orthopaed Res Soc. 2010;28:1252–6. https://doi.org/10.1002/jor.21110.

37. Hoekstra MJ, Westgate SJ, Mueller S. Povidone-iodine ointment demonstrates in vitro efficacy against biofilm formation. Int Wound J. 2017;14(1):172–9. https://doi.org/10.1111/iwj.12578. Epub 2016 Mar 10. PMID: 26968574; PMCID: PMC7949843

38. Lepelletier D, Maillard JY, Pozzetto B, Simon A. Povidone iodine: properties, mechanisms of action, and role in infection control and Staphylococcus aureus decolonization. Antimicrob Agents Chemother. 2020;64(9):e00682–20. https://doi.org/10.1128/AAC.00682-20. PMID: 32571829; PMCID: PMC7449185.

39. Hirsch T, Koerber A, Jacobsen F, Dissemond J, Steinau HU, Gatermann S, Al-Benna S, Kesting M, Seipp HM, Steinstraesser L. Evaluation of toxic side effects of clinically used skin antiseptics in vitro. J Surg Res. 2010;164(2):344–50. https://doi.org/10.1016/j.jss.2009.04.029. Epub 2009 May 18

40. Alves PJ, Barreto RT, Barrois BM, Gryson LG, Meaume S, Monstrey SJ. Update on the role of antiseptics in the management of chronic wounds with critical colonisation and/or biofilm. Int Wound J. 2021;18(3):342–58. https://doi.org/10.1111/iwj.13537. Epub 2020 Dec 13. PMID: 33314723; PMCID: PMC8244012.

41. Gwak HC, Han SH, Lee J, Park S, Sung KS, Kim HJ, Chun D, Lee K, Ahn JH, Kwak K, Chung HJ. Efficacy of a povidone-iodine foam dressing (Betafoam) on diabetic foot ulcer. Int Wound J. 2020;17(1):91–9. https://doi.org/10.1111/iwj.13236. Epub 2019 Nov 26. PMID: 31773882; PMCID: PMC7949421.

42. Davies B, Patel H. Systematic review and meta-analysis of preoperative antisepsis with combination chlorhexidine and povidone-iodine. Surg J. 2016;02:e70–7. https://doi.org/10.1055/s-0036-1587691.

43. Back DA, Scheuermann-Poley C, Willy C. Recommendations on negative pressure wound therapy with instillation and antimicrobial solutions – when, where and how to use: what does the evidence show? Int Wound J. 2013;10(Suppl 1):32–42. https://doi.org/10.1111/iwj.12183. PMID: 24251842; PMCID: PMC7950486

44. Armstrong DG, Edmonds ME, Serena TE. Point-of-care fluorescence imaging reveals extent of bacterial load in diabetic foot ulcers. Int Wound J. 2023;20(2):554–66. https://doi.org/10.1111/iwj.14080. Epub 2023 Jan 28. PMID: 36708275; PMCID: PMC9885466.

Catheter-Associated Urinary Tract Infection (CAUTI)

5

J. P. Geelhoed

Abstract

Catheter-associated urinary tract infection (CAUTI) is a common hospital-associated infection, seen in approximately 40% of hospitalised patients. CAUTI is caused by commensal and non-commensal bacteria which enter the bladder via the catheter. *E. coli* is the most frequent cause of CAUTI. Treatment of UTI is important when it is symptomatic, especially in vulnerable patients, with appropriate antibiotics, based on a urine culture. It is advised to follow up on local regulations.

To prevent CAUTI, removal of the catheter is the best way, when it is possible to remove. Assess on a daily basis the need of the catheter and remove as soon as possible. Approximately 69% of CAUTI is preventable, with approximately 9000 preventable deaths. Antibiotic resistance and multi-resistant bacteria are a great danger in treatment options of CAUTI, with 19.2% of all hospital-acquired infections.

Placement of the catheter and maintenance must be done in accordance with the (local) guidelines, including adequate hand hygiene. Problems with the catheter should be solved immediately and with the most adequate measures.

Keywords

Catheter · Indwelling catheter · Urinary catheter · Suprapubic catheter · Urinary tract infection · Catheter-associated urinary tract infection · Antibiotic treatment

J. P. Geelhoed (✉)
Nurse practitioner/CNS in urology/andrology, St. Antonius Hospital,
Nieuwegein, The Netherlands
e-mail: j.geelhoed@antoniusziekenhuis.nl

5.1   What Is CAUTI?

Catheter-associated urinary tract infection (CAUTI) is defined as germs entering the urinary tract through a urinary catheter and causing infection. It is one of the most common types of hospital-acquired infections (HAI) [1, 2]. Almost 40% of all hospital-acquired infections are related to CAUTI. This can occur through an indwelling urethral or suprapubic catheterisation. The risk of CAUTI can be reduced by increasing the knowledge of nurses in catheter care. It is estimated that 69% of CAUTI events are avoidable by following guidelines. A large cohort study estimated that 12% of patients who have a catheter inserted for 30 days will develop a CAUTI [3, 4].

5.1.1   Difference Between Bacteriuria and Urinary Tract Infection (UTI)

Patients having an indwelling urethral or suprapubic catheter will have bacterial colonisation. It increases by 5% per day, with almost 100% after 7–10 days. It can be found in urine analysis. If patients do not experience complaints from bacteriuria, treatment is not necessary. When having symptoms of UTI while having a catheter the patient has a CAUTI. The signs and symptoms are fever, suprapubic tenderness, costovertebral angle tenderness, urinary frequency or urgency, or dysuria [1, 4]. Beside the signs and symptoms, the urine culture must be positive having 10^5 CFU/ml or more of one bacterial species.

5.1.2   Complex UTI and Pyelonephritis

A CAUTI is always a complex UTI, since it is caused by an indwelling catheter [5]. Patients may have a greater risk of getting a pyelonephritis when having an indwelling catheter than patients who don't have an indwelling catheter. Pyelonephritis is a serious condition, coming with (high) fever illness, possible hydronephrosis and the risk of developing urosepsis. If a CAUTI is proven and causes complaints, an antibiotic treatment is required, preferably based on a urine culture. In that case, a targeted treatment with antibiotic sensitive for the bacteria can be started. If the patient is very ill, an antibiotic treatment has to start immediately following the culture and can be adapted after the result of the culture.

Suprapubic indwelling catheterisation has also a risk of getting skin infection at the insertion side, which can possibly cause abscess. This should be treated with antibiotic adequately. The most appropriate treatment is through oral or intravenous access.

5.1.3 Most Common Bacteriuria in UTI

UTI can be caused by different uropathogen bacteria. They can be commensal to the patient like the gram-negative *Escherichia coli* (E. coli) or come from other sources such as an indwelling catheter being a healthcare-associated UTI. *E. coli* is the most frequent cause of UTI with 65–75% followed by *Staphylococcus saprophyticus* [6]. With CAUTI, other gram-negative bacteria are more pronounced, like Proteus spp., Klebsiella spp., *Pseudomonas aeruginosa*, Streptococcus, aeruginosa, and *Staphylococcus aureus*.

5.2 Facts and Figures on Indwelling Catheters and CAUTI

Indwelling catheters are used very often in hospitals and elderly nursing homes. Exact figures and numbers are unknown. In intensive care units in hospitals the use of indwelling catheters is the highest.

5.2.1 Prevalence and Incidence of CAUTI (ECDC)

In the Netherlands the prevalence of indwelling catheter use is monitored by PREZIES. In their prevalence report 2021 they reported 18% of indwelling catheter use in hospitals, being 91% with the right indication [7]. CDC estimates that between 15% and 25% of hospitalised patients receive a short-term indwelling catheter [8], most of them for inappropriate reasons.

The prevalence of long-term indwelling catheters in nursing homes is estimated on approximately 5% in the USA.

The CAUTI infection rates from pooled data in 2006 showed 3.1–7.5 infections per 1000 catheter days. An estimated 69% of CAUTI can be preventable, with approximately 9000 preventable deaths with the recommended infection prevention control measures [8].

In urology patients, UTIs are even more common up to 47%, of which CAUTI is 71% [9]. It is more common in the southern and eastern parts of Europe with a growing part of multi-resistant bacteria with 19.2% of all hospital-acquired infections [10].

5.3 How to Perform Catheterisation (According to EAUN Guideline on Indwelling Catheter in Adults 2024)

The European Association for Urology Nurses (EAUN) has developed a guideline on indwelling catheterisation and updated the guideline in 2024 [4]. This guideline is evidence based developed. First PICO questions are formulated to help to answer the questions from the nurses. Based on these questions a literature search is performed to answer the PICO questions.

5.3.1   Urethral and Suprapubic Catheterisation

Transurethral indwelling catheterisation means that the urinary catheter is inserted into the bladder through the urethra. A suprapubic urinary catheter is inserted into the bladder through the abdominal wall.

The purpose is to drain the urine in case of urinary retention, voiding difficulties, to assist incontinent patients, and to improve end-of-life care. Other reasons are post-surgery in which the catheter placement is of short term, less than 14 days. Measurement of urinary production, mostly in critically ill patients. Specific indications for suprapubic indwelling catheterisation are infectious disease like Fournier's Gangrene, urethral trauma, acute prostatitis, urethral stricture, complex urethral, or abdominal (bladder) surgery. Relative preference for suprapubic indwelling catheterisation are wheel chair use, sexual issues, complication with urethral catheterisation or soiling of faeces with incontinence.

Relative contraindications for placing a urethral indwelling catheter are traumatic events to meatus or urethra in previous catheterisation.

Contraindication for suprapubic indwelling catheterisation are known or suspected bladder cancer, visible haematuria, absence of an easily palpable or by ultrasonography localised distended urinary bladder.

Relative contraindications are previous lower abdominal surgery [1] because of altered anatomy of the abdomen; prosthetic devices [2] like hernia mesh; anticoagulant [3] that can't be stopped for a short time; Ascites and pregnancy [4].

Suprapubic indwelling catheterisation has some advantages over urethral indwelling catheterisation:

- The risk of urethral trauma and traumatic hypospadias with a change of necrosis is less, including catheter-induced urethritis.
- Reduced risk of catheter contamination with bacteria from the bowel.
- Easier access to the entry site of the catheter for cleansing and changing the catheter.
- Sexual intercourse is easier with suprapubic catheter for both men and women.
- It can be blocked to regain urethral micturition again and measure residue after micturition easily.

Also, there are limitations and risks to the use of the suprapubic indwelling catheter. It is an invasive procedure with risks of bleeding, visceral injury, perforate bowel and peritoneal perforation. This can cause high fever rapidly, with a very small risk of cardiac arrest. Patients with comorbidity like mechanical heart valves require antibiotic prophylaxis and bridging of blood thinners prior to initial insertion. These patients also need antibiotic prophylaxis before every change of the catheter. Patients may still leak urine through the urethra.

5.3.2   Tips and Tricks

There are some differences between the urethral and suprapubic catheter in maintenance. The urethral catheter is the most common indwelling catheter, certainly for short-term use. For long-term use, the suprapubic catheter is used, when there is an advantage over the urethral catheter.

With both catheters, bladder spasm is a commonly seen problem causing disadvantages for the patient. This can be painful and cause leakage through the urethra and the insertion in the abdomen [11]. Spoolder et al. did a literature review on nursing interventions to reduce catheter-related bladder spasms [11]. Possible interventions they found were to reduce the balloon size, fixate the catheter in the right way, secure the urine bag to the leg or use a valve, treat constipation, advice a fibre-rich diet, and increase fluid intake if possible. Besides these advices, the tube of the urine bag should be free of kinking to guarantee a free passage of the urine to the urine bag. The urine bag should be placed below the bladder level.

By fixating the catheter in the right way, with enough space to move the leg or for the men to have nightly erections, prevents wounding of the urethra, meatus, or labia in women.

With the supra pubic catheter, the insertion opening should be kept clean and if leakage is present covered by a bandage, which is changed when necessary.

Changing the catheter is in the EAUN guideline advised with sterile gloves in an aseptic manner. In the Netherlands the newest guideline for catheterisation advices non-sterile gloves and insert the catheter with no-touch technique or an aid to guide the catheter [2]. The advice is based on similar chance of urethral infections with indwelling catheters with or without complaints of UTI. Therefore the safety of patients is similar to both ways of placing a urethral catheter.

5.4 Maintenance of Indwelling Catheters Based on EAUN Guideline

The maintenance of indwelling catheters is important. This can prevent serious bladder infections and provide more comfort for the patient with a higher quality of life.

Always reassess the reason for the indwelling catheter. The best way to prevent UTI and improve quality of life is to remove the indwelling catheter.

5.4.1 Placing an Indwelling Catheter and Problems During Placement

The insertion of the urethral catheter needs to be done using by the no-touch procedure. An aseptic field can be created if this is indicated. When using non-sterile gloves, change them after cleaning the meatus and use non-touch technique when inserting the catheter by using the sterile grip connected to the catheter or a separate one. Always apply by the local protocols before starting the procedure. Use a hydrogel in the urethra before inserting the catheter. Always check if urine is floating before filling the fixation balloon [2, 4]. Always use the smallest size catheter possible. In adult men this usually 14–16 ch and in women 12–14 ch. With indwelling catheters for women, sometimes shorter lengths are available. Do not use these in men!

After insertion of the indwelling catheter, the use of a leg bag with a volume of 500–750 ml or a valve can be considered. This depends on the indication for the indwelling catheter. For the night a night bag with a larger content of 1500–2000 ml is advised. Avoid as much as possible disconnecting the leg bag or valve from the catheter when in situ. A reflux valve is normally present in the leg bag to prevent reflux of urine with bacteria to the bladder.

Several problems can occur when placing an indwelling catheter. In men, when placing a urethral catheter, the catheter has to follow the urethra passing several possible obstructions. Due to the length and anatomy of the male, urethral problems can be expected such as meatal stretching, bulbar urethral stricture, fause route, bladder neck stenoses or spastic sphincter/overactive pelvic floor muscles. At all levels, there is a chance of damaging the urethra with placing the catheter. When hypospadias is present it can be difficult to determine which opening is the real one connected to the urethra. In case of urethral obstruction in men due to urethra stricture or enlarged prostate, a Thiemann catheter can be used. Sometimes another type of catheter is indicated, this can be determined by specialist urological healthcare providers.

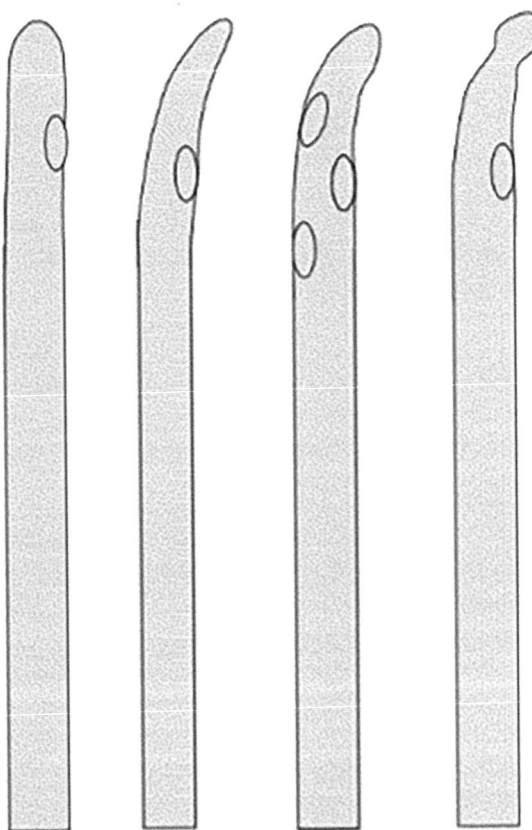

Picture of different catheter tips, with permission from Veronika Geng 17.2.2025

In female patients it can sometimes be difficult to find the meatus when spreading the labia. To make it easier to insert the catheter, a cushion can be placed beneath the pelvic floor of the woman to lift the bottom and have a better view at labia, vulva, and meatus. If the catheter is accidently placed into the vagina, you can leave it there and take another catheter to insert into the bladder. Another method is to guide the catheter over a finger placed into the vagina.

5.4.2 Problem Solving with Indwelling Catheters

Problems that can occur with indwelling catheters can be divers, for many reasons [12].

Leakage of urine is a well-known problem with decrease of quality of life for the patient. Reasons for occurrence of leakage are constipation, obstruction of the tube, small size of the catheter or balloon filing, and detrusor overactivity. Also, blockage inside the catheter due to encrustation or bladder stones is possible. To reslove thes issues, you need to identify the cause so that you can provide a solution. You start with the most common and easiest way to resolve problems, by assessing the placement of the tube and bag. Is kinking of the tube present? Solve this problem by good fixation of the tube. Special fixating material is available from different manufacturers. Empty the leg bag and advise the patient to do this as frequently as necessary. Place the bag always lower than the bladder level. In case of difficult stool, you can advise your patient to eat more fibres and drink more liquid. If this won't help enough, you can ask the physician or nurse practitioner to prescribe medication. With the next changing of the catheter, you can choose for a larger carrier to prevent leakage [4, 11].

The catheter can be blocked due to encrustation because of bacteria like *Proteus mirabilis* in the urine. This causes alkalinity resulting in development of crystals around the eyelets, and internal lumen of the catheter. Debris originates from the urothelial bladder wall, containing cells, blood, or mucus. Biofilm is a thin layer of microorganisms adhering to the surface of the catheter to prevent antibiotics to treat an infection. If the catheter is blocked due to debris or encrustation, it is advised to perform bladder washout with bladder irrigation.

You can start with a saline or advise the patient to drink more to increase the urine volume. In case of encrustation a specific solution with citric acid can be used to dissolve the encrustation. In case of debris and biofilm, a polyhexanide disinfectant can be used to wash out the microorganism and minimise the forming of a biofilm [4].

5.5 Infection Prevention Control

Infection prevention is an important part in prevention of CAUTI. The urinary tract is the most common source of nosocomial infections. CAUTI can be present in patients with a urinary catheter for >2 weeks. It means UTI infection with symptoms like fever, suprapubic tenderness, more dysuria and urgency, despite the catheter depsite the catheter, and a urine culture of 10^5 CFU/ml or more. Bacteriuria without symptoms of UTI are inevitable in patients with indwelling catheters. It is estimated that asymptomatic bacteriuria can grow by 5% of patients per day to 100% after 7–10 days colonisation risk. Asymptomatic Bacteriuria does not have to be treated with antibiotics. It is estimated that 69% of CAUTI events are avoidable by following guidelines and greater access to specialised nurses [4].

5.5.1 Hand Hygiene

Hand hygiene is the cornerstone of infection prevention. Transfer of bacteria, viruses, and other microbes is the most common and easiest by hands. We have seen during the COVID pandemic that reducing physical contact including hand shaking is the best way to reduce transfer of infectious diseases, besides keeping distance and wearing masks. Even Florence Nightingale promoted hand hygiene as one of the cornerstones in nursing to prevent spreading of infections between patients.

In current days, the rules when and how to perform hand hygiene are not for debate anymore. Maintenance and compliance are the most challenging. Everyone working in healthcare should be aware of the importance and oblige to hand hygiene.

The five moments of handhygiene are commenly accepted (Fig. 5.1), perform handhygiene before every contact with a patient and after each contact with a patient. Perform handhygiene between activities at the same patient. For example, when caring for someone, between activities from dirty to clean. To stimulate hand hygiene it is important to have immediate excess to hand alcohol pumps in the hospital, i.e., at each patient bed.

5.5.2 Performing a Urine Culture

Perform urine culture only if there is an indication or suspicion for UTI. Patients with an indwelling catheter should have systemic signs of an infection, like fever, feeling unwell, and lack of response to treatment. To perform a good culture, which gives a reliable answer to the question if an UTI is present, you must obey to the rules. To perform a correct urine culture, you must instruct your patient how to do this. These are the key elements for a patient without catheter:

- Wash your hands before starting.
- Wash the genitals with water.
  - Men should wash the penis, specifically the glans and meatus.
  - Women should wash the labia outer and inner and around vulva and meatus.
- Collect a mid-stream sample; the middle part of the urine portion. So let the first part flow in the toilet and then hold the collection container under the stream.
- Close the container with the lid and put a label on with all patient details.

Your 5 Moments
for Hand Hygiene

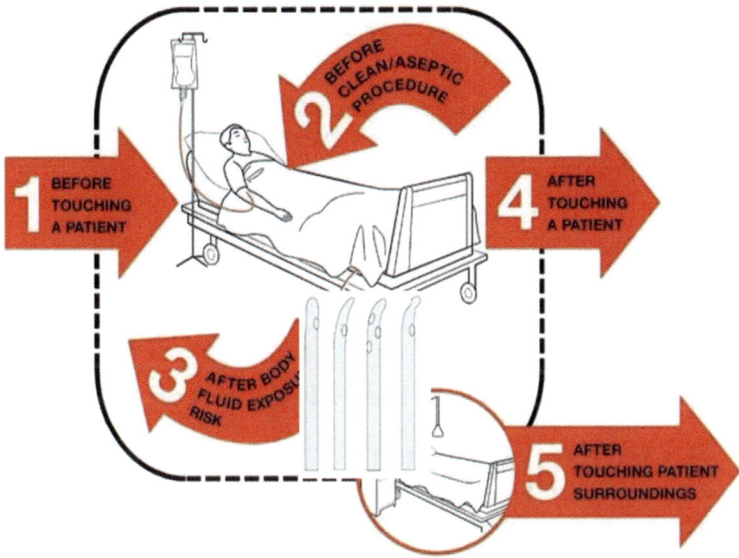

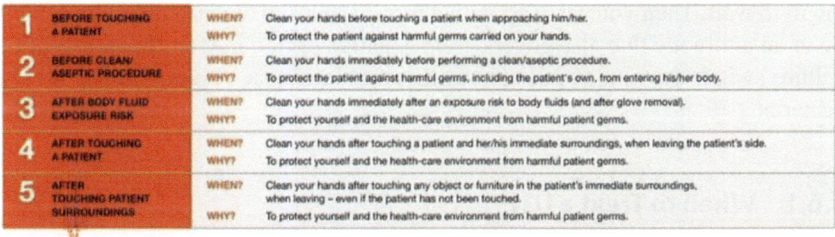

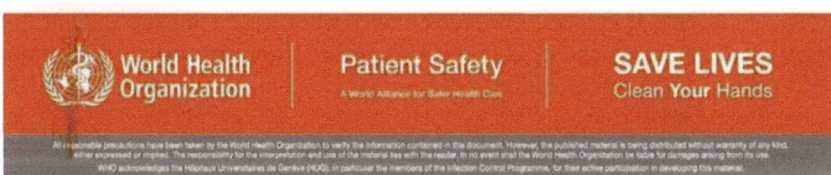

Fig. 5.1   The five moments of hand hygiene by World Health Organization

If a patient has an indwelling catheter, you should take the urine from the needle-free point in the upper part of the tube of the collection bag. If the catheter is in place >14 days, change the catheter first before taking a sample. You probably will only culture the bacteria inside the catheter (intraluminal). The culture should be obtained prior to the start of antibiotics.

Instruction to obtain a urine sample form an indwelling catheter—procedure:

1.	Obtain consent and ensure the procedure is performed maintaining patient dignity
2.	Wash your hands and put on an apron. Clean hands with alcohol hand rub.
3.	If there is no urine visible in the catheter tubing, a clamp may be placed a few centimetres distal to the sampling port
4.	Once there is sufficient urine visible in the drainage tube above the clamp, wipe the sampling port with an alcohol swab and allow to dry
5.	Insert a sterile syringe into the needle-free sampling port. Aspirate the required amount of urine
6.	Remove the syringe and transfer specimen into sterile specimen pot
7.	Wipe the sampling port with an alcohol swab and allow to dry
8.	Unclamp the drainage tubing
9.	Dispose of all waste materials
10.	Wash hands
11.	Complete documentation according to the organisational guidelines
12.	Dispatch the specimen to the laboratory

Adapted from EAUN guideline indwelling catheter, 2024 [4]

5.6   Treatment of UTI with Indwelling Catheter (CAUTI)

Treatment of the UTI in case of CAUTI is critical in ill patients, especially when they are compromised. Therefore, it is important to be able to distinguish between the available antibiotics, which one will be the most effective. If possible, to wait for the results of the culture you should do so, but most of the times the patient is too ill to wait. Then you can start with a broad spectrum of antibiotic, like penicillin or an antibiotic that also covers gram negative bacteria. After the results of the culture switch as soon as possible to the antibiotic that covers best the present bacteria.

5.6.1   When to Treat a UTI

An uncomplicated UTI should be treated only when symptoms are present, like urgency and frequency and dysuria. It can be treated with pain medication, ample fluid intake and frequent urination. Adequate antibiotic treatment should be administered if there are serious symptoms, including fever. Uncomplicated UTI is common in healthy females at adult age.

A complicated UTI is found in the following patient groups: Diabetes Mellitus, males, females with previous complicated UTI, pregnant women and elderly people. UTI should always be treated with antibiotics.

In patients with a catheter a CAUTI should be treated when complaints are present like fever, dysuria/pain, and illness. Colonisation of bacteria with catheterisation is inevitable and estimated to grow with 5% per day up to 100%. A symptomatic bacteriuria in patients with an indwelling catheter should not be treated with antibiotics. This cannot be prevented [4].

5.6.2 How to Treat a UTI

A UTI can be treated with antibiotics suitable for treatment of bacteria common for UTI, like *E. coli, K. pneumoniae, S. aureus*, etc. Most used antibiotics are nitrofurantoine, fosfomycine, and pivmecillinam. If these antibiotics are contrainidcated, Cephalosporins or trimethoprim (in the Netherlands first line), Co-tirmoxazole in countries with known resistance for *E. coli* < 20%. Amoxicillin/clavulanic acid, second generation cephalosporin + an aminopencillines are not recommended for experimental therapy [13, 14]. In the Netherlands, a third generation cephalosporin or amoxicillin + an aminoglycoside intravenously can be recommended as empirical treatment of UTI with systemic symptoms [13, 14]. A urine culture should be taken before start of antibiotic treatment to determine the uro-pathogens. Ciprofloxacin and other fluroquinolones are not suitable for empirical treatment of systemic UTI in patients admitted to the urology department. Empirical treatment with Ciprofloxacin is only suitable, when starting orally and patient do not require hospitalisation [13, 14]. According to the EAU guideline on UTI, the EU commission implemented stringent regulatory conditions regarding the use of fluorquinolones [14].

When a patient has an indwelling catheter with only local symptoms, it is recommended to wait for the results of a urine culture before starting treatment. When empirical treatment is required a regimen with an aminoglycoside is advised to cover less common bacteria like *P. aeroginosa*, Serratia spp., and Acinetobacter spp. Additional to cover enterococci co-amoxiclav can be added when a catheter is in place for at least ten days [13]. The NICE advises in uncomplicated UTI Nitrofurantoine, Trimethoprim, Amoxicillin. If not suitable they advise Pivmecillinam [15]. This is recently added to the Dutch guidelines as well.

When the catheter is in place for more then two weeks at onset of CAUTI, the catheter must be replaced to have better resolution of symptoms together with treatment [13]. When a urine culture is advised, always take one from the newly placed catheter [14]. It is important to treat according to local resistance to bacteria. This is known by the Medical microbiology and Immunological department of the hospital.

5.7 Measurements to Prevent CAUTI

The prevention of CAUTI is one of the cornerstones in treatment of CAUTI. A lot of preventive measures are possible. Nurses play a key role in prevention of CAUTI in hospitalised and non-hospitalised patients. Nurses most often insert the catheter and perform maintenance of the urinary catheters. Nurses should understand CAUTI and the attitude towards CAUTI prevention is considered essential for safe practice.

Educational interventions are essential to improve nurses' knowledge about infection control [16].

To effectively minimise the incidence of CAUTI, a combination of key preventive strategies must be implemented. The following measures outline essential steps that healthcare professionals, particularly nurses, can take to reduce the risk of infection and improve patient outcomes:

- The best prevention off CAUTI is the removal of the catheter!
- It is advised to assess daily if the reason for urinary catheterisation is appropriate [4].
- Is the indication of the indwelling catheter still present?
- Are there alternatives for catheterisation? Suprapubic may have less CAUTI than urethral catheterisation [4].
- An improper reason for catheterisation is the measurement of urine in incontinent patients. Remove the catheter as soon as possible, without delay.
- Take care of proper insertion of the catheter, correct securement of the bag to the leg or bed of the patient. Use the right drainage bag or use a valve [4].
- Use a closed drainage system to maintain reduction risk of CAUTI [4].
- Perform (hand)hygiene at appropriate moments in the correct way.
- Solve problems, like bladder spam, bladder pain, urinary extravasation, encrustation [4, 11, 12].

The nurse also has an important role in education of the patient on how to live with an indwelling catheter to maintain and improve quality of life for the patient, including sexuality with a catheter [4].

5.8   Conclusions

Catheter-associated urinary tract infections (CAUTI) remain a significant healthcare-associated infection in 15–25% of hospitalised patients. With urology patients, UTI is seen in 47%, of which is 71% CAUTI. The widespread use of urinary catheters increases the risk of infection, with a substantial proportion of cases being preventable through evidence-based practices. Adhering to international and local guidelines for catheter insertion, maintenance, and timely removal is paramount in reducing CAUTI incidence.

Effective prevention strategies include regular assessment of catheter necessity, proper hand hygiene, and adherence to aseptic techniques during insertion and handling. When CAUTI occurs, treatment should be guided by clinical symptoms and microbiological culture results, ensuring targeted antibiotic therapy to minimise the risk of antimicrobial resistance. Additionally, replacing or removing the catheter when appropriate enhances treatment efficacy and reduces infection recurrence.

Healthcare professionals, particularly nurses, play a critical role in CAUTI prevention and patient education. By implementing stringent infection prevention measures and fostering a culture of adherence to best practices, the burden of CAUTI can be significantly reduced, improving patient outcomes and overall healthcare quality.

References

1. Centres for disease control and prevention [Internet]. CDC. 2024. Available from: https://www.cdc.gov/uti/about/cauti-basics.html. Last access 27/01/2025.
2. Samenwerkingsverband Richtlijnen Infectiepreventie. Richtlijn Blaaskatheterisatie. Samenwerkingsverband Richtlijnen Infectiepreventie. 2023. Available at: https://www.sri-richtlijnen.nl/blaaskatheterisatie. Last Accessed 27 Jan 2025.
3. Letica-Kriegel AS, Salmasian H, Vawdrey DK, et al. Identifying the risk factors for catheter-associated urinary tract infections: a large cross-sectional study of six hospitals. BMJ Open. 2019;9:e022137. https://bmjopen.bmj.com/content/bmjopen/9/2/e022137.full.pdf
4. Geng V, Lurvink H, Pearce I, Vahr-Lauridsen S. Evidence-based Guidelines for Best Practice in Urological Health Care Indwelling catheterisation in adults Urethral and Suprapubic. European Association of Urology Nurses. 2024. Available at: https://nurses.uroweb.org/guideline/indwelling-catheterisation-in-adults-urethral-and-suprapubic/. Last Accessed 27 Jan 2025.
5. Federatie Medisch Specialisten. Urineweginfecties (UWI) bij volwassenen. Federatie Medisch Specialisten. 2024. Available at: https://richtlijnendatabase.nl/richtlijn/urineweginfecties_uwi_bij_volwassenen/startpagina_-_uwi_bij_volwassenen.html. Last Accessed 27 Jan 2025.
6. Zhou Y, Zhou Z, Zheng L, Gong Z, Li Y, Jin Y, et al. Urinary tract infections caused by Uropathogenic Escherichia coli: mechanisms of infection and treatment options. Int J Mol Sci. 2023;24(13):10537. https://doi.org/10.3390/ijms241310537.
7. PREZIES. Jaarcijfers 2021 thema urethrakathetergebruik: Alle basis ziekenhuizen. Rijksinstituut voor Volksgezondheid en Milieu (RIVM). Versie juli 2022. Available at: https://www.rivm.nl/sites/default/files/2022-07/Jaarcijfers%202021%20-%20alle%20basis%20ziekenhuizen%20thema%20UK.pdf. Last Accessed 27 Jan 2025.
8. Centres for disease control and prevention [Internet]. CDC. 2024. Available from: https://www.cdc.gov/infection-control/hcp/cauti/background.html#:~:text=Epidemiology,short%2Dterm%20indwelling%20urinary%20catheters. Last Accessed 27 Jan 2025.
9. European Centre for Disease Prevention and Control. Point prevalence survey of healthcare-associated infections and antimicrobial use in European hospitals. ECDC; 2013.
10. European Centre for Disease Prevention and Control. Point prevalence survey of healthcare-associated infections and antimicrobial use in European acute care hospitals. Stockholm: ECDC; 2024.
11. Spoolder DAE, Geelhoed JP. Management of bladder spasms in patients with indwelling urinary catheters: a systematic review. Continence. 2023;7:100713.
12. Beets M, Mulder H-J. Katheter management Handreiking bij katheter gerelateerde problemen. V&VN urologie Verpleegkundigen. Utrecht. 2022. Available at: https://www.venvn.nl/afdelingen/urologie-verpleegkundigen/kwaliteit/publicaties/. Last Accessed 27 Jan 2025.
13. Stichting Werkgroep AantibioticaBeleid. Guideline for antimicrobial therapy of urinary tract infections in adults. SWAB. 2020.
14. Bonkat G, Bartolettie R, Bruyère F, Cai, T, Geerlings SE, Köves B, et al. EAU guidelines on urological infections. European association of Urology. 2024.
15. NICE. Urinary tract infection (catheter-associated): antimicrobial prescribing. NICE; 2018.
16. Mong I, Ramoo V, Ponnampalavenar S, Chong MC, Nawawi WNFN. Knowledge, attitude and practice in relation to catheter-associated urinary tract infection (CAUTI) prevention: A cross-sectional study. J Clin Nurs 2022;31:209–219.

The Sepsis Challenge: Breaking the Chain with a Cohesive Multimodal Strategy—A Nursing Perspective

Camelia Bogaert

Abstract

Sepsis remains a leading cause of morbidity and mortality worldwide, requiring a structured, multidisciplinary approach to prevention, early detection, and intervention. This chapter explores the sepsis care continuum, emphasizing the crucial role of nurses in early warning detection, prevention strategies, and post-sepsis care.

While sepsis can arise from various infections, bloodstream infections (BSIs) are a significant and preventable contributor. Healthcare-associated BSIs, such as catheter-related infections and secondary BSIs from pneumonia or urinary tract infections, can escalate into sepsis if not promptly detected and treated. Preventing these infections is crucial to reducing sepsis cases.

Beyond prevention, early detection is essential. The Early Warning Score (EWS) and Nurse Intuition Patient Deterioration Score (NIPDS), combined with rapid response protocols improve healthcare workers ability to identify patients at risk and prevent progression to severe sepsis.

Sepsis prediction models in emergency and primary care are promising advancements. Their development could enhance early diagnosis and reduce in-hospital mortality.

Post-sepsis, survivors often face long-term impairments, necessitating structured rehabilitation. Strengthening frameworks and interdisciplinary collaboration ensures effective sepsis management, patient safety, and recovery. Nurses and infection prevention and control (IPC) teams have a key role in translating these strategies into practice.

C. Bogaert (✉)
Department of Infection Prevention and Control, AZ Sint Lucas, Ghent, Belgium
e-mail: camelia.bogaertmiclaus@azstlucas.be

© The Author(s), under exclusive license to Springer Nature Switzerland AG 2025
B. Oomen, S. Gastaldi (eds.), *Principles of Nursing Infection Prevention Control*,
Principles of Specialty Nursing, https://doi.org/10.1007/978-3-032-01446-7_6

Keywords

Sepsis · Infection prevention · Nurses · Early warning score · Multimodal strategy · Sepsis survivorship care

6.1   Introduction

6.1.1   "Why?"—The Race Against Time in Sepsis

Understanding the "Why" behind early clinical signs and symptoms is crucial for driving timely action and sustaining vigilance and motivation [1]. Sepsis does not develop suddenly; it often evolves from subtle warning signs that can be overlooked if their underlying significance is not recognized. Defined as life-threatening organ dysfunction caused by a dysregulated response to infection [2], sepsis is a time-critical emergency where every hour of delayed recognition and treatment increases the risk of death. Globally, sepsis affects 49 million people annually, and causes 11 million deaths worldwide [3], with mortality rates ranging from one in three to one in six [4]. Raising awareness and strengthening the healthcare response to sepsis are vital steps toward improving patient survival and long-term outcomes.

6.1.2   "How?"—Building the Key Pillars—The Crucial Role of Nurses

Preventing and managing sepsis requires a structured, multidisciplinary approach that integrates standardized screening tools, technological advancements, and evidence-based workflows [4]. A multimodal strategy, incorporating infection prevention and early recognition protocols, reduces healthcare-associated bloodstream infections [5–7]. Nurses play a central role by embedding early detection strategies into routine care, ensuring seamless coordination, and fostering proactive intervention [8]. The presence of clear escalation pathways and decision-support tools further strengthens the effectiveness and responsiveness of sepsis management [9]. By systematically integrating these elements, nurses strengthen interdisciplinary collaboration and contribute to improved patient outcomes.

6.1.3   "What?"—Navigating Nursing Challenges in Sepsis Care

Despite significant advancements, healthcare professionals continue to encounter substantial challenges in sepsis care, including difficulties in early recognition, inconsistent adherence to prevention protocols, and delays in initiating timely interventions [10]. Variability in compliance with early warning systems can impede prompt clinical escalation and contribute to adverse patient outcomes [11]. Further barriers include insufficient access to educational resources, as well as persistent staffing shortages and workforce constraints that restrict the delivery of optimal care [12]. Addressing these challenges requires targeted investment in education and training, with a particular focus on strengthening advanced nursing competencies in sepsis recognition and critical care response. Reinforcing educational infrastructure, ensuring adequate allocation of resources and fostering interprofessional teamwork grounded in mutual trust and expertise are equally essential to improving patient safety and outcomes [13]. Within this context, nurse-led screening tools have demonstrated particular value in enhancing early detection, especially when embedded into standardized clinical pathways [14].

6.2   Multimodal Strategy for Sepsis Prevention and Management

Effective sepsis management necessitates the use of structured, evidence-based frameworks that support consistent clinical decision-making and sustained outcomes. Rather than relying on different, fragmented approaches, Infection Prevention and Control (IPC) teams are responsible for implementing validated strategies that promote adherence and long-term impact, across all infection prevention training and improvement projects, fostering familiarity and consistency [5]. The World Health Organization's Multimodal Strategy (WHO MMS) [15] offers a comprehensive and framework to support IPC teams in translating the international guidelines to the local hospital context and realistic workflows, while ensuring that no vital component is overlooked, and serving as a cornerstone for harmonized practice. Rather than relying on different, fragmented approaches, IPC nurses could implement this trusted framework across all infection prevention training and improvement projects, fostering both familiarity and consistency [5].

A well-structured model strengthens nurses' ability to manage high-pressure environments with confidence and competence while simultaneously addressing system-level fragmentation and competing priorities that undermine continuity across disciplines [2, 10].

6.2.1   Build It—System Change: Ensuring the Availability of Basic Resources, Tools, and Conditions

Establishing a robust system for sepsis prevention and management—referred to as "Build It"—begins with ensuring the availability of essential structural components across all healthcare facilities. These include adequate staffing, comprehensive training, standardized screening protocols, integrated Electronic Health Record (EHR) support and strong infection prevention practices [4, 6]. Collectively, these foundational resources enable consistent identification and timely management of sepsis in daily clinical practice.

Adequate staffing and multidisciplinary team support are essential yet often underappreciated structural elements in sepsis management [12]. An alert is only as good as the team responding to it [9]. No tool or protocol can replace the need for enough trained professionals on the ground. Nurse staffing levels are particularly critical, as timely sepsis recognition and intervention rely on nurses' ability to closely monitor patients. Research has shown a strong link between higher nurse staffing and improved sepsis outcomes—a recent large study of U.S. hospitals found that "each additional registered nurse hour per patient day was associated with a 3% decrease in the odds of 60-day mortality" in sepsis patients [12]. In other words, well-staffed units see significantly lower sepsis mortality, likely because nurses can monitor patients more intensively and respond sooner. Sufficient staffing also allows for rapid response activation e.g. calling a physician or rapid response team at the first sign of sepsis. Several hospitals have created dedicated multidisciplinary sepsis response teams or coordinator roles as part of their structural preparedness [16]. Some centres also employ nurse sepsis navigators or designate "sepsis champions" on each unit to ensure adherence to protocols—interventions that have significantly improved bundle compliance and reduced sepsis mortality [17]. From a nursing perspective, these teams and roles mean backup and guidance: bedside nurses can call on experts like an ICU nurse or sepsis coordinator to assist with sepsis management decisions. Hospital leadership commitment is vital here—allocating the necessary human resources: nurse staffing, critical care consults, infection control practitioners, etc. and accountability structures e.g. a sepsis committee chaired by a nursing leader and physician creates an environment where sepsis care is prioritized [6]. Building on this foundation with current international guidelines, such as those from the Surviving Sepsis Campaign [18], emphasize the implementation of performance improvement programs in every hospital setting. These programs should include routine screening of high-risk patients and the use of standardized early treatment protocols [4]. In practice, this means having a systematic screening process e.g. incorporating criteria like Systemic Inflammatory Response Syndrome (SIRS) or an Early Warning Score (EWS) applied consistently to all acute patients, since "if you don't look for it, you might miss sepsis" [4]. A recent study notes these latest guidelines *"advocate that all hospitals use sepsis performance improvement programs"*, underlining that sepsis screening and protocols should be universally adopted [16]. Such programs formalize the expectation that nurses and clinicians check for sepsis at triage and during rounds, using validated triggers to flag potential sepsis early [19]. For example, the UK's National Early Warning Score (NEWS) is recommended across National Health Service (NHS) hospitals to provide a common language of illness severity and to trigger escalations [20]. Despite its impact on workload, its widespread adoption has enhanced the consistency of vital sign monitoring and facilitated timely interventions for patient deterioration [20].

Overall, integrating a standard screening tool into routine nursing assessments, together with a clear sepsis protocol or bundle e.g. the "Hour-1 bundle", enables nurses to trigger a rapid, standardized response-including labs, antibiotics, fluids and other measures-as soon as sepsis is suspected [2, 6, 12, 16, 17, 21]. In sum, a solid staffing plan and team approach are foundational so that when a septic patient is identified, the hospital has the *people* ready to deliver rapid, appropriate care [4, 12].

Since the best way to "treat" sepsis is to prevent it from occurring, every hospital must enforce rigorous infection prevention policies as a structural cornerstone [22]. Recent global data indicate that over half of all sepsis cases originate from preventable or manageable infections, such as those associated with respiratory, gastrointestinal, or device-related sources [3]. For nursing practice, this entails consistently applying high standards of hygiene and meticulous care for invasive devices—such as employing sterile techniques during IV line or catheter insertion, ensuring timely removal of unnecessary lines, maintaining strict hand hygiene, and following evidence-based protocols to prevent ventilator-associated pneumonia and catheter-related bloodstream infections [23]. To support these practices, hospitals must maintain comprehensive infection control programs encompassing active surveillance of healthcare-associated infections (HAI), effective isolation procedures, and robust antibiotic stewardship strategies to combat antimicrobial resistance [6, 24]. Interventions that reduce the incidence of surgical site infections, urinary tract infections, and pneumonia have demonstrated a substantial impact on lowering the risk of subsequent sepsis. Institutional policies—such as mandatory hand hygiene compliance, routine environmental decontamination, and the use of standardized checklists for central line insertions—have proven highly effective in interrupting the progression from infection to sepsis [25].

In the context of sepsis prevention, infection control is equally as critical as early detection. It ensures that nurses are not only prepared to recognize and respond to sepsis but are also actively engaged in preventing infection at the point of care. Although hospital-wide protocols for infection prevention are widely implemented, their role in mitigating the risk of sepsis remains foundational—contributing to safer care environments and decreasing the likelihood of deterioration into septic shock [4, 20]. These preventive efforts extend beyond the intensive care setting and begin with maintaining clean clinical environments, proper sterilization of equipment, and vigilant nursing oversight in all care areas [26]. Building upon this foundational framework, hospitals can further strengthen their approach by incorporating emerging technologies such as automated clinical alerts, artificial intelligence–driven decision support, continuous patient monitoring systems, and advanced diagnostic tools. These innovations offer new opportunities to enhance the timeliness and precision of sepsis detection and management [27].

6.2.2 Teach It—Training and Education: Knowledge and Awareness—Strengthening Sepsis Prevention

Continuous education and training are critical for enhancing early sepsis detection and response, particularly as bedside nurses are often the first to identify signs of patient deterioration. Despite their pivotal role, significant knowledge gaps persist. A 2021 multi-site cross-sectional study found that only 52% of nurses could accurately define sepsis, highlighting a widespread need for educational reinforcement [10]. These findings underscore the need for structured, comprehensive educational programs to strengthen recognition and response.

Current clinical guidelines emphasize that all healthcare personnel involved in sepsis care must possess strong foundational knowledge and a clear understanding of their roles within a team-based response framework [4, 6]. Standardized and recurring educational initiatives—including onboarding modules, regular competency assessments, and high-fidelity simulation training—equip nurses to recognize early indicators such as altered mental status, tachypnoea, and hypotension, thus facilitating timely intervention [28].

Several hospitals have successfully integrated sepsis-specific modules into their ongoing educational curricula. Programs such as "Sepsis Six" and sepsis care bundles reinforce clinical decision-making and assessment skills. The integration of case reviews, hands-on simulation training, and structured early recognition protocols has been shown to enhance adherence to sepsis guidelines [29]. Moreover, the concept of embedding sepsis awareness within nursing culture, such as through unit-based sepsis champions, has demonstrated improvements in early intervention and adherence to clinical pathways [17]. These champions undergo advanced sepsis training and serve as peer educators, further fostering a culture of continuous learning and vigilance [17].

6.2.2.1 Simulation—Based Training for Sepsis Recognition and Management

Simulation-based training has emerged as a pivotal strategy in advancing sepsis recognition and response among healthcare professionals. High-fidelity simulations using life-like manikins and scenario-based drills allow nurses to engage in real-world sepsis case management within a controlled environment. Through these exercises, nurses practice early identification, rapid assessment, and the implementation of key interventions such as the "Hour-1 bundle". Empirical evidence indicates that simulation-based training significantly enhances both sepsis knowledge and clinical performance, while also improving provider confidence in recognizing and managing sepsis cases [30].

The most effective simulation exercises involve interprofessional teams, mimicking real-world dynamics in which nurses, physicians, and allied healthcare professionals work in tandem to manage sepsis [14]. Notably, high-fidelity simulation has been associated with greater compliance with sepsis care bundles compared to traditional, case-based instructional methods [30]. Despite these proven benefits, many hospitals still rely heavily on didactic, lecture-based learning formats, even though studies demonstrate that active learning methods such as simulation yield superior knowledge retention and skill development [30].

6.2.2.2 E-learning and Digital Innovations in Sepsis Education

In addition to hands-on simulation training, digital learning platforms have revolutionized sepsis education, offering flexible, on-demand training for nurses. E-learning modules, interactive case scenarios, and virtual patient simulations provide accessible, scalable education that nurses can complete at their convenience. In one U.S. hospital initiative, the implementation of a longitudinal online sepsis curriculum for nurses and physicians resulted in notable knowledge gains and an increase in SEP-1 bundle compliance from 71% to 80% over 32 months [31]. Nurses completed nearly half of the 3616 modules, with most participants intending to apply the concepts in clinical practice, highlighting the effectiveness of structured digital education [14].

Innovative digital tools are transforming sepsis education, providing dynamic and interactive learning experiences. Simulations, virtual reality (VR), and telesimulation immerse nurses in realistic clinical scenarios, allowing them to refine decision-making skills without the need for a physical lab. Research has shown that telesimulation significantly enhances sepsis knowledge and team communication, with benefits persisting for at least two months [14]. Participants also reported a deeper understanding of interdisciplinary roles, improving team collaboration.

Expanding beyond simulations, mobile learning applications offer on-demand refreshers on sepsis screening and treatment protocols. Evaluations indicate high engagement and strong content validity, with one study reporting a clinical validation index of 0.99 [32]. These tools reinforce National Institute for Health and Care Excellence (NICE) and Surviving Sepsis Campaign guidelines and are especially valuable in resource-limited settings, ensuring equitable access to up-to-date training.

6.2.2.3 Mastering Early Warning Score Systems for Sepsis Detection

Effective sepsis prevention relies on early detection, making proficiency in EWS systems essential for nurses. Training in the NEWS has been particularly effective, as it translates vital sign deviations into a numerical score, signalling clinical deterioration. Many hospitals use NEWS thresholds e.g., ≥ 5 as triggers for sepsis screening or rapid response activation [9].

Beyond NEWS, emerging tools like the Nurse Intuition Patient Deterioration Scale (NIPDS) enhance early sepsis detection by incorporating clinical intuition into risk assessments. A European study found that combining NIPDS with NEWS achieved 90% sensitivity in detecting deterioration, far surpassing the 30% sensitivity of NEWS alone [8]. Integrating both objective scoring and nursing intuition can significantly improve recognition and response times.

Sustaining sepsis awareness requires more than initial training; it demands continuous education, professional engagement, and deliberate integration into nursing culture. Awareness is not a static concept—it must be actively sustained, nurtured, and embedded within the professional culture of nursing teams [11]. The intrinsic commitment of nurses to patient safety serves as a driving force for maintaining vigilance and adherence to best practices in infection prevention [33]. By fostering ongoing training, reflective practice, and proactive clinical behaviours, healthcare institutions empower nurses to deliver timely interventions that reduce sepsis-related morbidity and mortality [34].

6.2.3   Check It—Monitoring and Feedback: Ensuring Continuous Improvement in Sepsis Prevention

Effective sepsis prevention relies on rigorous adherence to infection prevention care bundles, encompassing both catheter-related and non-catheter-related interventions

[24]. These standardized protocols form the foundation of infection control and must be embedded in routine nursing practice. To ensure compliance, infection prevention programs should implement audits, checklists, and infection rate tracking, supplemented by structured feedback to refine practices [35].

6.2.3.1 Monitoring and Auditing of Infection Prevention Bundles

The systematic implementation and auditing care bundles represent an essential first step in mitigating complications that can escalate into sepsis. Consistent adherence to evidence-based catheter care protocols in daily clinical practice serves as a tangible and effective strategy for reducing HAIs and their potential progression to life-threatening bloodstream infections BSIs [4, 6]. Ongoing compliance monitoring is essential for maintaining infection control standards and preventing septic complications [35].

Advanced surveillance technologies, such as digital dashboards and wearable monitors, offer real-time tracking of infection-related metrics. These tools provide immediate insights into BSI incidence rates, enabling proactive infection control interventions. Data-driven methodologies enhance situational awareness, accountability, and bedside infection prevention efforts [36].

Real-time feedback mechanisms reinforce compliance by giving nurses access to unit-specific performance dashboards, detailing hand hygiene adherence, catheter bundle compliance, and infection rates. Structured discussions on infection incidents provide frontline staff with actionable insights, fostering a culture of accountability and reinforcing the impact of infection control practices on patient outcomes [36].

Empirical evidence supports integrating education with performance feedback, showing that structured training programs improve compliance and reduce infection rates [37]. Structured training programs, particularly when paired with routine auditing, have been associated with significant reductions in central line-associated bloodstream infections (CLABSIs) and catheter-associated urinary tract infections (CAUTIs) [22, 23]. Investing in ongoing education, competency validation, and performance monitoring strengthens safety culture and ensures sustained infection control adherence [2, 6].

6.2.3.2 Post-intervention Case Reviews and Continuous Improvement

Post-intervention case reviews offer a structured approach for analysing sepsis cases retrospectively, enabling healthcare teams to identify missed opportunities for early recognition, treatment delays, and deviations from established protocols. These review processes serve as valuable learning mechanisms for both nursing staff and multidisciplinary teams, highlighting areas requiring improvement while reinforcing adherence to best practices [25, 38].

Morbidity and mortality (M&M) reviews, specifically focusing on sepsis cases and hospital-acquired infections, have proven to be instrumental in refining infection prevention frameworks at an institutional level. By systematically evaluating patient trajectories, response timelines, and clinical decision-making processes, hospitals can develop targeted interventions to rectify systemic inefficiencies and enhance protocol adherence [19]. Such structured analyses facilitate the proactive identification of gaps in clinical workflows, allowing institutions to implement evidence-based solutions that improve sepsis prevention outcomes.

A critical component of effective post-intervention review is the integration of nursing perspectives into sepsis prevention frameworks. As frontline responders in the early detection of infection, nurses offer essential insights into workflow inefficiencies, barriers to timely sepsis recognition, and practical challenges with protocol implementation. Ensuring that these perspectives are incorporated into institutional learning processes helps keep infection prevention strategies dynamic, responsive, and clinically relevant—ultimately enhancing nursing engagement and improving hospital-wide infection control practices [28].

6.2.4   Sell It—Reminders in the Workplace

6.2.4.1 Frontline Reminders: Strengthening Adherence to Sepsis Protocols

Maintaining sepsis protocols at the forefront of clinical practice is essential—particularly for nurses, who are often responsible for initial patient assessments. Visual reminders, such as posters, bedside checklists, and reference cards, reinforce key sepsis criteria and bundles, minimizing reliance on memory and promoting early detection [39]. Digital alerts within electronic health records EHRs also play a crucial role in prompting timely sepsis care. Automated systems that monitor vital signs and laboratory parameters can identify high-risk patients in real time, prompting earlier antibiotic administration and contributing to decreased mortality [40]. Hospitals that have implemented EHR-based sepsis alerts, standardized order sets, and bedside checklists report increased compliance with sepsis protocols and reductions in ICU length of stay [18]. Additionally, mobile health technology extends these alerts to clinicians' smartphones or pagers, ensuring a coordinated team response to sepsis cases [18].

Early recognition is arguably the most critical link in the chain—and nurses are on the frontlines of detecting subtle patient deteriorations. Equipped with decision-support prompts, visual reminders, and clinical knowledge, nurses are empowered to identify sepsis earlier and initiate protocol-based care more rapidly. The implementation of triage screening tools, sepsis checklists, and automated alerts has been shown to improve early detection and accelerate care activation [39]. This proactive nursing role is reflected in outcome improvements; speeding up sepsis care has been shown to save lives [40].

Nurses also play a central role in protocol enforcement, ensuring that sepsis bundles are completed, antibiotics are administered on time, and escalation procedures are followed. A quality improvement initiative at a community hospital—featuring multidisciplinary collaboration, visual sepsis cues, data feedback, and innovative education strategies such as a sepsis escape room—led to a 23 percentage-point increase in bundle compliance, a 50% reduction in sepsis mortality, and improved nurse triage screening and order set utilization [39].

6.2.4.2 Sepsis Awareness Campaigns and Continuing Education

Sepsis awareness begins with reinforcing infection control practices, where reminders and educational initiatives reinforce hand hygiene, aseptic technique, and catheter care—critical steps in reducing HAIs. Beyond clinical protocols, awareness initiatives sustain engagement in sepsis prevention. A prominent example is World Sepsis Day (WSD), held annually on September 13 and spearheaded by the Global Sepsis Alliance. Through educational events, media outreach, and healthcare provider training, WSD promotes global awareness of sepsis and its prevention [41]. Although public engagement with sepsis education has increased since the launch of WSD, recent surveys indicate that population-level awareness remains suboptimal, with fewer than 50% of respondents accurately identifying sepsis or its symptoms [42].

To address knowledge gaps, hospitals often incorporate sepsis awareness into staff training via annual sepsis weeks, mock drills, and formal competency assessments. Interactive formats, such as sepsis-themed "escape room" simulations, have demonstrated effectiveness in reinforcing clinical knowledge and promoting team-based learning among nurses [39]. Despite ongoing efforts, surveys continue to reveal significant knowledge deficits in the definition and clinical criteria for sepsis, emphasizing the need for continuous education across disciplines [11]. National initiatives such as Sepsis Net Netherlands, the UK Sepsis Trust, and the U.S. Sepsis Alliance provide structured resources, including screening tools and symptom checklists, to support standardized sepsis recognition and timely intervention [43].

This ongoing cultural shift—driven by visual prompts like "Think Sepsis!", recurring awareness campaigns, and multidisciplinary education—forms a cornerstone of breaking the sepsis chain. Whether it is a poster on the wall, a screen alert, or a clinical huddle focused on early recognition, each intervention reinforces the critical importance of vigilance. In doing so, these strategies contribute to improved outcomes and lives saved from one of healthcare's most time-sensitive conditions.

6.2.5   Live It—Culture Change

6.2.5.1 Leadership Engagement in Sustaining Sepsis Protocols

Effective sepsis management extends beyond acute care; it requires sustained institutional commitment to a culture of safety that supports both early intervention and long-term recovery for survivors. Hospitals with active leadership involvement in sepsis prevention programs report higher compliance rates and improved long-term patient survival [4, 7]. Strategic investments by leadership in real-time data monitoring, quality dashboards, and interdisciplinary education are essential to maintaining effective sepsis management frameworks [26].

As part of structural preparedness, many hospitals have implemented dedicated multidisciplinary sepsis response teams or designated sepsis coordinator roles to enhance sepsis recognition and accelerate response. While exact global figures

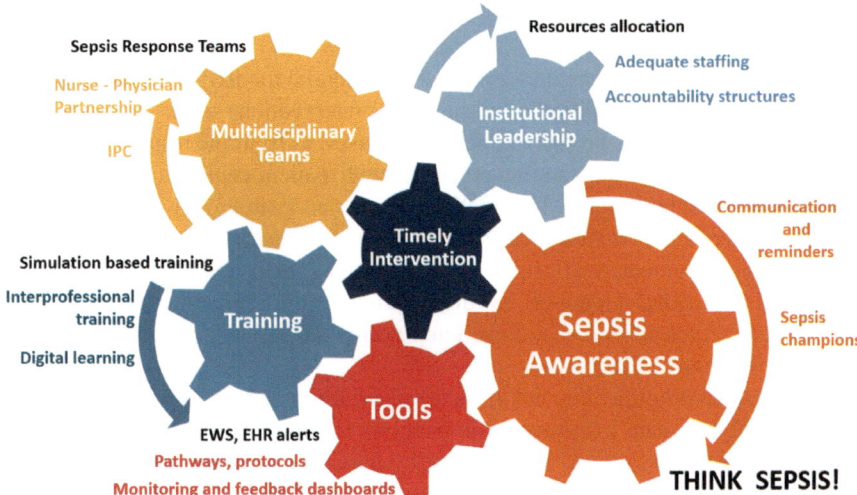

Fig. 6.1 Driving components of effective sepsis prevention (figure created by the author). This schematic illustrates the interconnected components required for effective sepsis prevention. At the centre is Timely Intervention, representing the critical point of clinical action that determines outcomes. Surrounding it are five essential gears: Multidisciplinary Teams, Training, Tools, Institutional Leadership, and most prominently, Sepsis Awareness. The highlighted gear of Sepsis Awareness, reinforced by the directive "THINK SEPSIS!", serves as the driving force that initiates and sustains all other components. It reflects the ongoing need for communication, visual reminders, and empowered roles such as sepsis champions to keep early recognition top of mind. (*IPC* Infection Prevention and Control, *EWS* Early Warning Score, *EHR* Electronic Health Record)

remain limited, a U.S.-based survey in 2022 reported that over 70% of acute care hospitals had a formal sepsis program, with participation increasing alongside hospital size [44]. These programs often integrate nurse-led coordination, education, and protocol monitoring as key components of care delivery. For example, a nurse-driven sepsis protocol in an inpatient rehabilitation facility reduced acute care transfer readmissions related to sepsis from 36.3 to 25% within eight weeks [13, 16] (Fig. 6.1).

6.2.5.2 Post-sepsis Syndrome PSS and Long-term Impact and Care Pathways

Sepsis survivors often experience persistent physical, cognitive, and psychological impairments, collectively termed Post-Sepsis Syndrome (PSS). This condition affects nearly 50% of sepsis survivors, manifesting as chronic fatigue, neurocognitive dysfunction, and PTSD-like symptoms [4, 45]. Addressing these long-term consequences necessitates comprehensive post-sepsis care extending beyond hospital discharge. Early, structured follow-up interventions, particularly those involving home health care and timely medical provider visits, have been associated with reduced hospital readmission rates among sepsis survivors [13, 46]. Implementing well-defined care pathways is essential for enhancing recovery outcomes and reducing the healthcare burden associated with PSS [47, 48].

6.3   Conclusion

Understanding the "Why" behind sepsis care is essential for driving effective action. As a life-threatening condition requiring rapid intervention, sepsis demands constant vigilance and strict protocol adherence. Nurses, as frontline responders, play a critical role in merging scientific precision with patient-centred care, and their engagement must be supported through education and institutional investment.

Standardized frameworks, such as the WHO's Multimodal Strategy, enforce IPC by replacing fragmented efforts with a consistent, evidence-based framework. Structured protocols, supported by digital monitoring, simulation training, and feedback, reinforce adherence to infection prevention bundles and promote continuous improvement.

Finally, extending care beyond the acute phase through defined post-sepsis pathways is vital to reduce long-term complications and improve survivors' quality of life. A strong safety culture, underpinned by nursing leadership and system-wide commitment, is key to breaking the sepsis cycle.

Key Messages

- Early sepsis recognition and rapid intervention are essential to reducing mortality and improving patient outcomes.
- Nurses play a pivotal role in sepsis detection, protocol adherence, and delivering patient-centred, evidence-based care.
- Standardized frameworks—such as the WHO Multimodal Strategy—strengthen infection prevention and foster consistent practice.
- Continuous training, simulation, and data-driven feedback are critical to sustaining long-term compliance and performance.
- "The eye sees only what the mind is prepared to comprehend."—Henri Bergson [49]. Sustained awareness is not just a task—it's a mindset that transforms vigilance into action.

References

1. Sinek S. Start with why: how great leaders inspire everyone to take action. Portfolio Penguin; 2011.
2. Singer M, Deutschman CS, Seymour CW, Shankar-Hari M, Annane D, Bauer M, et al. The third international consensus definitions for sepsis and septic shock (Sepsis-3). JAMA. 2016;315(8):801–10.
3. Rudd KE, Johnson SC, Agesa KM, Shackelford KA, Tsoi D, Kievlan DR, et al. Global, regional, and national sepsis incidence and mortality, 1990–2017: analysis for the global burden of disease study. Lancet. 2020;395(10219):200–11.
4. Evans LA-O, Rhodes A, Alhazzani W, Antonelli M, Coopersmith CM, French C, et al. Surviving sepsis campaign: international guidelines for management of sepsis and septic shock 2021. Intensive Care Med. 2021;47(11):1181–247.

5. Organization WH. Multimodal strategies for hand hygiene improvement. Geneva: WHO; 2023. [Available from: https://www.who.int/campaigns/world-hand-hygiene-day/key-resources-on-hand-hygiene.

6. (CDC) CfDCaP. Hospital Sepsis Program Core Elements 2024 [updated August 13]. 2024. Available from: https://www.cdc.gov/sepsis/core-elements.html.

7. Hansen SA-O, Remschmidt C, Schröder C, Behnke M, Gastmeier P. Strengthening the role of hospital leadership in infection control (LEAD-IC) – a multimodal educational intervention in German acute care hospitals. BMC Med Educ. 2021;21(1):29

8. Haegdorens F, Lefebvre J, Wils C, Franck E, Van Bogaert P. Combining the nurse intuition patient deterioration scale with the National Early Warning Score provides more net benefit in predicting serious adverse events: a prospective cohort study in medical, surgical, and geriatric wards. Intensive Crit Care Nurs. 2023;76:103361.

9. Chua WA-O, Rusli KDB, Aitken LM. Early warning scores for sepsis identification and prediction of in-hospital mortality in adults with sepsis: a systematic review and meta-analysis. J Clin Nurs. 2023;32(1–2):13–24.

10. Chua WA-O, Teh CS, Basri M, Ong ST, Phang NQQ, Goh EL. Nurses' knowledge and confidence in recognizing and managing patients with sepsis: a multi-site cross-sectional study. J Adv Nurs. 2023;79(1):370–81.

11. Regina J, Le Pogam MA-O, Niemi T, Akrour R, Pepe S, Lehn I, et al. Sepsis awareness and knowledge amongst nurses, physicians and paramedics of a tertiary care center in Switzerland: a survey-based cross-sectional study. PLoS One. 2019;14(12):e0226410.

12. Cimiotti JP, Becker ER, Li Y, Sloane DM, Fridkin SK, West AB, et al. Association of Registered Nurse Staffing with Mortality Risk of Medicare beneficiaries hospitalized with sepsis. JAMA Health Forum. 2023;4(6):e231491.

13. Jacobs JL. Implementation of an evidence-based, nurse-driven sepsis protocol to reduce acute care transfer readmissions in the inpatient rehabilitation facility setting. Rehabil Nurs. 2021;46(5):277–85.

14. Chua WA-O, Ooi SA-O, Chan GA-O, Lau TA-O, Liaw SA-O. The effect of a sepsis Interprofessional education using virtual patient Telesimulation on sepsis team Care in Clinical Practice: mixed methods study. J Med Internet Res. 2022;24(6):e35490.

15. World Health O. Hand hygiene self-assessment framework: infection prevention and control assessment tool (IPCAT)—Core component: multimodal strategy. Geneva: World Health Organization; 2024.

16. Schinkel M, Holleman F, Vleghels R, Brugman K, Ridderikhof ML, Dzelili M, et al. The impact of a sepsis performance improvement program in the emergency department: a before-after intervention study. Eur J Clin Microbiol Infect Dis. 2020;39(6):1105–12.

17. Grootendorst MAB, Bilyeu TE, Harris LA, Kreiser JB. Sepsis navigators and hospital outcomes. Amer Nurse J. 2024;19(3):42–8.

18. Warstadt NA-O, Caldwell JR, Tang N, Mandola S, Jamin C, Dahn C. Quality initiative to improve emergency department sepsis bundle compliance through utilisation of an electronic health record tool. BMJ open. Qual. 2022;11:e001624.

19. Kwok ESH, Calder LA, Barlow-Krelina E, Mackie C, Seely AJE, Cwinn AA, et al. Implementation of a structured hospital-wide morbidity and mortality rounds model. BMJ Open Qual. 2021;10(1):e000956.

20. Holland MA-O, Kellett JA-O. The United Kingdom's National Early Warning Score: should everyone use it? A narrative review. Ir J Med Sci. 2023;192(1):31–42.

21. Suh GJ, Shin TG, Kwon WY, Kim K, Jo YH, Choi SH, et al. Hemodynamic management of septic shock: beyond the surviving sepsis campaign guidelines. J Korean Med Sci. 2020;35(37):e314.

22. Kubde D, Badge AK, Ugemuge S, Shahu S. Importance of hospital infection control. Int J Health Sci Res. 2023;13(2):290–4.

23. Lucchini AA-OX, Giani MA-O, Rezoagli EA-O, Favata G, Andreani A, Spada M, et al. Impact of a 'catheter bundle' on infection rates and economic costs in the intensive care unit: a retrospective cohort study. Acta Biomed. 2020;91(12-S):e2020001.

24. Organization WH. Guidelines for the prevention of bloodstream infections and other infections associated with the use of intravascular catheters: Part I—Peripheral catheters. Geneva: World Health Organization; 2024.

25. Garcia R, Barnes S, Boukidjian R, Goss LK, Spencer M, Septimus EJ, et al. Recommendations for change in infection prevention programs and practice. Am J Infect Control. 2023;51(1):1–5.

26. King JC, Carol E, England PC, Heiler A, Kenes MT, Raghavendran K, Wood W, Zhou S. Early recognition and initial Management of Sepsis in adult patients. Ann Arbor (MI): Michigan Medicine, University of Michigan; 2023.

27. Li F, Wang S, Gao Z, Qing M, Pan S, Liu Y, et al. Harnessing artificial intelligence in sepsis care: advances in early detection, personalized treatment, and real-time monitoring. Front Med Technol. 2023;5:1223747.

28. Lourenço LA-O, Meszaros MA-O, Silva MA-O, São-João TA-O. Nursing training for early clinical deterioration risk assessment: protocol for an implementation study. JMIR Res Protoc. 2023;12:e47417.

29. Health EE. Getting it right: the current state of sepsis education and training for healthcare staff across England. Leeds: Health Education England; 2016. 2025-03-29

30. Cuesta-Montero P, Navarro-Martínez JA-O, Yedro M, Galiana-Ivars MA-O. Sepsis and clinical simulation: what is new? (and Old). J Pers Med. 2023;13(10):1475.

31. Heslin SA-O, Qadeer A, Kotarba AE, Ahmad S, Morley EJ. Click and learn: a longitudinal interprofessional case-based sepsis education curriculum. BMJ Open Qual. 2024;13(1):e002859.

32. Limeira JBR, Silva VC, Galindo Neto NM, Silva CRDT, Oliveira VL, Alexandre ACS. Development of a mobile application for health education about sepsis. Rev Esc Enferm USP. 2023;57:e20220269.

33. Vaismoradi MA-O, Tella S, Logan PA, Khakurel JA-O, Vizcaya-Moreno FA-O. Nurses' adherence to patient safety principles: a systematic review. Clin Infect Dis. 2011;52(9):e162–93.

34. Choy CL, Liaw SY, Goh EL, See KC, Chua WL. Impact of sepsis education for healthcare professionals and students on learning and patient outcomes: a systematic review. J Hosp Infect. 2022;122:84–95.

35. O'Grady NP, Alexander M, Fau-Burns LA, Burns La Fau-Dellinger EP, Dellinger Ep Fau-Garland J, Fau-Heard SO GJ, Heard So Fau-Lipsett PA, et al. Guidelines for the prevention of intravascular catheter-related infections. Lin. Infect Dis. 2011;52(9):e162–e93.

36. Chemparathy A, Seneviratne MG, Ward A, Mirchandani S, Li R, Mathew R, et al. Development and implementation of a real-time bundle-adherence dashboard for central line-associated bloodstream infections. NEJM Catal Innov Care Deliv. 2022;3(6)

37. Mogyoródi B, Skultéti D, Mezőcsáti M, Dunai E, Magyar P, Hermann C, et al. Effect of an educational intervention on compliance with care bundle items to prevent ventilator-associated pneumonia. Intensive Crit Care Nurs. 2022;70:103188.

38. Gustad LA-O, Bangstad IA-O, Torsvik MA-O, Rise MA-O. Nurses' and physicians' experiences after implementation of a quality improvement project to improve sepsis awareness in hospitals. J Multidiscip Healthc. 2021;14:271–8.

39. Kiser M. Improving sepsis compliance with human factors interventions in a community hospital emergency room. Patient Safety. 2023;5(1):26–37.

40. Kim HJ, Ko RE, Lim SY, Park S, Suh GY, Lee YJ. Sepsis alert systems, mortality, and adherence in emergency departments: a systematic review and meta-analysis. J Intensive Care Med. 2023;38(6):547–59.

41. Day WS. About WSD Global Sepsis Alliance. 2023. Available from: https://www.worldsepsisday.org/what-is-sepsis.

42. Fiest KM, Krewulak KD, Brundin-Mather R, Leia MP, Fox-Robichaud A, Lamontagne F, et al. Patient, public, and healthcare professionals' sepsis awareness, knowledge, and information seeking behaviors: a scoping review. Crit Care Med. 2022;50(7):e599–610.

43. European Sepsis A. European sepsis report—The Netherlands. 2023.

44. Bagchi S, Wise ME, Edwards JR, Srinivasan A, Pollock D. Sepsis program elements and hospital characteristics — National Healthcare Safety Network, United States, 2022. Morb Mortal Weekly Rep (MMWR). 2023;72(34):901–6.

45. van der Slikke EA-O, Beumeler LA-O, Holmqvist M, Linder A, Mankowski RT, Bouma HA-OX. Understanding post-sepsis syndrome: how can clinicians help? Patient Relat Outcome Meas. 2023;14:169–81.
46. Deb P, Murtaugh CM, Bowles KH, Mikkelsen ME, Khajavi HN, Moore S, et al. Does early follow-up improve the outcomes of sepsis survivors discharged to home Health care? Med Care. 2022;60(2):114–20.
47. Hartley P, Pelkmans J, Lott C, Higgins MK, Chen X, Reinhardt A, et al. Readmissions in sepsis survivors: discharge setting risks. Am J Manag Care. 2023;29(4):e132–e40.
48. Born S, Matthäus-Krämer C, Bichmann A, Boltz HS, Esch M, Heydt L, et al. Sepsis survivors and caregivers perspectives on post-acute rehabilitation and aftercare in the first year after sepsis in Germany. Front Public Health. 2023;11:1124543.
49. Bergson H. An introduction to metaphysics. New York: G.P. Putnam's Sons; 1912.

Integration of New Technology in Infection Control

Silvana Gastaldi ⓘD

Abstract

This chapter explores the transformative role of advanced technologies in infection control, focusing on robotics, artificial intelligence (AI), wearable devices, the Internet of Things (IoT), and innovative sterilization methods. Robotics, including UV-C disinfection systems and automated logistics solutions, have enhanced cleaning protocols and minimized healthcare worker exposure to pathogens. AI has revolutionized infection surveillance, leveraging predictive analytics for early intervention, while wearable devices offer real-time health monitoring to detect infections proactively. IoT-enabled smart environments integrate air filtration, automated disinfection, and disease tracking, creating safer healthcare facilities. The chapter also emphasizes sustainability through eco-friendly solutions like electrolyzed water and highlights ethical and economic considerations, including data privacy and accessibility in low-resource settings. While challenges such as cost, training, and infrastructure persist, the compelling benefits of these innovations are shaping the future of infection control, ensuring enhanced patient outcomes and operational effectiveness.

Keywords

Infection control · Advanced technologies · Robotics · Artificial intelligence · Wearable devices · Internet of Things (IoT) · Whole-genome sequencing · Sterilization · Healthcare-associated infections (HAIs) · Disinfection · Automated systems · Smart environments

S. Gastaldi (✉)
Independent Researcher, Mazzano, Italy

7.1   Introduction

The integration of advanced technologies in infection control represents a transformative shift in healthcare, with the potential to redefine traditional practices. Infection control has historically relied on manual protocols and chemical agents, but emerging technologies, such as robotics, wearable devices, artificial intelligence (AI), and Internet of Things (IoT), have introduced unprecedented opportunities to enhance effectiveness and efficiency. This chapter explores the application of these technologies, highlighting their contributions, challenges, and future directions in combating healthcare-associated infections (HAIs).

7.2   Robotics in Infection Control

Robotics has been a significant innovation in infection prevention, particularly during outbreaks of highly infectious diseases. Robots equipped with ultraviolet (UV) disinfection systems and autonomous navigation capabilities can perform thorough and consistent cleaning of healthcare environments. These systems, such as UV-C emitting robots, have been shown to reduce microbial load and prevent HAIs by accessing hard-to-reach areas often overlooked during manual cleaning [1, 2].

Robotics also extends to patient care, with teleoperated systems minimizing direct contact between patients and healthcare workers during diagnostic or treatment processes. During the COVID-19 pandemic, robots were used to assist with nasopharyngeal swabbing, temperature monitoring, and medication delivery, significantly reducing the risk of cross-infection [1].

Robots are increasingly employed in laboratory workflows for sample handling and testing, ensuring biosafety and efficiency. Automated guided vehicles and drones are being utilized for transporting specimens and medical supplies, reducing delays and minimizing exposure risks [1]. Additionally, robots are now designed to adapt to various healthcare settings, performing tasks such as bedside nursing assistance and surgical interventions in high-risk environments.

Robotic disinfection systems are also revolutionizing cleaning protocols in healthcare facilities. These robots autonomously navigate environments, using UV light or disinfectant sprays to eliminate pathogens effectively. By reducing human error and reaching areas often missed during manual cleaning, robotic systems play a pivotal role in curbing healthcare-associated infections. They also operate safely in unoccupied spaces, enhancing sanitation without compromising patient or staff safety.

Furthermore, advanced robotics systems are integrating sensor-based technologies to assess microbial contamination levels before and after cleaning, optimizing disinfection processes. These capabilities align with calls for data-driven and precision infection prevention methods that adapt to specific environmental challenges [3].

7.2.1   Challenges and Advantages

Challenges
The cost of implementing robotic systems remains a barrier for many healthcare facilities. Additionally, the need for training personnel to operate and maintain these robots poses logistical challenges. Compatibility issues with existing systems and the complexity of troubleshooting technical issues can also limit deployment, especially in resource-limited settings.

Advantages
Robotic systems enhance the thoroughness and consistency of cleaning protocols, significantly reducing microbial load. Their ability to operate autonomously minimizes human exposure to infectious agents, thereby protecting healthcare workers. Robots can also ensure precision in repetitive tasks, freeing staff for more complex duties and increasing overall efficiency. Furthermore, their use in laboratory and logistical tasks accelerates workflows, reduces human error, and enhances overall biosafety. Robotic disinfection systems, in particular, ensure consistent coverage, reach inaccessible areas, and optimize safety standards in infection control [1].

7.3   Artificial Intelligence and Big Data

AI-driven tools have revolutionized infection surveillance and prediction. Machine learning algorithms analyze vast datasets to identify patterns and predict outbreaks, enabling proactive interventions. For instance, AI systems have been used to forecast infection trends and identify patients at high risk of HAIs, thereby optimizing resource allocation and preventive measures [4, 5]. Additionally, AI has proven effective in outbreak detection, identifying clusters of HAIs more efficiently than traditional surveillance methods [6].

AI-powered diagnostic tools are also transforming early detection processes by analyzing real-time patient data to identify infections quickly and accurately. Predictive modeling techniques integrated into electronic medical records (EMRs) use machine learning algorithms to flag patients at higher risk of HAIs, such as central line-associated bloodstream infections and ventilator-associated pneumonia [4]. This proactive approach allows clinicians to implement targeted preventive measures, ultimately reducing infection rates.

AI also enhances diagnostic accuracy by integrating with wearable sensors to monitor patient vitals in real time. These systems provide early warnings of infections, facilitating timely interventions. Big data analytics further supports this by synthesizing information from electronic health records (EHRs), wearable devices, and laboratory results to improve infection control strategies [7].

7.3.1   Challenges and Advantages

Challenges
Data privacy concerns and the interoperability of various systems remain significant hurdles. Ethical considerations, such as potential biases in AI algorithms, also pose challenges. Additionally, integrating AI tools into existing healthcare workflows can be resource-intensive and require significant training for staff.

Advantages
AI-driven tools offer unparalleled capabilities in analyzing large datasets, enabling early detection and targeted intervention for infections. They improve diagnostic accuracy and resource allocation, reducing the spread of HAIs. By automating complex data analyses, AI significantly enhances decision-making processes, ultimately leading to better patient outcomes. Furthermore, AI systems for outbreak detection reduce the workload on healthcare staff and offer greater sensitivity and accuracy compared to manual methods. Predictive tools embedded in EMRs further streamline infection prevention efforts, ensuring high-risk patients receive timely interventions [4, 6].

7.4   Wearable and Smart Devices

Wearable technology, such as smartwatches and biosensors, has become integral in monitoring patient health and detecting early signs of infection. Devices measuring temperature, oxygen levels, and heart rate provide continuous data streams that can alert healthcare providers to deviations from normal parameters [4].

Smart devices also include automated hand hygiene compliance systems that use sensors and analytics to monitor adherence to handwashing protocols. These systems have demonstrated significant improvements in compliance rates, which are critical for reducing HAIs [8]. Additionally, digital health and e-health platforms have empowered patients, enabling them to actively monitor their health post-discharge, particularly in surgical site infection (SSI) management [6].

Novel experimental technologies have also been applied in clinical simulations to understand pathogen transmission better. For instance, fluorescent markers used in operating room simulations revealed how contaminated hands and gloves of healthcare providers contribute to environmental contamination, emphasizing the importance of robust infection prevention protocols [8].

7.4.1   Challenges and Advantages

Challenges
Despite their potential, wearable devices face adoption barriers, including high costs, data security issues, and the need for user-friendly interfaces. Concerns about data ownership and interoperability with existing systems can also hinder

implementation. Additionally, healthcare providers may need significant training to effectively utilize wearable technology.

Advantages
Wearable devices provide continuous, real-time monitoring of vital signs, allowing for early detection of infections. Their ability to seamlessly integrate into daily routines enhances compliance and user engagement. Wearable technology also facilitates remote monitoring, reducing the need for frequent in-person visits and enabling proactive healthcare. Moreover, these devices support patient empowerment by fostering active involvement in health management, contributing to better outcomes and overall satisfaction [6]. Furthermore, advanced simulation technologies highlight critical areas for intervention, such as better hand hygiene practices and enhanced cleaning protocols, to reduce environmental contamination [8].

7.5   Internet of Things in Infection Control

IoT technology connects devices and systems to create "smart environments" in healthcare facilities. For example, IoT-enabled air filtration systems monitor and adjust air quality in real-time to minimize airborne pathogens [9].

Smart hospital rooms incorporate IoT for automated disinfection and monitoring systems, providing a sterile environment and reducing the likelihood of pathogen transmission. These technologies have been pivotal in transforming hospital infrastructure to support infection control efforts [2]. IoT also plays a role in predictive infection control, using integrated sensors and data analytics to anticipate infection hotspots and streamline preventive measures [6].

IoT technologies such as wearable devices and sensors have also been used in nursing to improve infection prevention. Automated hand hygiene surveillance systems, which use IoT-based reminders, have enhanced compliance rates among healthcare workers, reducing the transmission of healthcare-associated infections [7]. Additionally, IoT devices combined with GPS systems have been employed to track and predict the spread of diseases such as Zika virus, showcasing their versatility in addressing public health challenges.

7.6   Ethical and Economic Considerations

While new technologies promise substantial benefits, they also raise ethical concerns, particularly around data privacy and equitable access. Digital technologies, such as AI, IoT, and whole-genome sequencing (WGS), must be designed and implemented to comply with robust data protection regulations to ensure public trust and usability [10]. Ensuring that technologies are accessible to low-resource settings is crucial to avoid exacerbating existing healthcare disparities [3]. Social and political barriers, such as unequal technological infrastructure and resource allocation, often hinder implementation in underprivileged areas.

Sustainability is another critical consideration. Technologies like electrolyzed water (EW) and other eco-friendly cleaning agents are being explored to reduce environmental impact while maintaining infection control efficacy. However, the short shelf life and limited evidence for EW's effectiveness in healthcare highlight the need for rigorous testing and evaluation before widespread adoption [11]. A balance must be struck between environmental goals and ensuring safe, high-quality care.

Ethical concerns specific to WGS include the implications of identifying individuals involved in transmission chains. Sequencing data could unintentionally reveal personal or occupational roles in outbreaks, which raises considerations for consent, privacy, and the potential emotional and professional impact on those identified [5].

Economically, while upfront costs can be high, the long-term savings from reduced infection rates and hospital stays may offset these expenses. A systematic analysis of cost-effectiveness is essential, especially for large-scale deployments of technologies like wearable devices, IoT systems, and WGS in healthcare facilities [4]. Additionally, lessons from pilot implementations of digital tools for surveillance and outbreak response underscore the importance of international collaboration and funding for sustainable healthcare innovation [10].

7.7   Conclusion

The integration of advanced technologies into infection control is reshaping the landscape of healthcare. Technologies like whole-genome sequencing (WGS) have provided unprecedented insights into the epidemiology and transmission of healthcare-associated infections, enabling more targeted and effective interventions. Innovations in sterilization and disinfection, including vaporized hydrogen peroxide, electrostatic sprayers, and electrolyzed water, are contributing to safer and more sustainable clinical environments. "No-touch" room decontamination technologies, such as UV-C and hydrogen peroxide systems, significantly reduce microbial contamination and HAIs. While challenges remain, including ethical considerations and the need for robust infrastructure, the potential benefits—from improved patient outcomes to enhanced operational efficiency—are compelling. Continued innovation, coupled with efforts to address ethical and practical barriers, will be key to leveraging these technologies effectively and equitably in the global fight against infectious diseases.

References

1. Gao A, Murphy RR, Chen W, et al. Progress in robotics for combating infectious diseases. Sci Robotics. 2021;6:eabf1462.

2. Piaggio D, et al. The use of smart environments and robots for infection prevention control: a systematic literature review. Am J Infect Control. 2023;51:1175–81. https://doi.org/10.1016/j.ajic.2023.03.005.
3. Birgand G, Ahmad R, Holmes A. Innovation for infection prevention and control—revisiting Pasteur's vision. Lancet. 2022;400:2250–60.
4. Pryor R, Bearman G. Latest advancements in infection prevention technology. Infect Control Today. 2022;26(7)
5. Eyre DW, et al. Infection prevention and control insights from a decade of pathogen whole-genome sequencing. J Hosp Infect. 2022;122:180–6. https://doi.org/10.1016/j.jhin.2022.01.024.
6. Arzilli G, De Vita E, Pasquale M, Carloni LM, Pellegrini M, Di Giacomo M, Esposito E, Porretta AD, Rizzo C. Innovative techniques for infection control and surveillance in hospital settings and long-term care facilities: a scoping review. Antibiotics. 2024;13:77. https://doi.org/10.3390/antibiotics13010077.
7. Huang F, Brouqui P, Boudjema S. How does innovative technology impact nursing in infectious diseases and infection control? A scoping review. Nurs Open. 2021;8:2369–84.
8. Birnbach DJ, Rosen LF, Fitzpatrick M, Carling P, Munoz-Price LS. The use of a novel technology to study dynamics of pathogen transmission in the operating room. Anesth Analg. 2015;120(4):844–7. https://doi.org/10.1213/ANE.0000000000000226.
9. Li C, Wang J, Zhang Y. A review of IoT applications in healthcare. Neurocomputing. 2024;565:127017.
10. ECDC. Digital technologies for infectious disease surveillance, prevention and control: a scoping review of the research literature 2015–2019. Europ Centre Disease Prev Control. 2021; https://doi.org/10.2900/086179.
11. Jain S, Dempsey K, Clezy K, Mitchell BG, Kiernan MA. Sustainability and novel technologies to improve environmental cleaning in healthcare: implications and considerations. Infection, Disease & Health. 2024;30 https://doi.org/10.1016/j.idh.2024.07.002.

Infection Control and Artificial Intelligence—AI

8

Tihana Gašpert

Abstract

Artificial Intelligence (AI) revolutionizes infection control by improving diagnostic precision, preventive measures, and treatment approaches. AI-driven systems oversee adherence to hand hygiene protocols and enhance infection control in medical environments. The capacity of AI to differentiate between inflammation and bacterial infection enhances diagnostic accuracy, hence minimizing antibiotic usage. Moreover, AI methods facilitate the evaluation of infection transmission risk, allowing for preemptive actions to avert outbreaks. In combating antimicrobial resistance, AI aids in discovering new medicines and forecasting resistance patterns. The incorporation of AI in infection control presents substantial ethical and safety issues, such as data privacy, algorithmic bias, and the necessity for human supervision. IPC specialists must address these difficulties to guarantee the safe and ethical implementation of AI technologies while improving infection prevention and control initiatives.

Keywords

Artificial Intelligence · Infection control · Hand hygiene · Inflammation · Bacterial infection · Antibacterial resistance · AI ethics · Healthcare safety · Transmission prevention · Diagnostics

T. Gašpert (✉)
University Hospital Rijeka, Rijeka, Croatia

Faculty of Health Sciences, University of Maribor, Maribor, Slovenia

8.1   Introduction

Artificial intelligence (AI) demonstrates the potential to improve healthcare-associated infection surveillance, possibly optimizing duties and liberating healthcare personnel for patient-centered activities. Optimal utilization of AI necessitates user education and continuous development of AI models [1]. The swift progression of AI has profoundly influenced infection prevention and management, especially during the COVID-19 pandemic [2]. Artificial intelligence methodologies, including machine learning (ML), deep learning, and natural language processing (NLP), have effectively revolutionized infection prevention and control (IPC) measures (Table 8.1). These technologies have augmented our comprehension of infectious diseases, enabled the prediction of disease propagation, and refined public health emergency responses [3].

Artificial intelligence is crucial to the monitoring and forecasting of infectious disease epidemics. The capacity to analyze various kinds of data enables healthcare authorities to implement proactive interventions. A multitude of deep learning models has been created to forecast the antigenic development of several viruses, including severe acute respiratory syndrome coronavirus 2 (SARS-CoV-2), influenza, human immunodeficiency virus (HIV), Lassa, and Nipah viruses [4, 5]. These accomplishments highlight the critical role of AI in global disease management systems [6].

Table 8.1 Common AI Terms and Models in Healthcare [1–3]

AI Term/model	Description	Application in healthcare
Machine learning (ML)	Algorithms that learn from data and improve performance over time	Predicting disease outcomes and optimizing antibiotic therapy
Deep learning (DL)	A subset of ML using neural networks to analyze complex patterns	Image analysis for diagnostics
Natural language processing (NLP)	AI that understands and processes human language	Extracting medical insights from clinical notes and research papers
Neural networks (NNs)	Algorithms mimic the human brain to recognize patterns	Detecting abnormalities in medical images and identifying pathogens
Convolutional neural networks (CNNs)	Specialized NNs for image and spatial data processing	Medical imaging (X-rays, MRIs, CT scans)
Transformer models	Advanced DL models for sequence data, such as text	AI-driven diagnostics, drug discovery, and chatbots for healthcare
Generative AI	AI that creates new data or content based on learned patterns	Drug discovery, medical report generation
Support vector machines (SVMs)	ML models that classify data points	Disease detection and classification
Gradient boosting machines (GBM)	ML technique that improves predictive accuracy	Identifying antibiotic resistance patterns
Reinforcement learning (RL)	AI that learns by trial and error with rewards and penalties	Personalized treatment recommendations, robotic surgery

Advanced technology could potentially influence standard nursing duties, including vital sign assessment, drug administration, and infection control methods, thereby altering the function of nurses within the healthcare system. This alteration may raise apprehensions among nurses as they transition from their established practices, coupled with the worry that AI-integrated technology could facilitate surveillance and monitoring, thereby infringing upon the privacy of both practitioners and patients [7–9]. Nonetheless, nursing informatics, about breakthroughs in AI, has experienced significant progress during the past 20 years [10].

Notwithstanding these advantages, AI technologies face issues regarding ethics, biosafety, and privacy, particularly with commercial organizations' management of medical data and the risk of its exploitation [11, 12]. Successfully employing AI in infection prevention and control necessitates balancing technical capabilities and ethical, policy, and societal factors [6].

8.2   Hand Hygiene

Hand hygiene is an essential element of an IPC program, and artificial intelligence technologies for hand hygiene teaching and assessment present prospects to enhance compliance and optimize IPC procedures [13].

Computer vision is a domain of artificial intelligence that examines the automatic interpretation of picture and video input in a manner akin to human perception. In a simulated clinical setting utilizing computer vision with depth images (where individuals are represented as outlines devoid of distinct features) for hand hygiene auditing, the system demonstrated greater efficacy in detecting alcohol hand rub dispensing and the initial moment than identifying hand rubbing [14]. In a survey of technological behavior monitoring systems, hand hygiene enhancement ranged from 6% to 54%, while the findings on the sustainability of this increase were less certain [15]. Given that wearable technologies necessitate constant use by staff, user attitude, device functionality, and usability are critical considerations before advancing the development of associated AI applications. For instance, if a gadget is designed to provide aural or visual reminders, the capacity to suppress this feature in specific clinical contexts, such as palliative care, is crucial. Similarly, the design, dimensions, or mass of devices may be regarded as impediments to patient care or, in fact, an infection prevention and control risk, particularly considering that most commercially available wearables are intended for wrist application [16].

8.3   Distinguishing Inflammation from Bacterial Infection

From an antibiotic stewardship perspective, the most challenging yet consequential distinction is whether the patient has a genuine infection or merely systemic inflammation absent of infection. Distinguishing between these two illness states necessitates the amalgamation of various data types, none of which exhibit high sensitivity or specificity, as abnormal values for these variables are prevalent in both conditions, and there is a deficiency of highly discriminative tests at present. Machine-learning method utilizing random forests with eight normally available parameters surpasses existing biomarkers in distinguishing between infectious and non-infectious conditions in critically unwell infants [17]. When the goal was to detect all sepsis cases, the model correctly identified 28% of non-infectious cases. If further validation and clinical trials confirm its accuracy, this model could help reduce unnecessary antibiotic use. A recent example of the challenge in distinguishing inflammation from bacterial infection was seen during the COVID-19 pandemic when diagnosing bacterial co-infections was particularly difficult [18].

8.3.1   Commencing Antimicrobial Treatment

Currently, antimicrobials are provided either empirically or supplemented with data from surveillance cultures when accessible. AI and machine learning play a crucial role in improving rapid diagnostics by enabling the early identification of multidrug-resistant organisms (MDROs). By analyzing genomic and microbiological data, AI can predict antimicrobial resistance patterns more quickly and accurately than traditional culture-based methods. Machine learning algorithms also help optimize antimicrobial therapy by integrating patient data, infection patterns, and resistance trends to recommend the most effective treatment. The causal pathogen remains unidentified in both scenarios. The antibiotic susceptibility of the causal organism is determined only after the initiation of antimicrobial therapy. Optimal rapid diagnostics would facilitate the identification of the pathogen and its antimicrobial susceptibility directly from clinical samples within approximately 30 minutes, significantly reducing the necessity for empirical treatment or enabling modifications to antimicrobial therapy before the administration of a second dose, thus resulting in more timely and appropriate treatment. Additionally, studies have demonstrated that AI and machine learning can contribute to this domain [19].

8.3.2   Antimicrobial Dosage and Administration Interval

Pharmacometrics has traditionally determined dosage and dosing intervals by linear regression, population pharmacokinetic models, and Bayesian forecasting. The developed models remain predominantly in the research phase, attempting to integrate into clinical settings as dosage software; nevertheless, extensive deployment in clinical practice is insufficient [20, 21].

8.3.3   Support for Antimicrobial Stewardship

In recent years, significant efforts have been dedicated to the development and maintenance of hospital-specific antimicrobial stewardship programs. The implementation of antimicrobial stewardship programs has significantly affected both the duration of hospital stays and antimicrobial costs [22]. A critical component of these strategies is the review of antimicrobial prescriptions and feedback to prescribers, assessing many key factors for prescribed antimicrobials, such as indication, dosage, method of administration, and duration. Due to the labor-intensive nature of this task, electronic tools are frequently employed to assist in identifying patients for review. It is important to acknowledge that clinical decision support systems (CDSS) typically rely on an expert and rule-based knowledge base, necessitating that their development and maintenance by evolving recommendations is both time-consuming and resource-intensive. Moreover, resource limitations result in the prioritization of specific antibiotics of interest rather than assessing all given antibiotics [23].

8.4   Enhanced Diagnosis and Prevention of Transmission Assessment

The apprehension regarding the transfer of infectious diseases has prompted authorities to establish protocols for identifying at-risk individuals. Contemporary methodologies employing mathematical modeling are enhancing this form of surveillance. A comparable technique was established to identify infected individuals through classification based on vital signs [24]. Consequently, respiration rate, heart rate, and face temperature were employed to effectively classify patients at elevated risk for influenza utilizing neural network and fuzzy clustering methodologies. Due to the protracted procedure of reaching a definitive diagnosis, early signs of the infection were investigated. Current systems, such as the artificial immune recognition system (AIRS), are utilized for the diagnosis of many diseases. AIRS was designed utilizing the characteristics of the immune system. The immune system's function is to identify dangers and retain them in memory. Immunological memory is arguably the most critical aspect of immunity, as it enables a more effective response upon subsequent encounters with the infectious agent. This aligns with the development of AI tools grounded in human cognitive function; the sole distinction is that intelligence is delegated to the periphery blood [25].

8.5   Therapies and Antibacterial Resistance

Despite proficient malaria diagnostic capabilities and anticipated advancements, resistance remains a significant issue with antibacterial and antiparasitic medications [26]. The implementation of artemisinin-based combination therapy two decades ago is currently being contested by the advent of *Plasmodium falciparum* malaria parasites exhibiting reduced resistance to these medications [27]. The presence of databases documenting antibiotic resistance can enhance efforts to combat this issue [28].

The Comprehensive Antibiotic Resistance Database (CARD) provides high-quality reference material regarding the molecular mechanisms of antimicrobial resistance. CARD is ontologically organized, model-centric, and encompasses various antimicrobial resistance medication classes and processes. The database is a structured and interconnected system that facilitates efficient data sharing and organizing. This underscores the significance of appropriate architecture for the database (big data architecture) [29].

Current and prior investigations indicate that machine learning offers substantial accuracy, corroborating recent research that validates in silico methods for screening extensive datasets to uncover prospective anti-infectious options [30]. Shen et al. have demonstrated how therapies can be enhanced through the application of mathematical models. Shen et al. suggested a decision support system that may recommend antibiotic medication tailored to the patient, considering criteria such as body temperature, infection locations, symptoms/signs, complications, antibacterial spectrum, contraindications, and drug–drug interactions. This was possible due to the extensive dataset used to develop the model. The system includes a vast range of infectious diseases, pathogens, symptoms, complications, treatment options, and antibiotic interactions. By incorporating detailed relationships between infections, bacteria, and medications, the model effectively supports accurate diagnosis and treatment decisions [31].

In addition to antibiotics, antibodies are highly effective in safeguarding against viral infections. The principle of vaccination is to elicit a robust memory response for future encounters with the virus. This occurs through the generation of antibodies that inhibit the virus's reproduction. Research indicates that machine learning has a crucial role in identifying optimal candidate vaccinations by antigen selection, predicting potential mutations, and personalizing vaccine recommendations based on genetic and demographic factors [32].

All facets of therapy response are contingent upon a critical parameter: compliance. There are limited systems for large-scale verification of compliance with infection-related treatments. To monitor the progression of HIV infection, one can assess the blood concentration of HIV RNA. This method is highly effective for therapeutic adjustment but is seldom financially feasible in resource-limited environments. The evolution of HIV infectivity is significantly influenced by antiretroviral medication, making it crucial to ensure proper adherence to the therapy and to prevent fluctuations in viral loads due to inconsistent treatment compliance [33].

In groups susceptible to virological failure, employing a sensitive strategy may facilitate the identification of patients with inconsistent drug adherence, thereby enhancing their health outcomes, decreasing the expenses associated with repetitive testing, and increasing awareness of the importance of adhering to treatment regimens [34].

8.6   Ethical and Safety Considerations

Recent breakthroughs in artificial intelligence, particularly in generative AI models, have profoundly influenced multiple industries. Artificial intelligence has proved important in forecasting epidemics and enhancing resource distribution during the pandemic. It has transformed drug design and disease management by offering rapid and precise predictions for diagnosis, disease progression, and treatment development. Artificial intelligence is anticipated to assume a progressively significant role in the management of future public health emergencies, especially in tackling infectious disease epidemics [35, 36].

The increasing utilization of AI in medicine and public health highlights its vital function in improving disease surveillance, early identification of infectious diseases, resource distribution, and crisis management. Nonetheless, this expansion also presents considerable ethical and safety issues [6].

The utilization of AI in vaccine development presents ethical concerns around data privacy, prejudice, and equity. Artificial intelligence is extensively employed to evaluate data, encompassing personal health records and genetic information, so highlighting the imperative of safeguarding data privacy. Moreover, the disproportionate allocation of healthcare resources results in skewed data in vaccine research, frequently privileging individuals with enhanced healthcare access [37]. This disparity, coupled with possible biases, may lead to vaccines being less effective and safe for diverse populations. This disparity can intensify the divergence in healthcare standards between industrialized and developing nations on a national scale. Consequently, it is imperative to employ AI ethically in vaccine research to guarantee that communities with restricted healthcare access also gain from developing technology and mitigate global health inequities [6].

8.6.1   Obstacles

AI offers numerous potential benefits for IPC, including rapidity, uniformity, and the ability to manage indefinitely huge datasets; yet certain problems persist. AI relies heavily on the quality and completeness of data, the existence of rigorous reference standards (which often are lacking in IPC), and close coordination with IPC experts to interpret results and assure clinical applicability. Otherwise, errors made during the machine learning training process may lead to false negatives, misclassification, or inapplicability. IPC practitioners must also comprehend the limitations of AI within a specific application and context. Machine learning outcomes might inadequately classify fresh data (underfitting) or fail to identify analogous patterns in new data (overfitting), contingent upon the methods of data collection and the design of learning algorithms. They may also indicate the inherent bias present in the training data [16].

Currently, health data is stored in several locations, including hospitals, community settings, and on patient devices like smartphones and wearables. Numerous healthcare facilities and specific departments have established customized data infrastructures utilizing various vendors. For AI to provide a complete picture, it needs access to data from multiple healthcare institutions, rather than being limited to isolated data sources. However, most research on AI in healthcare focus on specific, easier-to-manage areas rather than the bigger picture. To fully benefit from AI, infection prevention and control (IPC) and healthcare systems need to be more connected. It's also essential to train AI models in ways that ensure they work reliably across different patient groups, especially those that are often underrepresented in the data [16].

Additional problems encompass data ownership, privacy, and the exploitation of data for economic or political gain [38, 39]. A potential approach is allowing patients to manage their own data and grant approval for its use in developing AI applications [39]. Public discourse, regulatory frameworks, and future legislation will be necessary to facilitate the secure development, utilization, and supervision of AI applications, ensuring that individual privacy is prioritized while allowing healthcare systems access to inform public health and infection prevention and control measures [16].

8.6.2   Opportunities

To properly tackle these difficulties, it is essential to foster international collaboration, implement stringent rules, uphold ethical oversight, and enhance public information literacy. These procedures are crucial for optimizing the advantages of AI while alleviating related concerns. The effective implementation of AI's revolutionary influence on human civilization relies on a coordinated endeavor of global public health organizations, research institutes, and scientists, all dedicated to advancing universal human welfare. Regulators must consistently evaluate and address the ethical and safety issues related to the application of AI in IPC.

The AI Act categorizes AI systems based on risk levels, with the highest-risk applications facing strict regulations while lower-risk systems have lighter requirements or remain unregulated. High-risk AI systems, such as those used in law enforcement, healthcare, and infrastructure, must meet transparency, safety, and accountability standards. General-purpose AI (GPAI) models must follow documentation and cybersecurity guidelines, with stricter measures for those posing systemic risks. For policymakers, this is crucial because it ensures AI is developed and deployed responsibly, preventing unethical uses like social scoring and manipulative AI while fostering innovation. The Act also establishes governance structures, including an AI Office, to oversee compliance, making it essential for shaping AI policy, protecting fundamental rights, and maintaining public trust in AI technologies (41). Policymakers must proactively confront future difficulties by implementing legislation and regulations that ensure information security and maintain medical ethics. This strategy will cultivate an environment suitable for AI's stable advancement [6].

8.7   Conclusion

The potential for AI applications to enhance IPC is substantial; yet AI alone will not enhance IPC. Enhancing sustainability in IPC necessitates a transformation in culture and behavior, underpinned by suitable governance frameworks. The principle that "correlation does not imply causation" is especially pertinent in the context of AI utilization in healthcare. Artificial intelligence is propelled by extensive datasets to uncover correlations that may signify medically pertinent disorders or to detect potential danger factors. Nonetheless, AIs may occasionally neglect minor clusters that could be clinically significant and cannot currently apply a profound understanding of the underlying mechanisms to analyze tiny datasets. The emphasis should be on the IPC issue that requires resolution through the formulation of strategies, objectives, and processes, which may incorporate AI techniques. Organizations that have effectively executed digital transformations have prioritized understanding of culture and drivers before selecting suitable technical tools. Furthermore, engaging insiders who understand the culture, recognizing that a uniform approach is inadequate for all contexts, and implementing a flat hierarchy to facilitate swift iterative changes are critical factors [40]. IPC practitioners must recognize the constraints and biases inherent in AI, as well as the propensity of personnel to delegate jobs to AI and exhibit excessive confidence in its capabilities. Concerns about privacy and data ownership necessitate meticulous examination; AI applications must be evaluated and incorporated into actual clinical practice, and for the majority of healthcare environments, substantial investment in data infrastructure is essential to fully actualize its promise.

References

1. Wiemken TL, Carrico RM. Assisting the infection preventionist: use of artificial intelligence for health care–associated infection surveillance. Am J Infect Control. 2024;52(6):625–9.
2. Syrowatka A, Kuznetsova M, Alsubai A, Beckman AL, Bain PA, Craig KJT, et al. Leveraging artificial intelligence for pandemic preparedness and response: a scoping review to identify key use cases. NPJ Digital Med. 2021;4(1):96.
3. Jia Z, Yan X, Li Y, Ma J. Internet data for improving prevention and control of global infectious diseases. China CDC Weekly. 2020;2(52):1009.
4. Han W, Chen N, Xu X, Sahil A, Zhou J, Li Z, et al. Predicting the antigenic evolution of SARS-COV-2 with deep learning. Nat Commun. 2023;14(1):3478.
5. Thadani NN, Gurev S, Notin P, Youssef N, Rollins NJ, Ritter D, et al. Learning from prepandemic data to forecast viral escape. Nature. 2023;622(7984):818–25.
6. Yang L, Lu S, Zhou L. The implications of artificial intelligence on infection prevention and control: current Progress and future perspectives. China CDC Weekly. 2024;6(35):901.
7. Clancy TR. Artificial intelligence and nursing: the future is now. JONA. J Nurs Adm. 2020;50(3):125–7.
8. Robert N. How artificial intelligence is changing nursing. Nurs Manag. 2019;50(9):30–9.
9. Haleem A, Javaid M, Singh RP, Suman R. Medical 4.0 technologies for healthcare: features, capabilities, and applications. Internet Things Cyber-Phys Sys. 2022;2:12–30.
10. Alruwaili MM, Abuadas FH, Alsadi M, Alruwaili AN, Elsayed Ramadan OM, Shaban M, et al. Exploring nurses' awareness and attitudes toward artificial intelligence: implications for nursing practice. Digital Health. 2024;10:20552076241271803.
11. Bélisle-Pipon J-C, Vayena E, Green RC, Cohen IG. Genetic testing, insurance discrimination and medical research: what the United States can learn from peer countries. Nat Med. 2019;25(8):1198–204.
12. Wan Z, Hazel JW, Clayton EW, Vorobeychik Y, Kantarcioglu M, Malin BA. Sociotechnical safeguards for genomic data privacy. Nat Rev Genet. 2022;23(7):429–45.

13. Higgins A, Hannan M. Improved hand hygiene technique and compliance in healthcare workers using gaming technology. J Hosp Infect. 2013;84(1):32–7.

14. Awwad S, Tarvade S, Piccardi M, Gattas DJ. The use of privacy-protected computer vision to measure the quality of healthcare worker hand hygiene. Int J Qual Health Care. 2019;31(1):36–42.

15. Meng M, Sorber M, Herzog A, Igel C, Kugler C. Technological innovations in infection control: a rapid review of the acceptance of behavior monitoring systems and their contribution to the improvement of hand hygiene. Am J Infect Control. 2019;47(4):439–47.

16. Fitzpatrick F, Doherty A, Lacey G. Using artificial intelligence in infection prevention. Curr Treat Options Infect Dis. 2020;12:135–44.

17. Lamping F, Jack T, Rübsamen N, Sasse M, Beerbaum P, Mikolajczyk RT, et al. Development and validation of a diagnostic model for early differentiation of sepsis and non-infectious SIRS in critically ill children-a data-driven approach using machine-learning algorithms. BMC Pediatr. 2018;18:1–11.

18. Rawson TM, Hernandez B, Wilson RC, Ming D, Herrero P, Ranganathan N, et al. Supervised machine learning to support the diagnosis of bacterial infection in the context of COVID-19. JAC Antimicrobial Resis. 2021;3(1):dlab002.

19. De Corte T, Van Hoecke S, De Waele J. Artificial intelligence in infection management in the ICU. In: Annual Update in Intensive Care and Emergency Medicine, vol. 2022; 2022. p. 369–81.

20. Roggeveen LF, Fleuren LM, Guo T, Thoral P, de Grooth HJ, Swart EL, et al. Right dose right now: bedside data-driven personalized antibiotic dosing in severe sepsis and septic shock—rationale and design of a multicenter randomized controlled superiority trial. Trials. 2019;20:1–13.

21. Chai MG, Cotta MO, Abdul-Aziz MH, Roberts JA. What are the current approaches to optimising antimicrobial dosing in the intensive care unit? Pharmaceutics. 2020;12(7):638.

22. Nathwani D, Varghese D, Stephens J, Ansari W, Martin S, Charbonneau C. Value of hospital antimicrobial stewardship programs [ASPs]: a systematic review. Antimicrob Resist Infect Control. 2019;8:1–13.

23. Bystritsky RJ, Beltran A, Young AT, Wong A, Hu X, Doernberg SB. Machine learning for the prediction of antimicrobial stewardship intervention in hospitalized patients receiving broad-spectrum agents. Infect Control Hosp Epidemiol. 2020;41(9):1022–7.

24. Sun G, Matsui T, Hakozaki Y, Abe S. An infectious disease/fever screening radar system which stratifies higher-risk patients within ten seconds using a neural network and the fuzzy grouping method. J Infect. 2015;70(3):230–6.

25. Cuevas E, Osuna-Enciso V, Zaldivar D, Perez-Cisneros M, Sossa H. Multithreshold segmentation based on artificial immune systems. Math Probl Eng. 2012;2012(1):874761.

26. Blasco B, Leroy D, Fidock DA. Antimalarial drug resistance: linking plasmodium falciparum parasite biology to the clinic. Nat Med. 2017;23(8):917–28.

27. Saralamba S, Pan-Ngum W, Maude RJ, Lee SJ, Tarning J, Lindegårdh N, et al. Intrahost modeling of artemisinin resistance in plasmodium falciparum. Proc Natl Acad Sci. 2011;108(1):397–402.

28. Jia B, Raphenya AR, Alcock B, Waglechner N, Guo P, Tsang KK, et al. CARD 2017: expansion and model-centric curation of the comprehensive antibiotic resistance database. Nucleic Acids Res. 2016:gkw1004.

29. Wang Y, Yang Y-J, Chen Y-N, Zhao H-Y, Zhang S. Computer-aided design, structural dynamics analysis, and in vitro susceptibility test of antibacterial peptides incorporating unnatural amino acids against microbial infections. Comput Methods Prog Biomed. 2016;134:215–23.

30. Zhang X, Amin EA. Highly predictive support vector machine (SVM) models for anthrax toxin lethal factor (LF) inhibitors. J Mol Graph Model. 2016;63:22–8.

31. Shen Y, Yuan K, Chen D, Colloc J, Yang M, Li Y, et al. An ontology-driven clinical decision support system (IDDAP) for infectious disease diagnosis and antibiotic prescription. Artif Intell Med. 2018;86:20–32.

32. Choi I, Chung AW, Suscovich TJ, Rerks-Ngarm S, Pitisuttithum P, Nitayaphan S, et al. Machine learning methods enable predictive modeling of antibody feature: function relationships in RV144 vaccinees. PLoS Comput Biol. 2015;11(4):e1004185.
33. Petersen ML, LeDell E, Schwab J, Sarovar V, Gross R, Reynolds N, et al. Super learner analysis of electronic adherence data improves viral prediction and may provide strategies for selective HIV RNA monitoring. JAIDS J Acq Immun Deficiency Syn. 2015;69(1):109–18.
34. Bisson GP, Gross R, Bellamy S, Chittams J, Hislop M, Regensberg L, et al. Pharmacy refill adherence compared with CD4 count changes for monitoring HIV-infected adults on antiretroviral therapy. PLoS Med. 2008;5(5):e109.
35. Brownstein JS, Rader B, Astley CM, Tian H. Advances in artificial intelligence for infectious-disease surveillance. N Engl J Med. 2023;388(17):1597–607.
36. Wong F, de la Fuente-Nunez C, Collins JJ. Leveraging artificial intelligence in the fight against infectious diseases. Science. 2023;381(6654):164–70.
37. Smith J, Lipsitch M, Almond JW. Vaccine production, distribution, access, and uptake. Lancet. 2011;378(9789):428–38.
38. Scott IA, Cook D, Coiera EW, Richards B. Machine learning in clinical practice: prospects and pitfalls. Med J Aust. 2019;211(5):203–5.
39. Rajkomar A, Dean J, Kohane I. Machine learning in medicine. N Engl J Med. 2019;380(14):1347–58.
40. Tabrizi B, Lam E, Girard K, Irvin V. Digital transformation is not about technology.[online] Harv Bus Rev. 2019.

Healthcare-Associated Infection Surveillance and AI

Silvana Gastaldi [ID]

Abstract

Healthcare-associated infections (HAIs) continue to exert a heavy toll on patient outcomes and healthcare system costs worldwide. Traditional surveillance methods, relying on manual chart review and administrative data, are limited by delays, under-reporting, and inconsistencies. The advent of artificial intelligence (AI) and the digital transformation of health records have opened new frontiers for infection prevention and control (IPC), enabling real-time monitoring, risk stratification, and predictive interventions. This chapter traces the evolution of HAI surveillance from early rule-based systems to current machine learning and deep learning applications, highlighting the shift from reactive detection to proactive risk prediction. Comparative studies demonstrate that AI-driven surveillance outperforms manual methods in sensitivity, timeliness, and operational efficiency. Nonetheless, significant barriers persist, including data integration challenges, high infrastructure costs, limited AI literacy among healthcare professionals, and regulatory and ethical concerns surrounding data privacy and algorithmic bias. Despite these hurdles, economic analyses suggest that AI surveillance can offer substantial long-term savings through reduced infection rates and optimized resource allocation. Adoption patterns vary by setting, with high-income hospitals pioneering full automation while lower-resource environments explore semi-automated and open-source models. Sustainability and scalability hinge on continuous model updates, interoperability standards, cloud-based infrastructures, and international collaboration. Looking ahead, priorities include multi-center validation trials, explainable AI development, integrated antimicrobial stewardship, and comprehensive cost-effectiveness evaluations. Ultimately, AI-driven surveillance stands poised to transform IPC practice, moving from

S. Gastaldi (✉)
Independent Researcher, Mazzano, Italy

retrospective identification to proactive prevention, and offering a promising pathway to enhance patient safety and healthcare quality globally.

Keywords

Healthcare-associated infections · Surveillance · Artificial intelligence · Machine learning · Real-time monitoring · Predictive analytics · Infection prevention and control · Ethical considerations

9.1 Introduction

In acute-care hospitals, approximately 7% of patients in high-income countries and 15% in low- and middle-income countries develop at least one healthcare-associated infection (HAI) during their stay. A 2022–2023 point-prevalence survey spanning 28 EU/EEA Member States and three Western Balkan territories reported that 8% of patients in acute-care settings had acquired at least one HAI [1]. Beyond human toll, HAIs inflate healthcare expenditures by billions of dollars each year through prolonged hospital stays, additional diagnostics, antimicrobial treatments, and complication management [2]. Early detection underpins effective infection prevention and control (IPC), yet traditional surveillance—relying on manual chart review, laboratory reporting, and administrative codes—suffers from delays, underreporting, and variable accuracy [3]. In parallel, the digital transformation of health records and the advent of artificial intelligence (AI) offer transformative potential: automated, real-time monitoring of patient data streams, risk stratification, and predictive alerts that can preempt outbreaks and optimize resource allocation [4, 5]. This chapter narrates the evolution, capabilities, challenges, and future directions of AI-driven HAI surveillance, weaving quantitative evidence seamlessly into a technical yet accessible account for IPC professionals.

9.2 Evolution of Surveillance: From Rule-Based to Predictive AI

Early electronic surveillance systems relied on rule-based algorithms, generating alerts from combinations of fever, leukocytosis, positive cultures, or device use to identify potential HAIs for infection control teams [6]. While they reduced manual workload, their rigidity limited adaptation to emerging infection patterns or clinical nuance.

The next advancement came through machine learning models, which utilized historical clinical datasets to recognize complex interactions between features. For example, algorithms trained on vital signs, laboratory results, and medication orders were shown to effectively identify patterns indicative of emerging infections [7, 8]. Deep learning, particularly through convolutional neural networks (CNNs), further enhanced the ability to interpret unstructured data, enabling the analysis of free-text clinical narratives with greater sensitivity and specificity compared to traditional ML methods [9].

As technological integration deepened, real-time surveillance systems emerged, combining continuous electronic health record (EHR) data with laboratory and pharmacy records. These platforms demonstrated the capacity to detect multidrug-resistant organisms (MDROs) with impressive reliability and timeliness [5]. In addition, predictive analytics introduced dynamic risk scoring based on patient trajectories, allowing healthcare providers to anticipate infections before clinical symptoms fully emerged [10]. This evolution from reactive to proactive surveillance marks a fundamental shift in IPC strategies, aiming to not only detect but also prevent infections.

Comparative evaluations of AI-driven surveillance versus traditional methods consistently demonstrate the superiority of AI. Multi-center studies have shown that electronic surveillance identifies significantly more HAIs than manual chart reviews. In particular, the use of machine learning algorithms capable of mirroring established definitions such as those of the National Healthcare Safety Network (NHSN) has been associated with a considerable increase in detected infections [7]. Furthermore, neural network approaches have successfully reduced infection control workload by automating preliminary case detection, thus freeing IPC staff for higher-order tasks such as outbreak management and staff education [4].

Real-world impacts have been substantial. AI implementations in hospital settings have been associated with notable reductions in HAI incidence, supporting earlier interventions and improving patient safety [11]. Cluster detection algorithms utilizing AI have also enhanced outbreak identification compared to traditional single-indicator systems [12]. These outcomes suggest that AI-driven surveillance does not merely match traditional systems but exceeds them in sensitivity, timeliness, and actionable intelligence.

9.3 Barriers and Challenges

However, the adoption of AI in HAI surveillance faces significant barriers. Data integration challenges persist due to the heterogeneity of EHR systems, where differing formats and standards complicate the seamless sharing and analysis of data [13]. High costs of technical infrastructure—including servers, cloud storage, cybersecurity, and licensing—further inhibit adoption, particularly in low- and middle-income settings where budget constraints are a critical concern [14]. Beyond technological hurdles, cultural and educational barriers emerge. Surveys highlight that a significant proportion of healthcare workers remain skeptical about AI, often citing concerns over the opacity of "black-box" algorithms and the risk of deskilling clinical judgment [15, 16].

Legal and ethical challenges compound these technical difficulties. AI systems that process patient data must comply with stringent privacy laws such as the General Data Protection Regulation (GDPR) in Europe and Health Insurance

Portability and Accountability Act (HIPAA) in the United States. These regulations demand data anonymization, traceability, and accountability, adding layers of complexity to the development and deployment of AI solutions [10, 13]. Moreover, centralized AI systems storing massive volumes of sensitive data present lucrative targets for cyber-attacks, amplifying the importance of robust cybersecurity measures.

Ethical risks extend beyond data privacy. Algorithmic bias remains a major concern, particularly when AI models trained on incomplete or unrepresentative datasets systematically underperform in vulnerable populations, such as pediatric or immunocompromised patients [8]. Over-reliance on automated alerts can also erode critical clinical oversight, as demonstrated by studies showing increased rates of missed infections when clinicians deferred entirely to AI outputs [12]. Furthermore, the opacity of deep learning models complicates issues of accountability in the event of diagnostic errors, raising difficult questions about whether responsibility lies with the clinician, the hospital, or the AI vendor [13].

9.4 Economic Implications and Adoption Readiness

Despite these concerns, the economic case for AI-driven surveillance remains compelling. Institutions that have implemented AI systems have reported significant reductions in infection rates, leading to substantial savings through shortened hospital stays, reduced antimicrobial use, and lowered litigation risks [5, 11]. Automating surveillance processes also optimizes human resource allocation, allowing infection preventionists to focus on direct patient care, education, and strategic interventions [4, 10]. However, comprehensive economic analyses, especially in low- and middle-income countries, are still limited and should be prioritized to validate the broader return on investment.

The readiness for AI adoption varies greatly between healthcare settings. High-income tertiary hospitals often lead in piloting and deploying fully automated real-time surveillance systems, leveraging their greater IT infrastructure and specialized personnel [5]. Middle-income settings tend to adopt semi-automated models that require a balance between automated alerts and manual case validation [7, 15]. Meanwhile, low-resource environments focus on simpler, rule-based solutions, experimenting with scalable open-source platforms but facing persistent challenges related to infrastructure and workforce capacity [17]. Success in these settings will likely depend on governmental support, public–private partnerships, and sustained investment in AI literacy among healthcare professionals.

9.5 Levels of Automation

Current surveillance models in healthcare-associated infection monitoring vary widely in their level of automation and clinical integration. Semi-automated systems remain the most common in practice, where artificial intelligence (AI) algorithms generate alerts based on structured data inputs such as laboratory results, vital signs, or medication prescriptions. However, these preliminary outputs still require human interpretation and validation by infection prevention and control (IPC) teams, ensuring that clinical nuance and contextual factors are not overlooked. This collaborative model balances the efficiency gains of AI with the critical judgment of experienced healthcare professionals.

On the other end of the spectrum, fully automated pipelines are now capable of conducting end-to-end surveillance processes. These systems can ingest data in real time from electronic health records (EHRs), analyze it through machine learning models, and autonomously generate alerts or infection risk reports without immediate human intervention. In highly digitized hospital environments, such systems offer the promise of continuous, scalable, and rapid infection monitoring. However, they also raise concerns about algorithm transparency, reliability in complex clinical scenarios, and the potential deskilling of IPC personnel if human oversight is minimized too aggressively.

Beyond current deployments, there is a growing interest in advanced predictive models that not only detect active infections but anticipate the likelihood of infection development before clinical symptoms arise. These models analyze dynamic patient data streams, incorporating real-time changes in physiological parameters, laboratory results, and treatment courses to update individual risk profiles continuously. Although initial studies demonstrate promising capabilities, the application of predictive surveillance remains largely confined to research settings and pilot programs. Challenges such as model generalizability, integration into clinical workflows, and ethical considerations around early intervention thresholds must be addressed before such tools can be widely adopted into routine healthcare practice [10].

9.6   Sustainability and Scalability

Sustainability and scalability of AI surveillance depend on several factors. Continuous model retraining is necessary to account for the evolving landscape of pathogens, antibiotic resistance, and clinical practices [7]. Interoperability standards are essential to facilitate cross-institutional data sharing and multi-center validation efforts [10]. Cloud-based solutions offer scalable analytics capabilities, although they must navigate complex legal frameworks surrounding data sovereignty [14]. International collaborations, such as the European "Providing a Roadmap for Automated Infection Surveillance in Europe" (PRAISE) network, demonstrate the potential for harmonized governance and shared learning across different healthcare systems [13].

Looking ahead, several priorities emerge. Multi-center clinical trials are needed to rigorously assess the real-world performance of AI surveillance systems across diverse populations and settings. Development of explainable AI models is critical to build clinician trust and meet emerging regulatory demands for transparency. Economic modeling should be expanded to guide decision-makers in assessing the cost-effectiveness of AI adoption. Finally, greater integration of AI-based surveillance with antimicrobial stewardship programs could amplify the benefits of early infection detection while simultaneously mitigating antibiotic resistance.

9.7 Conclusion

In conclusion, AI-driven surveillance is poised to fundamentally transform infection prevention and control. Its ability to move the field from reactive case-finding toward proactive risk management is supported by growing evidence from diverse healthcare settings. However, the full realization of this potential demands overcoming persistent technical, regulatory, economic, and ethical challenges. With sustained investment, standardized frameworks, and close collaboration between technologists and clinicians, AI can evolve from a promising tool into an indispensable component of global healthcare quality improvement.

References

1. World Health Organization. Global report on infection prevention and control 2024. World Health Organization; 2024. https://iris.who.int/handle/10665/379632.
2. Classen DC, Rhee C, Dantes RB, Benin AL. Healthcare-associated infections and conditions in the era of digital measurement. Infect Control Hosp Epidemiol. 2024;45(1):3–8. https://doi.org/10.1017/ice.2023.139.
3. Freeman R, Moore LSP, García Álvarez L, Charlett A, Holmes A. Advances in electronic surveillance for healthcare-associated infections in the 21st century: a systematic review. J Hosp Infect. 2013;84(2):106–19. https://doi.org/10.1016/j.jhin.2012.11.031.
4. dos Santos RP, Silva D, Menezes A, Lukasewicz S, Dalmora CH, Carvalho O, Giacomazzi J, Golin N, Pozza R, Vaz TA. Automated healthcare-associated infection surveillance using an artificial intelligence algorithm. Infection Prev Pract. 2021;3(3):100167. https://doi.org/10.1016/j.infpip.2021.100167.
5. Wen R, Li X, Liu T, Lin G. Effect of a real-time automatic nosocomial infection surveillance system on hospital-acquired infection prevention and control. BMC Infect Dis. 2022;22(1):857. https://doi.org/10.1186/s12879-022-07873-7.
6. Woeltje KF, Lin MY, Klompas M, Wright MO, Zuccotti G, Trick WE. Data requirements for electronic surveillance of healthcare-associated infections. Infect Control Hosp Epidemiol. 2014;35(9):1083–91. https://doi.org/10.1086/677623.
7. Lukasewicz Ferreira SA, Franco Meneses AC, Vaz TA, da Fontoura Carvalho OL, Hubner Dalmora C, Pressotto Vanni D, Ribeiro Berti I, Pires Dos Santos R. Hospital-acquired infections surveillance: the machine-learning algorithm mirrors National Healthcare Safety Network definitions. Infect Control Hosp Epidemiol. 2024;45(5):604–8. https://doi.org/10.1017/ice.2023.224.
8. Chen Y, Zhang Y, Nie S, et al. Risk assessment and prediction of nosocomial infections based on surveillance data using machine learning methods. BMC Public Health. 2024;24:1780. https://doi.org/10.1186/s12889-024-19096-3.
9. Rabhi S, Jakubowicz J, Metzger MH. Deep learning versus conventional machine learning for detection of healthcare-associated infections in French clinical narratives. Methods Inf Med. 2019;58(1):31–41. https://doi.org/10.1055/s-0039-1677692.
10. van Mourik MSM, van Rooden SM, Abbas M, Aspevall O, Astagneau P, Bonten MJM, Carrara E, Gomila-Grange A, de Greeff SC, Gubbels S, Harrison W, Humphreys H, Johansson A,

Koek MBG, Kristensen B, Lepape A, Lucet JC, Mookerjee S, Naucler P, Palacios-Baena ZR, Presterl E, Pujol M, Reilly J, Roberts C, Tacconelli E, Teixeira D, Tängdén T, Valik JK, Behnke M, Gastmeier P, PRAISE network. PRAISE: providing a roadmap for automated infection surveillance in Europe. Clin Microbiol Infect. 2021;27(Suppl 1):S3–S19. https://doi.org/10.1016/j.cmi.2021.02.028.

11. Radaelli D, Di Maria S, Jakovski Z, Alempijevic D, Al-Habash I, Concato M, Bolcato M, D'Errico S. Advancing patient safety: the future of artificial intelligence in mitigating healthcare-associated infections: a systematic review. Healthcare. 2024;12(19):1996. https://doi.org/10.3390/healthcare12191996.

12. Fan Y, Wu Y, Cao X, Zou J, Zhu M, Dai D, Lu L, Yin X, Xiong L. Automated cluster detection of health care-associated infection based on the multisource surveillance of process data in the area network: retrospective study of algorithm development and validation. JMIR Med Inform. 2020;8(10):e16901. https://doi.org/10.2196/16901.

13. van Rooden SM, Aspevall O, Carrara E, Gubbels S, Johansson A, Lucet JC, Mookerjee S, Palacios-Baena ZR, Presterl E, Tacconelli E, Abbas M, Behnke M, Gastmeier P, van Mourik MSM, PRAISE network. Governance aspects of large-scale implementation of automated surveillance of healthcare-associated infections. Clin Microbiol Infect. 2021;27(Suppl 1):S20–8. https://doi.org/10.1016/j.cmi.2021.02.026.

14. Mølbak K, Andersen CØ, Dessau RB, Ellermann-Eriksen S, Gubbels S, Jensen TG, Knudsen JD, Kristensen B, Lützen L, Coia J, Olesen BRS, Pinholt M, Scheutz F, Sönksen UW, Søgaard KK, Voldstedlund M. Mandatory surveillance of bacteremia conducted by automated monitoring. Front Public Health. 2024;12:1502739. https://doi.org/10.3389/fpubh.2024.1502739.

15. Scardoni A, Balzarini F, Signorelli C, Cabitza F, Odone A. Artificial intelligence-based tools to control healthcare associated infections: a systematic review of the literature. J Infect Public Health. 2020;13(8):1061–77. https://doi.org/10.1016/j.jiph.2020.06.006.

16. Chen WS, Zhang WH, Li ZJ, Yang Y, Chen F, Ge XS, Wang TR, Fang P, Feng CY, Liu J, Liu SS, Pan HX, Zhu TL, Tian YY, Wang WY, Xing H, Yao J, Yuan YM, Jiang P, Tang HP, Zhou J, Zang JC, Lu S, Huang HP, Lei XH, Huang BH, Wang SH, Huang FY, Tao HY, Zhang YX, Liu B, Li HF, Li SQ, Hu BJ, Liu Y. Evaluation of manual and electronic healthcare-associated infections surveillance: a multi-center study with 21 tertiary general hospitals in China. Anna Trans Med. 2019;7(18):444. https://doi.org/10.21037/atm.2019.08.80.

17. Arzilli G, De Vita E, Pasquale M, Carloni LM, Pellegrini M, Di Giacomo M, Esposito E, Porretta AD, Rizzo C. Innovative techniques for infection control and surveillance in hospital settings and long-term care facilities: a scoping review. Antibiotics (Basel). 2024;13(1):77. https://doi.org/10.3390/antibiotics13010077. PMID: 38247635; PMCID: PMC1081275.

Education and Communication Strategies

10

Tihana Gašpert

Abstract

Effective educational and communicative strategies are essential for advancing infection prevention and control. Patient and family education is a fundamental component, highlighting the importance of clear, concise, and culturally sensitive guidance to enable persons in infection prevention. Healthcare practitioners must implement customized communication strategies, ensuring information is conveyed with empathy and efficacy, so cultivating trust and compliance with preventative measures. Public health initiatives and community outreach are essential for enhancing awareness on a larger scale, utilizing several media platforms to engage different groups.

By synchronizing communication tactics with the cultural and language requirements of varied populations, healthcare systems can attain enhanced engagement, understanding, and behavioral results. These activities enhance individual patient outcomes and advance public health goals by mitigating the transmission of illnesses. An integrated approach to education and communication, utilizing customized, multilingual, and culturally sensitive tactics, is essential for cultivating a knowledgeable and proactive society adept at effectively tackling infection prevention issues.

T. Gašpert (✉)
University Hospital Rijeka, Rijeka, Croatia

Faculty of Health Sciences, University of Maribor, Maribor, Slovenia

© The Author(s), under exclusive license to Springer Nature Switzerland AG 2025
B. Oomen, S. Gastaldi (eds.), *Principles of Nursing Infection Prevention Control*,
Principles of Specialty Nursing, https://doi.org/10.1007/978-3-032-01446-7_10

Keywords

Infection prevention · Patient education · Family education · Healthcare communication · Public health campaigns · Community outreach · Multilingual strategies · Cultural considerations · Healthcare professionals · Infection control

10.1 Introduction

10.1.1 Patient and Family Education on Infection Prevention

Effective infection prevention frequently necessitates teamwork among healthcare
providers, patients, and caregivers. Education for patients and caregivers is essential
for the transmission and execution of infection prevention strategies [1]. Patients
should receive training materials on infection prevention, covering invasive device
management, removal of unnecessary devices, and the importance of reminding
staff to follow standard protocols [2]. Patient-centered educational initiatives have
enhanced staff adherence to hand hygiene and reduced outpatient central-line-
associated bloodstream infections (CLABSIs). To formulate strategies that enhance
infection prevention for patients, it is crucial to tackle communication hurdles and
errors across preadmission, inpatient, and outpatient care [3]. Communication difficulties encompass the absence of interpreters and the shortage of healthcare professionals proficient in the patient's language. Communication errors include
relying on family members as interpreters and failing to provide written materials in
the patient's or caregiver's language [4].

Currently, limited information exists regarding the effective engagement of
patients and families in IPC, a critical aspect of patient safety [5–7]. The involvement of patients and families in infection prevention is ambiguous and faces previously identified obstacles [5]. Furthermore, the COVID-19 pandemic has highlighted
significant trade-offs between patient safety and infection prevention/control methods on one side, and patient and family engagement as vital collaborators on the
other side [8]. Formulating focused solutions to address the obstacles related to
patient engagement is essential for integrating patient as a fundamental element of
IPC programs. Involving patients in infection prevention and control helps mitigate
the incidence of healthcare-associated infections in clinical environments and
healthcare facilities. This study aims to delineate the "optimal" roles of patients in
infection prevention and control (IPC) and to identify targeted strategies that are
acceptable to stakeholders, including patients, family caregivers, healthcare professionals, managers, and other nonclinical personnel, due to the intricate reactions
and obstacles associated with patient engagement in patient safety [9].

To date, infection prevention and control (IPC) strategies in healthcare settings
have predominantly concentrated on the practices of healthcare professionals
(HCPs), such as nurses, physicians, and allied health professionals, as well as other
staff members, including housekeepers, transport attendants, and unit managers,
without delineating the role of patients and their relatives in mitigating infections.

Patient and family participation is broadly acknowledged as an effective approach for enhancing healthcare quality and patient safety [10, 11]. Numerous recent research studies have investigated patient participation in integrated primary care [12]. The literature indicates a consensus that patients, family caregivers, and health professionals should collaboratively participate in the IPC. Nonetheless, the degree to which patients and families can be effectively involved and their particular roles and obligations in IPC remains ambiguous [5]. Evidence indicates that patients may experience anxiety or discomfort when inquiring about or engaging in their safety [13]. Research indicates that healthcare workers frequently recognize patients as vulnerable, yet do not necessarily hold them co-responsible for preventing the transmission of infections [5]. Several studies have highlighted current techniques to involve patients and family caregivers in IPC; nevertheless, formulating specific strategies to facilitate patient and family engagement may increase IPC activities [9].

Implementing active IPC programs and best practices is an established method for safeguarding patients, healthcare personnel, and visitors in medical facilities by preventing preventable infections, including those caused by antimicrobial-resistant and epidemic- or pandemic-prone pathogens [14].

Infection prevention/control education is increasingly crucial for healthcare professionals and medical, nursing, physical therapy, occupational therapy, and other program students [15]. Methods of infection protection and control instruction for students include simulation, role-play, skill training, electronic learning, and in-person lectures. A study on infection education indicated that simulation training with a standardized patient was markedly more successful than role-play for nursing students [16]. The efficacy of simulation education in infection control for pupils is inadequately understood. Simulation education on infection control emphasizes the prevention of healthcare-associated infections (HAIs) for healthcare practitioners. Healthcare-associated infections (HAIs) encompass catheter-associated bloodstream infections, catheter-associated urinary tract infections, surgical site infections, and ventilator-associated pneumonia; 60–70% of these infections are preventable [17–19]. Consequently, it can be deduced that simulation-based education on infection prevention and control has been administered to healthcare personnel. Simulation education for students employed several ways, ranging from low-tech to high-fidelity simulators, to enhance their knowledge, critical thinking skills, satisfaction, and confidence [20, 21]. Systematic reviews indicated that simulation education for students in medical, nursing, and physical therapy programs markedly enhanced their learning regarding knowledge retention, clinical reasoning, practical skills, confidence, and satisfaction relative to conventional learning methods [21–23]. Consequently, it is imperative to implement simulation-based education on infection prevention and control for students, as well as to assess and elucidate the efficacy of this teaching [15].

Education in infection prevention and control offers numerous advantages, such as safeguarding healthcare staff, managing nosocomial infections, decreasing infection rates, and lowering medical costs associated with infections [17, 18, 24]. The WHO advocates for sufficient training, education on infection prevention and control, and the provision of personal protective equipment to ensure the occupational safety of healthcare professionals [25].

10.2   WHO Program

The "Infection Prevention and Control In-Service Education and Training Curriculum" addresses critical challenges in global health including pandemics and antimicrobial resistance (AMR). This curriculum is crafted to provide systematic, structured education for healthcare workers (HCWs) to reduce healthcare-associated infections (HAIs) and prevent AMR transmission [26]. The curriculum aims to train all HCWs, from clinical to auxiliary staff, in infection prevention skills. It defines three key competency levels based on WHO's IPC core components, which underpin the structured education approach for health service workers. The adaptable framework is grounded in evidence-based strategies, supporting local and national IPC policies to improve safety in healthcare. The foundational level provides basic IPC training applicable across all healthcare roles. Topics include microbiology, infection transmission, hand hygiene, use of personal protective equipment (PPE), and effective waste management. This baseline knowledge empowers HCWs to reduce infectious spread and supports a clean, safe healthcare environment [26].

10.2.1 Intermediate Competency Level

The intermediate level expands on foundational skills for clinical practitioners, introducing comprehensive risk assessments, advanced PPE handling, antimicrobial stewardship, and infection surveillance. Practitioners learn to manage devices such as catheters and adopt specialized techniques for minimizing HAIs [26].

10.2.2 Advanced Competency Level

The advanced level targets specialized practitioners and facility managers. This level delves into complex IPC areas, including outbreak investigation, leadership in infection control, medical device reprocessing, and cost-effectiveness assessments. Advanced training prepares HCWs for high-risk procedures and management roles [26].

10.2.3 Key IPC Practices and Teaching Methods

WHO's curriculum promotes essential IPC practices, notably hand hygiene, respiratory hygiene, environmental cleaning, and waste management. To enhance learning outcomes, it incorporates simulation, hands-on, and risk-based training. Such methods ensure that HCWs can efficiently implement IPC practices within various settings [26].

10.2.4 Assessment and Evaluation

Ensuring high IPC standards requires ongoing assessment of HCWs' competencies. The curriculum suggests structured knowledge and skill assessments, simulation exercises, and regular feedback. Annual and induction evaluations reinforce HCW readiness to uphold IPC practices and patient safety in diverse clinical environments [26].

10.3 ECDC Communication Toolkit to Support Infection Prevention in Schools

The European Centre for Disease Prevention and Control (ECDC) has created a comprehensive communication toolkit to support health authorities, nurses, educators, and school communities in preventing and managing gastrointestinal diseases in primary school settings. The toolkit emphasizes a whole-school approach, integrating policy, education, and practical measures to foster healthier behaviors among students and staff. It provides tools and guidelines to implement hygiene practices, address barriers to compliance, and promote disease prevention as part of a coordinated effort [27].

The toolkit highlights the importance of a collaborative approach to ensure the effectiveness and sustainability of hygiene measures. Gastrointestinal diseases are particularly concerning in school environments due to the close contact and shared spaces among children, which facilitate the rapid spread of contagious illnesses. These diseases, often caused by viruses such as norovirus, bacteria, or parasites, can lead to severe symptoms, significant absenteeism, and even school closures. Thus, fostering a culture of hygiene and prevention within the school community is crucial [27].

The toolkit offers various resources designed to support school-based efforts to prevent infections. These include an implementation handbook that outlines steps for planning and evaluating programs, as well as communication materials such as posters, slogans, and pictograms to disseminate hygiene messages effectively. PowerPoint presentations are also provided to educate specific groups, including parents, teachers, and local authorities. The materials are adaptable, allowing schools to tailor them to their specific needs and cultural contexts [27].

10.3.1 Steps for Implementation

The ECDC proposes a structured five-step process for implementing the toolkit. The first step is engaging stakeholders, such as school administrators, health officials, and parents, to form a project team that ensures active participation from all relevant parties. The second step involves assessing the current situation by identifying knowledge gaps, barriers, and specific objectives. This is followed by developing an action plan, which includes outlining activities, assigning roles, and creating a timeline for implementation. The fourth step is taking action by rolling out communication campaigns, hygiene programs, and preventive measures within the school. Finally, the evaluation step involves monitoring and measuring outcomes to determine the program's effectiveness and identify areas for improvement [27].

10.3.2 Preventive Measures and Communication Strategies

A cornerstone of the toolkit is its focus on preventive measures based on evidence-based practices. These include hand hygiene, isolation of affected individuals, proper cleaning and disinfection of school facilities, and adherence to food safety standards. The communication strategies embedded in the toolkit aim to ensure a broad understanding and adoption of these measures. By employing engaging and accessible formats, such as interactive activities, visual aids, and direct messaging, the toolkit seeks to resonate with diverse audiences within the school community [27].

10.4 Multilingual Communication Strategies for Healthcare Professionals and Cultural Considerations in Infection Prevention Education

Cultural competency has been characterized in numerous manners. A comprehensive definition provided by Betancourt et al. states: "Cultural competence in healthcare involves recognizing the significance of social and cultural influences on patients' health beliefs and behaviors; assessing the interaction of these factors across various levels of the healthcare delivery system; and ultimately, formulating interventions that address these considerations to ensure quality healthcare delivery to diverse patient populations [28]." This definition is characterized by several notable features: a focus on social and cultural context, indicative of a holistic or biopsychosocial approach to patient care; and the multilevel aspect of cultural competence, functioning at both interpersonal levels (e.g., interactions between patients and providers) and organizational/systemic levels (e.g., resources for interpreter services) [29].

The rationale for emphasizing cultural competence and humility in infection practice and research is persuasive. The primary and most significant concept is "justice." The 2019 Infectious Diseases Society of America (IDSA) Inclusion, Diversity, Access and Equity (IDE&A) Roadmap and Strategies articulates, "Infectious Diseases as a specialty is uniquely tilted toward social justice by the very nature of the conditions we treat." Cultural competency must be prioritized to advocate for those with intellectual disabilities, who are disproportionately represented among racial, ethnic, sexual, and gender minorities, as well as those of lower socioeconomic levels. There are additional, more pragmatic justifications for prioritizing cultural competence. Improving cultural competence at both the individual and organizational levels is expected to enhance care quality, potentially affecting costs. Patient happiness, which health systems increasingly promote, is associated with patients' assessments of providers' cultural competence [30]. Cultural competence transcends mere jargon; it represents an orientation and methodology that embodies respect for the lived experiences of others in an increasingly interconnected world, alongside a continual process of refining one's skills to enhance patient care irrespective of their background [31].

10.4.1   The Necessity for Cultural Competence and Humility in Infectious Disease Research

Considering the factors above, individuals from underrepresented backgrounds should ideally participate in research at rates comparable to their counterparts, and it may be argued that minorities should be deliberately overrepresented in numerous instances. It is regrettable that, despite the significant prevalence of infectious diseases such as HIV, TB, and viral hepatitis among racial and ethnic minorities, they represent a disproportionately small percentage of clinical trial participants [32, 33]. There is limited knowledge regarding individuals belonging to minority groups other than race, such as sexual and gender minorities, individuals with impairments, and those of lower socioeconomic standing. Nonetheless, these populations probably encounter analogous obstacles to study involvement. Considering the significant public health and ethical ramifications of nonrepresentative research enrollment, it appears that while cultural competency and humility are frequently addressed in clinical contexts, there is also a necessity to apply this essential perspective to research environments [31].

10.4.2   Strategies for Enhancing Cultural Competence and Humility

Strategies for enhancing cultural competence and humility have been analyzed at both the individual and systemic levels. Individual-level interventions focus on enhancing practitioners' awareness, knowledge, and abilities, whereas institutional-level interventions seek to incorporate cultural competency into policies and procedures. Certain tactics have been beneficial in enhancing patient satisfaction [30]; nevertheless, the correlation between cultural competency interventions and subsequent patient outcomes or their effect on health inequalities is little documented [34, 35]. Healthcare personnel and organizations need to enhance their cultural competency and humility, as accumulating data indicates that culturally competent care enhances patient outcomes [34].

A prevalent individual-level intervention is the training of providers. Cultural competence training has demonstrated efficacy in enhancing healthcare personnel's cultural knowledge, awareness, attitudes, and abilities [36]. Alongside enhancing providers' cultural awareness, comprehension of multiculturalism, and communication skills with minority patients, training also improved patients' utilization of social resources and overall functional capacity without escalating healthcare costs. A constraint of cultural competence training is the absence of a standardized framework for technique, frequency, or duration, constraining the widespread adoption and generalization of its benefits [37].

Interventions at the individual level may focus on enhancing multicultural patients' ability to navigate the healthcare system [38]. Patient-centered interventions, such as health literacy initiatives and culturally customized disease-specific programs, have demonstrated efficacy in enhancing patients' clinical outcomes [31].

10.4.3 Language Barriers

Both written and verbal patient education are crucial for infection prevention; however, educational materials and treatments have not been extensively researched in languages other than English. Patients are typically provided with training materials regarding infection prevention, including the management of invasive devices, the significance of removing superfluous devices and encouraging patients to prompt staff to adhere to standard infection prevention protocols [2]. Patient-centered educational programs have enhanced staff compliance with hand hygiene protocols [39] and have reduced outpatient central-line-associated bloodstream infections (CLABSIs) [40]. Assessing the execution and effectiveness of non-English resources is crucial for pinpointing areas needing enhancement in infection prevention communication. Enhancing the breadth of resources and increasing the number of languages in which these materials are accessible is essential for advancing healthcare education for all patients [3].

To formulate strategies that enhance infection prevention for patients, it is crucial to tackle communication hurdles and errors across preadmission, inpatient, and outpatient care. Communication constraints encompass the absence of interpreters and the scarcity of healthcare professionals proficient in the relevant language. Communication errors include employing a family member as a translator, failing to supply written information in the patient's or caregiver's preferred language, and neglecting to identify patients [4].

10.4.3.1 Communication with Migrants
The Six-Factor Model of Medical Communication 9 delineates six objectives: (1) cultivating a relationship, (2) collecting information, (3) disseminating information, (4) making decisions, (5) facilitating disease and treatment-related behaviors, and (6) addressing emotions that assist healthcare professionals in fulfilling patients' cognitive and emotional needs cohesively to achieve effective medical communication. When healthcare professionals effectively achieve these six

objectives, they are likely to satisfy patients' requirements; they can assist patients in comprehending their conditions and the necessary activities (i.e., cognitive needs), while also ensuring that patients feel understood, supported, and appreciated (i.e., affective needs). The assessment of whether each goal is achieved is contingent upon the observable outcomes stemming from the instrumental and affective communication strategies employed, specifically the behaviors exhibited by healthcare professionals to disseminate information (e.g., reiterating or rephrasing medical terminology) and foster rapport (e.g., engaging in casual conversation [41].

Employing these communication tactics independently is inadequate. Merely reiterating and rephrasing information in healthcare professionals' terminology will not enhance the comprehension of low language proficient (LLP) migrant patients, as these instrumental communication tactics fail to address the primary obstacle— the language barrier [42, 43]. Research on the communication tactics employed by healthcare professionals in low-development countries to fulfill the six objectives of limited language proficiency migrant patients and alleviate language obstacles is insufficient, as the existing framework was designed for language-concordant consultations. This is a challenge, since healthcare professionals currently lack explicit guidelines on the combinations of communication tactics that can be employed to effectively engage with migrant patients in low-development countries and enhance the quality of care [44].

To alleviate language obstacles in LDCs, healthcare professionals can collaborate with interpreters (professional, ad hoc, and informal) and utilize digital tools [45, 46]. Among the three categories of interpreters, professional interpreters deliver the most precise medical interpretations, enhance the safety of migrant patients, and elevate the overall quality of communication for patients in less-developed countries (LDCs) [47]. But, healthcare professionals frequently engage families as unofficial interpreters [48, 49]. While family members can offer supplementary medical histories, advocate for the patient, and deliver substantial emotional support, they are inadequate interpreters. Their absence of medical training leads to erroneous translations and may result in the omission of information for personal motives, hence posing ethical difficulties [50].

In addition to employing translators, healthcare professionals can utilize digital resources (e.g., Google Translate) to convert basic medical information into the patient's native language. The exclusive reliance on digital tools frequently results in clinical errors, as healthcare professionals are unable to verify translated documents, and these tools typically offer literal translations rather than culturally appropriate ones [51, 52]. Digital tools may impede the fulfillment of migrant patients' emotional needs when healthcare professionals overlook nonverbal signs, such as maintaining eye contact, due to their reliance on technology during medical interactions [53]. The reliance on ad hoc interpreters, informal interpreters, and digital means instead of professional interpreters diminishes the likelihood of addressing migrant patients' cognitive and emotional needs [54, 55].

To achieve effective medical communication in LDCs, healthcare professionals should collaborate with interpreters and employ digital tools alongside instrumental and affective communication tactics as recommended by the Six Function Model of Medical Communication, suited to cultural and linguistic contexts [41].

10.5 Conclusion

Education and communication methods are fundamental components of infection prevention and control, involving individual, community, and systemic levels of participation. Patient and family education empowers individuals with the knowledge and resources necessary to actively engage in protecting their health, promoting a culture of prevention both at home and elsewhere. Global frameworks, such as the World Health Organization's (WHO) initiatives, deliver essential leadership and standardization, supplying resources that accommodate various healthcare systems and community requirements globally.

The European Centre for Disease Prevention and Control (ECDC) communication toolkit exemplifies the significance of targeting specific environments, such as schools, where infection prevention education can influence behaviors from an early age and yield extensive effects on public health. Concurrently, multilingual communication tactics guarantee that essential messages overcome linguistic obstacles, rendering health information accessible to everyone. Incorporating cultural concerns, these solutions honor the diversity of beliefs and behaviors among people, thereby enhancing trust, participation, and adherence to preventive interventions.

Expanding the extent of education and communication necessitates utilizing collaborations among healthcare practitioners, public health entities, educators, and policymakers. This cooperative strategy improves resource allocation, fosters creativity, and customizes treatments to address both local and global requirements. By tackling structural disparities and promoting extensive awareness, infection prevention initiatives can attain lasting impact. A comprehensive emphasis on inclusive and adaptable communication converts infection prevention initiatives into a collective pursuit, fostering health equity and resilience among all societal sectors.

Literature

1. Yokoe DS, Anderson DJ, Berenholtz SM, Calfee DP, Dubberke ER, Ellingson KD, et al. A compendium of strategies to prevent healthcare-associated infections in acute care hospitals: 2014 updates. Infect Control Hosp Epidemiol. 2014;35(8):967–77.
2. MacEwan SR, Beal EW, Gaughan AA, Sieck C, McAlearney AS. Perspectives of hospital leaders and staff on patient education for the prevention of healthcare-associated infections. Infect Control Hosp Epidemiol. 2022;43(9):1129–34.
3. Prochaska EC, Caballero TM, Fabre V, Milstone AM. Infection prevention requires attention to patient and caregiver language: removing language barriers from infection prevention education. Infect Control Hosp Epidemiol. 2023;44(11):1707–10.
4. Yeheskel A, Rawal S. Exploring the 'patient experience' of individuals with limited English proficiency: a scoping review. J Immigr Minor Health. 2019;21(4):853–78.

5. Agreli HF, Murphy M, Creedon S, Bhuachalla CN, O'Brien D, Gould D, et al. Patient involvement in the implementation of infection prevention and control guidelines and associated interventions: a scoping review. BMJ Open. 2019;9(3):e025824.

6. Bishop AC, Macdonald M. Patient involvement in patient safety: a qualitative study of nursing staff and patient perceptions. J Patient Saf. 2017;13(2):82–7.

7. Abbasgholizadeh Rahimi S, Zomahoun HTV, Légaré F. Patient engagement and its evaluation tools–current challenges and future directions; comment on "metrics and evaluation tools for patient engagement in healthcare organization-and system-level decision-making: a systematic review". Int J Health Policy Manag. 2019;8(6):378–80.

8. Improvement CFfH. Better together: re-integration of family caregivers as essential partners in care in a time of COVID-19. Ottawa: The Canadian Foundation for Healthcare Improvement; 2020.

9. Clavel NC, Lavoie-Tremblay M, Biron A, Briand A, Paquette J, Bernard L, et al. Patient and family engagement in infection prevention in the context of the COVID-19 pandemic: defining a consensus framework using the Q methodology–NOSO-COVID study protocol. BMJ Open. 2022;12(7):e056172.

10. Berger Z, Flickinger TE, Pfoh E, Martinez KA, Dy SM. Promoting engagement by patients and families to reduce adverse events in acute care settings: a systematic review. BMJ Qual Saf. 2014;23(7):548–55.

11. Pomey M-P, Clavel N, Aho-Glele U, Ferré N, Fernandez-McAuley P. How patients view their contribution as partners in the enhancement of patient safety in clinical care. Patient Exp J. 2018;5(1):35–49.

12. Seale H, Chughtai AA, Kaur R, Phillipson L, Novytska Y, Travaglia J. Empowering patients in the hospital as a new approach to reducing the burden of health care–associated infections: the attitudes of hospital health care workers. Am J Infect Control. 2016;44(3):263–8.

13. Alzyood M, Jackson D, Brooke J, Aveyard H. An integrative review exploring the perceptions of patients and healthcare professionals towards patient involvement in promoting hand hygiene compliance in the hospital setting. J Clin Nurs. 2018;27(7–8):1329–45.

14. World Health Organization. Global report on infection prevention and control. World Health Organization; 2022.

15. Yoshikawa A, Tashiro N, Ohtsuka H, Aoki K, Togo S, Komaba K, et al. Protocol for educational programs on infection prevention/control for medical and healthcare student: a systematic review and meta-analysis. PLoS One. 2022;17(10):e0276851.

16. Kim E, Kim SS, Kim S. Effects of infection control education for nursing students using standardized patients vs. peer role-play. Int J Environ Res Public Health. 2021;18(1):107.

17. Zingg W, Holmes A, Dettenkofer M, Goetting T, Secci F, Clack L, et al. Hospital organisation, management, and structure for prevention of health-care-associated infection: a systematic review and expert consensus. Lancet Infect Dis. 2015;15(2):212–24.

18. Mauger B, Marbella A, Pines E, Chopra R, Black ER, Aronson N. Implementing quality improvement strategies to reduce healthcare-associated infections: a systematic review. Am J Infect Control. 2014;42(10):S274–S83.

19. Umscheid CA, Mitchell MD, Doshi JA, Agarwal R, Williams K, Brennan PJ. Estimating the proportion of healthcare-associated infections that are reasonably preventable and the related mortality and costs. Infect Control Hosp Epidemiol. 2011;32(2):101–14.

20. Cant RP, Cooper SJ. Simulation-based learning in nurse education: systematic review. J Adv Nurs. 2010;66(1):3–15.

21. Kim J, Park J-H, Shin S. Effectiveness of simulation-based nursing education depending on fidelity: a meta-analysis. BMC Med Educ. 2016;16:1–8.

22. McGaghie WC, Issenberg SB, Cohen ER, Barsuk JH, Wayne DB. Does simulation-based medical education with deliberate practice yield better results than traditional clinical education? A meta-analytic comparative review of the evidence. Acad Med. 2011;86(6):706–11.

23. Shinnick MA, Woo MA. The effect of human patient simulation on critical thinking and its predictors in prelicensure nursing students. Nurse Educ Today. 2013;33(9):1062–7.
24. Moralejo D, El Dib R, Prata RA, Barretti P, Corrêa I. Improving adherence to standard precautions for the control of health care-associated infections. Cochrane Database Syst Rev. 2018;2
25. World Health Organization. Laboratory testing for 2019 novel coronavirus (2019-nCoV) in suspected human cases: interim guidance. World Health Organization; 2020.
26. Bifa KT, Bedane HA, Adnew AD, Senbato FR. Education and training programs for infection prevention and control professionals. In: Global infection prevention and management in healthcare; 2024. p. 229.
27. Control ECfDPa. ECDC communication toolkit to support infection prevention in schools focus: gastrointestinal diseases. 2013.
28. Betancourt JR, Green AR, Carrillo JE, Owusu Ananeh-Firempong I. Defining cultural competence: a practical framework for addressing racial/ethnic disparities in health and health care. Public Health Rep. 2003;
29. Spicer CM, Ford MA. Monitoring HIV care in the United States: a strategy for generating national estimates of HIV care and coverage. 2013.
30. Govere L, Govere EM. How effective is cultural competence training of healthcare providers on improving patient satisfaction of minority groups? A systematic review of literature. Worldviews Evid-Based Nurs. 2016;13(6):402–10.
31. Hussen SA, Kuppalli K, Castillo-Mancilla J, Bedimo R, Fadul N, Ofotokun I. Cultural competence and humility in infectious diseases clinical practice and research. J Infect Dis. 2020;222(Supplement 6):S535–S42.
32. Castillo-Mancilla JR, Cohn SE, Krishnan S, Cespedes M, Floris-Moore M, Schulte G, et al. Minorities remain underrepresented in HIV/AIDS research despite access to clinical trials. HIV Clin Trials. 2014;15(1):14–26.
33. Huamani KF, Metch B, Broder G, Andrasik M. A demographic analysis of racial/ethnic minority enrollment into HVTN preventive early phase HIV vaccine clinical trials conducted in the United States, 2002-2016. Public Health Rep. 2019;134(1):72–80.
34. Truong M, Paradies Y, Priest N. Interventions to improve cultural competency in healthcare: a systematic review of reviews. BMC Health Serv Res. 2014;14:1–17.
35. Bhui K, Aslam RhW, Palinski A, McCabe R, Johnson M, Weich S, et al. Interventions designed to improve therapeutic communications between black and minority ethnic people and professionals working in psychiatric services: a systematic review of the evidence for their effectiveness. 2015.
36. Chipps JA, Simpson B, Brysiewicz P. The effectiveness of cultural-competence training for health professionals in community-based rehabilitation: a systematic review of literature. Worldviews Evid-Based Nurs. 2008;5(2):85–94.
37. Majumdar B, Browne G, Roberts J, Carpio B. Effects of cultural sensitivity training on health care provider attitudes and patient outcomes. J Nurs Scholarsh. 2004;36(2):161–6.
38. Fernández-Gutiérrez M, Bas-Sarmiento P, Albar-Marín MJ, Paloma-Castro O, Romero-Sánchez J. Health literacy interventions for immigrant populations: a systematic review. Int Nurs Rev. 2018;65(1):54–64.
39. McGuckin M, Taylor A, Martin V, Porten L, Salcido R. Evaluation of a patient education model for increasing hand hygiene compliance in an inpatient rehabilitation unit. Am J Infect Control. 2004;32(4):235–8.
40. Møller T, Borregaard N, Tvede M, Adamsen L. Patient education – a strategy for prevention of infections caused by permanent central venous catheters in patients with haematological malignancies: a randomized clinical trial. J Hosp Infect. 2005;61(4):330–41.
41. Chan BM, Suurmond J, van Weert JC, Schouten BC. Uncovering communication strategies used in language-discordant consultations with people who are migrants: qualitative interviews with healthcare providers. Health Expect. 2024;27(1):e13949.
42. Czapka EA, Gerwing J, Sagbakken M. Invisible rights: Barriers and facilitators to access and use of interpreter services in health care settings by Polish migrants in Norway. Scand J Public Health. 2019;47(7):755–64.

43. Landmark AMD, Svennevig J, Gerwing J, Gulbrandsen P. Patient involvement and language barriers: problems of agreement or understanding? Patient Educ Couns. 2017;100(6):1092–102.
44. Schouten BC, Cox A, Duran G, Kerremans K, Banning LK, Lahdidioui A, et al. Mitigating language and cultural barriers in healthcare communication: toward a holistic approach. Patient Educ Couns. 2020;103(12):2604–8.
45. Chang H, Hutchinson C, Gullick J. Pulled away: the experience of bilingual nurses as ad hoc interpreters in the emergency department. Ethn Health. 2021;26(7):1045–64.
46. Hadziabdic E, Albin B, Heikkilä K, Hjelm K. Family members' experiences of the use of interpreters in healthcare. Prim Health Care Res Dev. 2014;15(2):156–69.
47. Flores G. The impact of medical interpreter services on the quality of health care: a systematic review. Med Care Res Rev. 2005;62(3):255–99.
48. Kale E, Syed HR. Language barriers and the use of interpreters in the public health services. a questionnaire-based survey. Patient Educ Couns. 2010;81(2):187–91.
49. Meeuwesen L, Ani E, Cesaroni F, Eversley J, Ross J. Inequalities in health care for migrants and ethnic minorities. 2012.
50. Zendedel R, Schouten BC, van Weert JC, van den Putte B. Informal interpreting in general practice: Comparing the perspectives of general practitioners, migrant patients and family interpreters. Patient Educ Couns. 2016;99(6):981–7.
51. Downie J, Dickson A. Unsound evaluations of medical machine translation risk patient health and confidentiality. JAMA Intern Med. 2019;179(7):1001.
52. Turner AM, Choi YK, Dew K, Tsai M-T, Bosold AL, Wu S, et al. Evaluating the usefulness of translation technologies for emergency response communication: a scenario-based study. JMIR Public Health Surveill. 2019;5(1):e11171.
53. Vieira LN, O'Hagan M, O'Sullivan C. Understanding the societal impacts of machine translation: a critical review of the literature on medical and legal use cases. Inf Commun Soc. 2021;24(11):1515–32.
54. Heath M, Hvass AMF, Wejse CM. Interpreter services and effect on healthcare-a systematic review of the impact of different types of interpreters on patient outcome. J Migr Health. 2023;7:100162.
55. Panayiotou A, Gardner A, Williams S, Zucchi E, Mascitti-Meuter M, Goh AM, et al. Language translation apps in health care settings: expert opinion. JMIR Mhealth Uhealth. 2019;7(4):e11316.

Advanced Nursing Practice in IPC and AMS

11

Enrique Castro-Sánchez

Abstract

Advanced nursing practice in infection prevention and control (IPC) and antimicrobial stewardship (AMS) is increasingly recognised as pivotal in combating healthcare-associated infections and antimicrobial resistance. This chapter explores the multifaceted roles of advanced practice nurses in IPC and AMS implementation. These roles encompass leadership in policy development, autonomous clinical decision-making, implementation of innovative interventions, influencing institutional policies, leading multidisciplinary teams, and driving practice changes aimed at enhancing patient outcomes. The autonomy of advanced nurse practitioners in making infection-related clinical decisions, from initiating isolation protocols to optimising antibiotic therapy, is highlighted, alongside their contributions to education and professional development for the healthcare workforce. Challenges such as resource limitations, role ambiguity, and interprofessional barriers are discussed, and key facilitators such as strong leadership support and targeted training are identified. Case studies from Europe illustrate successful nurse-led IPC and AMS initiatives, with comparisons to practices in the United States and low- and middle-income countries (LMICs). This chapter emphasises that empowering nurses in IPC and AMS fosters more resilient and effective responses to infection threats, while underscoring the need for continued professional development and supportive policy frameworks.

E. Castro-Sánchez (✉)
Department of Infectious Diseases, Imperial College London, London, UK

Global Health Research Group, University of Balearic Islands, Palma de Mallorca, Spain
e-mail: e.castro-sanchez@imperial.ac.uk

Keywords

Infection prevention · Antimicrobial stewardship · Advanced nursing practice ·
Healthcare-associated infections · Multidisciplinary collaboration

11.1   Introduction

Infections and antimicrobial resistance present an urgent threat to global health,
demanding robust infection prevention and prudent antibiotic use [1]. Recent estimates attribute ~1.27 million deaths per year worldwide directly to antibiotic-
resistant infections [2], underscoring the critical need for effective IPC and AMS
strategies and optimal involvement of the health workforce. This chapter discusses
the challenges and enabling factors influencing the introduction of advanced nursing practice roles and provides case examples from Europe with comparisons to the
United States and low- and middle-income countries (LMICs) to illustrate global
successes, challenges, and variations in implementation and practice.

11.2   What Is Advanced Nursing Practice?

Nurses in Advanced Nursing Practice (ANPs), such as nurse practitioners, clinical
nurse specialists, and nurse consultants, have emerged as key players in healthcare
delivery and, by extension, IPC and AMS programs [3]. These nurses possess expert
knowledge and clinical skills and often have the authority to prescribe medications,
enabling them to lead initiatives that prevent healthcare-associated infections
(HAIs) and promote appropriate antimicrobial use. In line with expectations regarding these roles since their implementation more than 50 years ago [4], ANP roles in
IPC/AMS encompass a broad range of competencies, from leadership in policymaking and autonomous clinical decision-making in scenarios characterised by
uncertainty and staff and patient education to the implementation of innovations, all
undertaken in close collaboration with other health professionals within multidisciplinary teams (Fig. 11.1). This chapter explores the multifaceted contributions of
ANP to IPC and AMS, examining policy and leadership functions, clinical autonomy, education and training roles, and interprofessional collaboration.

11.2.1 Autonomously Managing Complex Clinical
Decision-Making, Key Feature of ANPs

A defining feature of advanced nursing practice is the high level of clinical autonomy in decision-making [5]. All models of advanced clinical practice recognise
how APNs apply their skills and expertise to resolve clinical situations surrounded
by uncertainty and complexity [6]. Importantly, complexity here does not denote the
need to consider many factors, but rather the lack of information, certainty, or

Key Domains of Advanced Nursing Practice

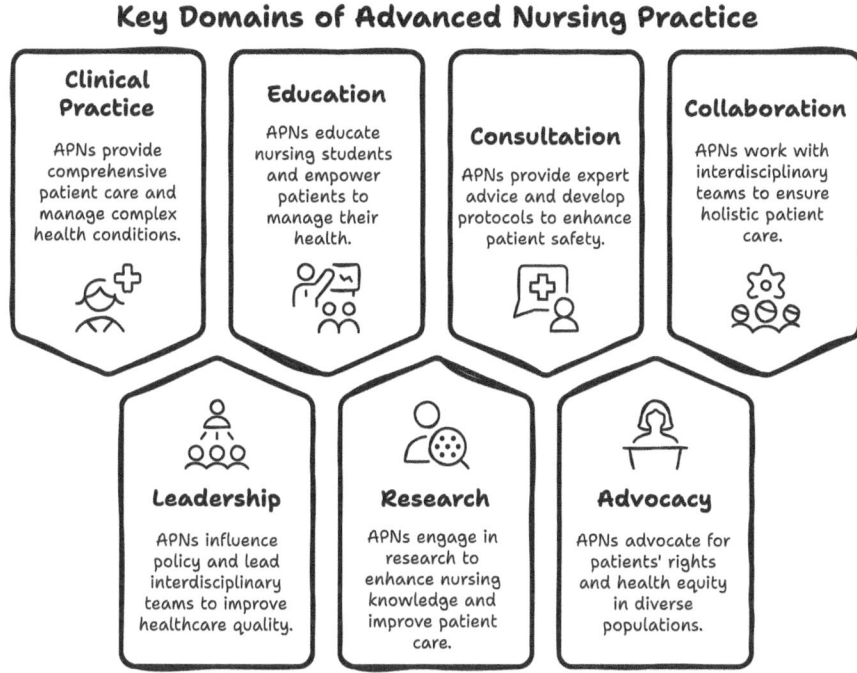

Fig. 11.1 The key domains of advanced nursing practice. (Author's own)

evidence relevant to an event or patient. In IPC and AMS, APNs are equipped to make independent judgements on infection prevention measures and antimicrobial therapy within the scope of their professional registration and competencies [7]. During the COVID-19 pandemic, for example, IPC nurse practitioners often independently led ward-based interventions (such as implementing PPE compliance audits and cohorting plans) as part of rapid response teams, demonstrating trust in their clinical judgment at the organizational level [8].

Regarding AMS, ANPs, particularly nurse practitioners and other nurse prescribers, make direct contributions to antibiotic decision-making [9]. In many countries, NPs are licenced as independent prescribers who practice autonomously, meaning they can initiate, adjust, or discontinue antibiotic therapy in accordance with stewardship principles. Studies have shown that ANPs play a key role in outpatient antibiotic management. For instance, a study of primary care nurse practitioners in the United States Veterans Affairs system found that these healthcare professionals actively engaged in stewardship: they emphasised patient education and demonstrated prudent prescribing behaviours, with a decline in antibiotics prescribed for viral respiratory infections over a 3-year period [10]. Nurse practitioners in the study reported that building patient trust and understanding was essential to their prescribing decisions, highlighting the autonomous yet patient-centred approach these nurses bring to AMS [11].

Advanced practice nurses also implement nurse-driven stewardship protocols that leverage their autonomy in interdisciplinary teams to improve patient outcomes. Examples from hospital practice include nurses independently initiating an "antibiotic timeout" 48–72 h after therapy start to reassess need, prompting IV-to-PO switch of antibiotics when patients stabilise, or verifying allergy histories and culture results to ensure appropriate antibiotic selection [3]. These actions often occur as part of best practice guidelines and protocols, but they still rely on the nurse's judgement at the bedside. Bedside nurses have described such stewardship activities as a natural extension of their advocacy role for patients [12].

Notably, the degree of autonomy can vary by region and setting. In the United States, some states allow nurse practitioners to prescribe medications without supervision, while others require varying degrees of collaboration with physicians [13]. In the United Kingdom and parts of Europe, qualified nurse independent prescribers have the authority to manage medications, including antimicrobials. Regardless of jurisdiction, successful IPC/AMS nursing practice requires institutional policies that grant nurses the autonomy to act promptly on infection prevention and stewardship issues. When these policies are place, APNs can significantly influence the clinical outcomes. Indeed, one integrative review observed that nurses view involvement in stewardship as enhancing the value of their role rather than an added burden, and they can integrate stewardship activities into routine care without compromising their other duties [14]. By profiting from their autonomy, whether implementing isolation precautions or changing an antibiotic due to a microbiology report, APNs function as pivotal decision-makers for safe, high-value care.

11.2.2 Education, Training, and Professional Development

To fulfil advanced roles in IPC and AMS, nurses require specialised education and ongoing professional development. High-level competency in IPC and antimicrobial management is supported by formal training programs, continuous learning, and certification. Education and training not only equip nurses with technical knowledge but also empower them to take the initiative and innovate in their practice and address the challenges of uncertainty and ambiguity [15].

Many countries have established postgraduate programs focusing on infection control or infectious diseases for nurses to address this issue. In Europe, for example, a dedicated Infection Prevention and Control certificate program (60 European Credit Transfer System credits over 2 years) was developed under the European Union's training network to standardise expertise across countries [16]. Such programs cover advanced IPC/AMS practices, epidemiology, microbiology, and leadership skills, preparing nurses for specialist and leadership roles. However, the availability of formal IPC/AMS education is uneven globally. A recent mapping of IPC training in 14 countries of the WHO Eastern Mediterranean Region found that less than half (42.9%) offered postgraduate degrees in IPC, although approximately 71% provided structured in-service IPC training through national programs [17]. Many IPC nurses in resource-limited settings are trained on the job via short courses or mentoring rather than through lengthy formal education [18]. Although this on-the-job training could be accepted as akin to a residency, it would be necessary for these learners to be adequately supported by formal education mechanisms and structures to achieve the threshold usually expected by ANP programs [19]. This highlights the need for broader access to advanced IPC curricula, especially but not solely in low-resource contexts, and for continued reflection on the direction advanced nursing practice in AMS and IPC should take.

Given the evolving nature of infectious threats and emerging patterns of drug resistance, ongoing education is critical. Advanced IPC/AMS nurses frequently attend workshops, conferences (such as those by association for professionals in infection control and Epidemiology, Infection Prevention Society, or ESCMID), and in-house training to remain current with best practices. The emerging body of literature stresses the need for engagement in lifelong learning; an integrative review identified education engagement as a core theme for nurses in stewardship roles [20]. Many healthcare facilities are mandated to incorporate IPC and AMS topics into nursing continuing education. For instance, training on new guidelines (e.g. updated isolation precautions or antibiotic prescribing and management protocols) is often led by the IPC or AMS nurse for all clinical staff. ANPs often become educators, conducting sessions on hand hygiene, aseptic techniques, and antimicrobial protocols for other nurses and interdisciplinary colleagues. This dual role of learner and educator ensures that advanced nurses both maintain their expertise and disseminate knowledge to frontline staff, thus magnifying their impact not only at the clinical level but also at the health system transformation level.

In terms of advanced education and professional practice, there is still a need to develop and implement competency validation and professional certification in advanced practice in IPC and AMS. Certifications such as the Certification in Infection Control (CIC) credential, administered by the Certification Board of Infection Control and Epidemiology, validate a nurse's knowledge and skills in IPC [21]. Whether such certification suggests that the clinician is now able to practice at an advanced level may not be that straightforward, as advanced practice does not take place merely when professionals are educated at that level, but there is an established normative framework which recognises such practice, employers authorise and endorse the roles thus accepting vicarious liability for any undesired consequences of such advanced practice (when *lex artis* maintained), and there are pathways for support and quality assurance [22].

Nonetheless, achieving certification has been linked to improved patient outcomes; certified infection preventionists tend to be effective champions of key IPC practices, and there is evidence of better clinical outcomes (e.g. lower infection rates) in settings with certified IPC professionals [23]. Similarly, in AMS, some nurses pursue specialised credentials or advanced degrees (such as an MSc in antimicrobial stewardship or infectious diseases) to deepen their expertise. Employers increasingly recognise or demand these qualifications; job descriptions for advanced IPC/AMS roles often list a master's degree or certification as preferred or required, particularly as the starting education point for ANPs is widely requested to be a master [24], although in setting with longstanding tradition of the role there are calls for doctoral education to be the minimum entry point to this level of practice [25].

11.2.3 Health System Transformation, a Fundamental Pillar of Advanced Practice

In addition to areas of practice focused on clinical work, nurses in advanced practice are designated health systems leaders and must contribute to mentoring and development of the clinical workforce [26] to ensure the capacity and resilience of the system. For this reason, training ANP leaders in IPC/AMS goes beyond clinical knowledge and includes developing soft skills in leadership, change management, negotiation, communication skills, implementation, and policy advocacy [27]. Programs such as the world health organization (WHO) Advanced IPC training course and national leadership workshops focus on cultivating nurses' ability to influence organizational culture and behaviours [28]. The importance of mentorship is also frequently noted: novice IPC or stewardship nurses benefit from mentoring by experienced practitioners [29]. Such mentorship accelerates skill acquisition in conducting infection surveillance, analysing antibiograms, and negotiating with prescribers. Structured mentoring and fellowship programs (e.g. 1-year fellowship for AMS nurses) have started to appear in some health systems to build a pipeline of skilled practitioners [12]. The personal support and growth offered by mentorship are even more important for dealing with the uncertainty surrounding advanced practice, an uncertainty for which best practice guidelines and protocols may not be of any use (as ambiguous scenarios and clinical episodes may, by definition, not be addressed by the steps reflected in the guidelines) [30].

11.2.4 Multidisciplinary Collaboration and Interprofessional Working

IPC and AMS, like most aspects of current healthcare provision, are inherently collective efforts that require seamless collaboration among multiple health professionals. Advanced practice nurses in these fields can act as 'knowledge brokers' within multidisciplinary teams [31], leveraging their communication skills and holistic perspective to bring disciplines together for the common goal of reducing infections and optimising antimicrobial use. The success of IPC and AMS programs often hinges on how well nurses collaborate with physicians, pharmacists, microbiologists, epidemiologists, and other stakeholders [32].

Nurses spend more time at the point of care than most other professionals do, and traditionally serve as patient care coordinators [33]. In IPC/AMS teams, APNs use this vantage status to facilitate information flow between patients and the healthcare team and ensure team actions are aligned [34], which is vital in stewardship. For example, a nurse communicates a patient's antibiotic allergies or symptom changes to the prescribing clinician, influencing the antibiotic choices. Effective AMS requires real-time communication of lab results and patient status; nurses routinely bridge the lab and clinician by alerting teams to positive cultures or monitoring for side effects, thereby closing the loop on stewardship recommendations. One qualitative study identified "communication and relationship" as a key theme impacting nurses' involvement in AMS, emphasising that good collaboration and dialogue with physicians and pharmacists empower nurses to participate actively [35]. When interprofessional relationships are strong, nurses feel more confident in voicing concerns (such as querying seemingly inappropriate antibiotic prescriptions) and contributing suggestions.

Advanced nurses in IPC and AMS often chair or participate in infection control committees that include members from nursing, medicine, surgery, microbiology, environmental services and hospital administration. These committees formulate policies on a broad range of issues, such as improving hand hygiene rates, optimal catheter use, and outbreak management. Nursing input is crucial, as nurses can speak to practical workflow considerations and frontline challenges, and in many settings, they lead IPC activities [36]. Similarly, AMS programs are typically overseen by multidisciplinary stewardship committees. An ideal ASP team, as recommended by guidelines, includes an infectious disease physician, clinical pharmacist, microbiologist, and infection control professional or nurse [12]. In practice, many hospitals have expanded their AMS rounds to multidisciplinary "antibiotic rounds" where a pharmacist, physician, and stewardship nurse review patients on broad-spectrum antibiotics together. Nurses contribute insights into patient preferences (e.g. ability to tolerate oral medications for IV-PO switch) and ensure that any changes in therapy are communicated and implemented at the bedside. This collaborative rounding approach has been credited with more comprehensive stewardship, as each professional brings unique expertise to the table [37].

Collaboration extends beyond formal meetings, and *ad hoc* interactions occur daily to progress the care and healing of patients. For example, in a complex surgical case with an infection, the APN in the IPC would work closely with the surgical team for proper wound care, with the microbiologist to interpret culture results, and with the pharmacist to adjust antibiotic dosing. This interprofessional synergy is essential for managing HAIs, such as surgical site infections and ventilator-associated pneumonia. The systematic review by Davey mentioned before about nurses' roles in stewardship noted that successful AMS is multidisciplinary, and nurses' partnership with other professionals is now recognised as critical [20]. Nurses acknowledge that they are part of a wider team addressing patient safety issues, and clarity in team roles helps them engage more effectively.

Historically, however, hierarchical cultures and ingrained traditions regarding clinical roles and healthcare professions could hamper open and effective collaboration in IPC and AMS, with nurses' input sometimes feeling unnecessary or undervalued [38]. However, this is changing as evidence grows that hierarchical barriers undermine IPC and AMS outcomes [39]. Many institutions encourage a flattened team structure for quality improvement projects. APNs in IPC and AMS can benefit from their leadership's 'pillar of practice' [40] and play a vital role in breaking down silos. In one hospital's ICU, lack of collaboration was identified as a barrier to nurses' AMS role (nurses were not included in decision-making or feedback discussions) [41]. Addressing this by formally including ICU nurses in stewardship rounds and discussions led to more effective implementation of the guidelines. Thus, fostering an environment of mutual respect and open communication is a key facilitator of interprofessional work, enabling advanced nurses to contribute maximally.

11.2.5 Policy and Leadership Roles in IPC and AMS

Closely related to their role as leaders and change agents, APNs drive policy development, implementation, and adoption [42]. In many health facilities, senior IPC nurses or nurse consultants help develop and enforce infection control policies by translating national guidelines into practice. Strong nursing leadership can directly improve infection outcomes – for example, a recent systematic review found that head nurses' transformational leadership was associated with reduced rates of device-associated infections and better adherence to preventive practices [43]. Empowering nurses in leadership positions is essential for a robust infection prevention program. Global guidelines also emphasise leadership support; the WHO's Core Components in IPC call for dedicated leadership and a trained IPC team at each facility [44], roles frequently filled by advanced nurses.

In AMS programs, advanced nurses are increasingly taking on leadership roles traditionally held by physicians or pharmacists, who may chair or coordinate these programs, lead the development of antibiotic guidelines, and monitor the use of antimicrobials. However, expanding nursing leadership in stewardship could enhance program impact and send a strong message to policymakers. Visibility matters, and involving nurse leaders in AMS program committees would ensure that nursing perspectives inform policy decisions. There is also a growing acknowledgement that stewardship efforts are more effective when nurses are formally included and empowered; one review reinforced that formally including nurses in AMS is associated with improved nursing confidence and even better patient outcomes [34]. These leadership efforts are particularly crucial in community settings and long-term care facilities, where the team mix is usually very different from that in hospital facilities and where there may be even less availability of relevant and appropriate guidelines [45].

There are already excellent examples of APN leadership in IPC/AMS in European healthcare systems. In the United Kingdom, for example, senior nursing roles, such as the Director of Infection Prevention and Control (DIPC) or IPC Nurse Consultant, are established to lead hospital infection prevention programs. These roles carry significant authority: in NHS Scotland, the nurse DIPC holds board-level responsibility for the IPC programme, including oversight of AMS initiatives, and provides strategic clinical leadership across the organization. At the policy level, European professional bodies advocate for advanced nursing leadership in this arena. The European Specialist Nurses Organisation (ESNO) has called for funded projects to train nurse leaders in AMR and IPC, reflecting a high-level commitment to strengthening nursing capacity in these areas [46]. Such policies and advocacy efforts support the recognition of advanced IPC/AMS nursing roles and facilitate their development.

11.3   Challenges, Barriers, and Facilitators for APN Roles in IPC and AMS

Advanced IPC and AMS nurses operate within complex healthcare systems, and their effectiveness can be limited or enabled by several factors. Understanding the common challenges and barriers they face, as well as the key facilitators for success, is crucial for strengthening these roles (Fig. 11.2).

One persistent challenge is the unclear definition or under-recognition of nurses' roles in IPC/AMS. Historically, stewardship programs focused on physicians and pharmacists, often leaving nurses' contributions informal or peripheral [47]. Although this is changing, some advanced nurses still struggle with full integration

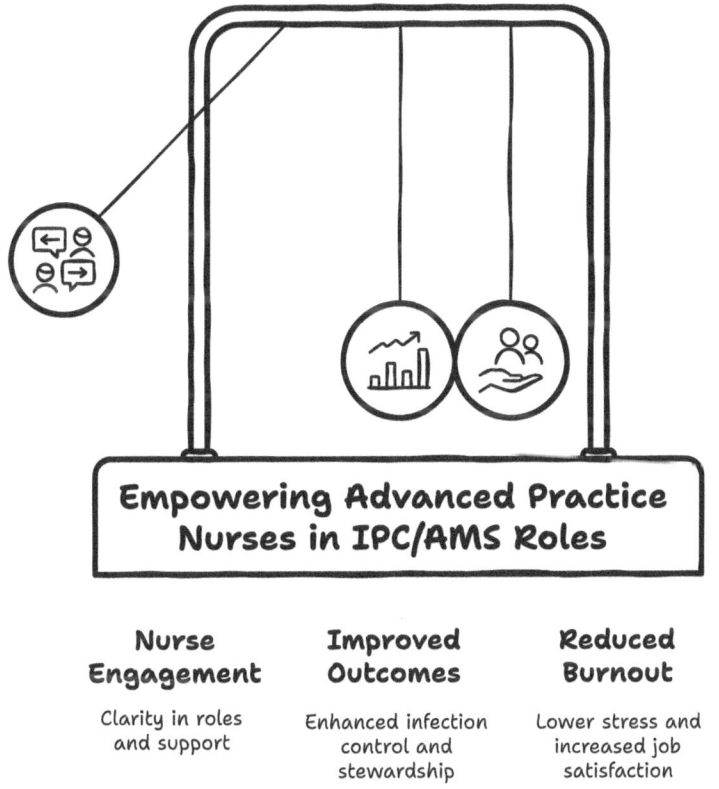

Fig. 11.2 Key barriers for the increased implementation of APN roles in IPC/AMS. (Author's own)

into decision-making processes. For example, the qualitative study by Rout et al. in an ICU in South Africa found that nurses were not routinely included in stewardship decision-making or feedback discussions, reflecting a lack of collaboration that impeded their role [41]. When nurses are not part of the information loop, their ability to contribute is hindered. This highlights the need for clearly defined responsibilities and the inclusion of nurses in IPC/AMS structures. Conversely, a facilitator is explicit organisational support for the nursing role – hospitals that formally appoint nurses to lead or co-lead IPC and AMS initiatives send a message that encourages nurse engagement. Clarity in expectations (such as including stewardship activities in job descriptions and performance metrics) can empower nurses to take ownership of these tasks.

Many barriers are structural, as is experienced in other areas of clinical practice across health systems. Inadequate staffing or resources can severely limit the achievements of APNs in IPC/AMS. If an IPC nurse is responsible for an overwhelming number of patients or multiple sites, the surveillance and interventions may be suboptimal. The ICU study above pointed out the shortage of experienced nurses and insufficient staffing for training as barriers to nurses' stewardship role. A high workload can force nurses to prioritise immediate clinical tasks over stewardship activities, such as auditing or data analysis. Similarly, the lack of dedicated time for AMS rounds or IPC surveillance can curtail proactive work [48]. Facilitators include ensuring optimal nurse-to-patient ratios and providing protected time for IPC/AMS duties. Some institutions have addressed these generalised shortages and deficits by creating additional advanced practice roles (e.g. a dedicated advanced AMS nurse for a hospital) to distribute the workload [49]. Access to resources is another factor; any IPC or AMS nurse without data analytics support or decision support tools will be less effective.

Knowledge and training gaps are longstanding barriers. Although advanced nurses are highly trained, specific gaps in AMS or IPC knowledge can exist, especially when nurses are new to these roles. Insufficient training and education in AMS for nurses have been consistently identified in the literature [50, 51]. Some nurses may feel uncomfortable reviewing antibiotic regimens if they lack a pharmacology background, or they may not fully understand microbiology reports [52], which limits their confidence to intervene. This barrier is closely tied to the facilitator of education, as targeted training programs and continuous professional development greatly enhance nurses' effectiveness. For instance, when nurses attend workshops on antibiotic mechanisms or infection control certification courses, their ability to contribute meaningfully increases [53]. The presence of experienced mentors can also mitigate knowledge gaps, as noted above. The formal inclusion of nurses in AMS has been shown to improve their knowledge and confidence [54], indicating that overcoming educational gaps is feasible with structured involvement and support.

External and system-level challenges, particularly in LMICs or resource-challenged environments, such as a lack of national policy support, limited access to data, or poor laboratory infrastructure, affect IPC/AMS efforts [55]. Advanced nurses in these contexts may find it challenging to implement guidelines when essential support (such as microbiology labs for cultures or sufficient PPE supplies for infection control) is lacking. A facilitator factor in these scenarios is networking and external support; for instance, international partnerships (like the WHO's AMS toolkit rollout or the CDC's international infection control training programs) can provide resources and frameworks that empower nurses locally [56]. Additionally, professional networks, such as the Infection Prevention Society in the UK or international nursing associations, offer platforms for knowledge exchange and advocacy, helping nurses in under-resourced settings to scale up the many creative and effective solutions they develop.

Finally, the psychological burden on APNs in IPC/AMS can be significant. They are responsible for preventing negative outcomes (infections, resistance), which are often invisible until they occur, and this can be stressful. Burnout is a risk, especially during COVID-19, when IPC teams were under immense pressure [57]. Without recognition and support, experienced nurses might leave or hesitate to embrace these roles. Providing recognition, ensuring a manageable scope, and fostering a sense of community and accomplishment (celebrating successes, such as reduced infection rates attributable to the team's work) would be effective in mitigating this psychological burden.

11.4   Case Studies and Examples: Europe, US, and LMICs

Examining real-world examples across different health system contexts illustrates how advanced nursing practice in IPC and AMS is implemented and the factors that drive its success.

In Europe, many countries have well-established roles for nurses in IPC and AMS. For instance, in the UK, every NHS hospital trust has an IPC program led by a DIPC, often a senior nurse. In Scotland, nurses hold strategic oversight of IPC and AMS, as seen in the nurse DIPC, who manages infection control for the entire health board. The UK has also been a leader in nurse prescribing, with thousands managing common infections in primary care and applying antimicrobial guidelines [58]. In the Netherlands, Infection Control Practitioners, often nurses with specialised training, monitor and advise clinicians on IPC measures. Their proactive approach, such as MRSA prevention through the "Search and Destroy" policy, is a model for success [59]. In France, some healthcare facilities include a nurse referent for antibiotic use who works with infectious disease specialists and pharmacists to audit prescriptions and provide feedback [47]. These examples underline that Europe's relatively strong institutional support (policies, training programs like European Committee on Infection Control, and nurse empowerment in clinical roles) facilitates advanced nursing practice in IPC/AMS, yielding measurable improvements in practice and patient outcomes.

In the US, both IPC and AMS roles for nurses are prominent, although the integration of AMS is recent. Most US hospitals have infection preventionists (IPs) on staff, usually nurses or epidemiology-trained professionals, who manage IPC activities, such as surveillance, staff training, and outbreak control. On the AMS side, US hospitals are increasingly including nurses in stewardship committees, guided by CDC and Joint Commission standards. The ANA-CDC White Paper (2017) [60] outlines how nurses can be leveraged in stewardship efforts. Many hospitals have started nurse-focused stewardship education; for example, a large academic hospital assigned a clinical nurse specialist to its AMS team, who championed the "48-hour antibiotic time-out", training nurses to prompt physicians to reassess antibiotics at 48 h. Over a year, the hospital saw a rise in appropriate de-escalation of therapy due to consistent nursing reminders [61].

Low- and middle-income countries face resource constraints and high infectious disease burdens, leading to the emergence of APNs in IPC and AMS. South Africa exemplifies this, with IPC nurses and growing nurse involvement in stewardship, as seen in an ICU study in which nurses identified barriers and expressed willingness to take on AMS roles. Private hospital groups in South Africa have established AMS nurse positions to collaborate with pharmacists, resulting in improved antibiotic prescription reviews [62]. In Kenya, a nurse-led infection prevention program improved hand hygiene compliance and reduced surgical site infections by implementing WHO guidelines, leading to the nurse becoming a regional mentor [63]. However, LMIC case studies highlight challenges, such as the shortage of specialised IPC nurses in India, where general duty nurses often lack extra training and experience inconsistent outcomes [64, 65]. International initiatives have been crucial, with the WHO developing a practical AMS toolkit for LMIC hospitals and recommending that stewardship teams build on existing structures and maximise teamwork, including nurse champions. This stepwise approach was piloted in Nigeria, where a tertiary hospital formed an AMS committee with a nursing services representative, implemented an antibiotic prescription form requiring justification, and observed a significant drop in the use of restricted antibiotics without justification within six months [66].

Common threads emerge across these settings. Strong leadership support and targeted training empower nurses to excel in IPC/AMS roles, whether in a high-resource European hospital or a resource-limited African clinic setting. Multidisciplinary collaboration is universal; in all contexts, when nurses are embraced as equal partners, programs flourish. Conversely, barriers such as under-resourcing and hierarchical cultures can stunt progress anywhere, though they are often more pronounced in LMICs. Structured approaches (with formal roles, certifications, and cross-country training programs) provide a template that can be adapted to all regions. There is an untapped benefit in robustly demonstrating the value of professional advocacy and research to quantify the impact of nurses, which helps drive policy changes (such as Joint Commission standards now implicitly expecting nurse involvement) [67]. LMIC examples highlight adaptability; nurses often innovate within constraints, such as using simple checklists or educational campaigns to achieve IPC gains when technology is not available.

11.5   Conclusion

Advanced practice nurses are crucial for IPC and AMS efforts. They bring clinical expertise, leadership, and collaboration to address healthcare challenges. This chapter highlights how they shape policy, lead teams, protect patients, educate the workforce, and embrace innovations. It also addresses challenges, such as limited resources and cultural hurdles. A panel of case studies has illustrated measurable improvements in care quality and patient outcomes when advanced nurses practice in IPC and AMS, and further empowering nurses in these areas will remain essential for effective healthcare delivery in the twenty-first century.

References

1. World Health Organization. Antimicrobial resistance. Geneva: WHO; 2020. https://www.who.int/news-room/fact-sheets/detail/antimicrobial-resistance
2. Murray CJL, Ikuta KS, Sharara F, Swetschinski L, Robles Aguilar G, Gray A, et al. Global burden of bacterial antimicrobial resistance in 2019: a systematic analysis. Lancet. 2022;399(10325):629–55. https://doi.org/10.1016/S0140-6736(21)02724-0.
3. Carter EJ, Greendyke WG, Furuya EY, Srinivasan A, Shelley AN, Larson EL. Exploring the role of advanced practice nurses in antimicrobial stewardship: a multisite qualitative study. Am J Infect Control. 2018;46(7):680–4. https://doi.org/10.1016/j.ajic.2017.11.005.
4. Australian Commission on Safety and Quality in Health Care. Role of nurses, midwives and infection control practitioners in antimicrobial stewardship. In: Antimicrobial Stewardship in Australian Health Care. Sydney: ACSQHC; 2018. p. 275–92. https://www.safetyandquality.gov.au/sites/default/files/migrated/Chapter12-Role-of-nurses-midwives-and-infection-control-practitioners-in-antimicrobial-stewardship.pdf.
5. Lowe G, Plummer V, O'Brien AP, Boyd L. Time to clarify – the value of advanced practice nursing roles in health care. J Adv Nurs. 2012;68(3):677–85. https://doi.org/10.1111/j.1365-2648.2011.05790.x.
6. International Council of Nurses. Guidelines on advanced practice nursing 2020. Geneva: ICN; 2020. https://www.icn.ch/system/files/documents/2020-04/ICN_APN%20Report_EN_WEB.pdf
7. Olans RN, Olans RD, DeMaria A Jr. The critical role of the staff nurse in antimicrobial stewardship – unrecognized, but already there. Clin Infect Dis. 2016;62(1):84–9. https://doi.org/10.1093/cid/civ697.
8. Whitehead L, Seaton P, Graham K, et al. The role of infection prevention and control nurse specialists in the COVID-19 pandemic: a mixed-methods study. J Hosp Infect. 2022;121:130–8.
9. Courtenay M, Stenner K, Carey N. Nurse prescribing in antimicrobial stewardship: a mixed-methods study. J Antimicrob Chemother. 2011;66(12):2869–76.
10. Knobloch MJ, Musuuza J, Baubie K, Saban KL, Suda KJ, Safdar N. Nurse practitioners as antibiotic stewards: examining prescribing patterns and perceptions. Am J Infect Control. 2021 Aug;49(8):1052–7. https://doi.org/10.1016/j.ajic.2021.01.018.
11. Latter S, Blenkinsopp A, Smith A. Evaluating nurse prescribing: findings from a national study. Nurse Educ Today. 2007;27(8):832–41.
12. Barlam TF, Cosgrove SE, Abbo LM, et al. Implementing an antibiotic stewardship program: guidelines by the Infectious Diseases Society of America and the Society for Healthcare Epidemiology of America. Clin Infect Dis. 2016;62(10):e51–77.

13. American Association of Nurse Practitioners. Nurse Practitioner (NP) State Practice Environment. [Internet]. Austin: AANP; 2024. https://www.aanp.org/advocacy/state/state-practice-environment

14. Schuts EC, Hulscher ME, Adriaenssens PV, et al. Current evidence for effective interventions to improve antimicrobial use in hospitals: a systematic review and meta-analysis. Antimicrob Agents Chemother. 2011;55(6):2312–21.

15. World Health Organization. Global competency and outcomes framework for infection prevention and control programmes. Geneva: WHO; 2023.

16. European Centre for Disease Prevention and Control. Training Programme on Prevention and Control of Healthcare-Associated Infections. Stockholm: ECDC; 2013.

17. Moghnieh R, Al-Maani AS, Berro J, Ibrahim N, Attieh R, Abdallah D, Al-Ajmi J, Hamdani D, Abdulrazzaq N, Omar A, Al-Khawaja S, Al-Abadla R, Al-Ratrout S, Gharaibeh M, Abdelrahim Z, Azrag H, Amiri KM, Berry A, Hagali B, Kadhim J, Al-Shami H, Khan MA, Husni R, Heweidy I, Zayed B. Mapping of infection prevention and control education and training in some countries of the World Health Organization's Eastern Mediterranean Region: current situation and future needs. Antimicrob Resist Infect Control. 2023;12(1):90. https://doi.org/10.1186/s13756-023-01299-9.

18. World Health Organization. Antimicrobial stewardship programmes in low- and middle-income countries: a practical approach. Geneva: WHO; 2018.

19. Bryant-Lukosius D, DiCenso A, Browne AJ, Pinelli J. Advanced practice nursing roles: development, implementation and evaluation. J Adv Nurs. 2004;48(5):451–65.

20. Davey K, Aveyard H. Nurses' perceptions of their role in antimicrobial stewardship within the hospital environment. An integrative literature review. J Clin Nurs. 2022;31(21–22):3011–20. https://doi.org/10.1111/jocn.16204.

21. Certification Board of Infection Control and Epidemiology. CIC Certification. [Internet]. Washington (DC): CBIC; 2024. https://www.cbic.org/Certification/CIC

22. Schober M, Affara FA, Bryant-Lukosius D. Advancing nursing practice: a new concept for a new era. Int Nurs Rev. 2004;51(2):129–37.

23. Pogorzelska M, Stone PW. Impact of infection prevention and control programs on healthcare-associated infection: a meta-analysis. Am J Infect Control. 2015;43(7):665–71.

24. International Council of Nurses. Advanced Nursing Practice. Geneva: ICN; 2020.

25. Hamric AB, Hanson CM, Tracy MF, O'Grady ET. Advanced practice nursing: an integrative approach. 6th ed. St. Louis: Elsevier Saunders; 2018.

26. World Health Organization. Strengthening nursing and midwifery: report of the strategic directions on nursing and midwifery development for the South-East Asia Region (2016–2020). New Delhi: WHO Regional Office for South-East Asia; 2017.

27. World Health Organization. Transforming and scaling up health professionals' education and training: towards universal health coverage. Geneva: WHO; 2013.

28. World Health Organization. Infection prevention and control in healthcare settings. Geneva: WHO; 2022.

29. Stone PW, Larson E, Kawar LN. Organizational climate and infection prevention and control: lessons learned. Am J Infect Control. 2006;34(5):294–301.

30. Rolfe G, Freshwater D. Evidence-based practice in nursing: a sceptical approach. Edinburgh: Churchill Livingstone; 2005.

31. Monsees E, Goldman J, Popejoy L. Staff nurses as antimicrobial stewards: an integrative literature review. Am J Infect Control. 2017;45(8):917–22. https://doi.org/10.1016/j.ajic.2017.04.286.

32. Schmid S. Interprofessional collaboration between ICU physicians, staff nurses, and hospital pharmacists optimizes antimicrobial treatment and improves quality of care and economic outcome. J Multidiscip Healthc. 2022;15:123–32. https://doi.org/10.2147/JMDH.S345678.

33. Michel O, Garcia Manjon AJ, Pasquier J, Ortoleva BC. How do nurses spend their time? A time and motion analysis of nursing activities in an internal medicine unit. J Adv Nurs. 2021;77(11):4459–70. https://doi.org/10.1111/jan.14935.
34. Gotterson F, Buising K, Manias E. Nurse role and contribution to antimicrobial stewardship: an integrative review. Int J Nurs Stud. 2021;117:103787. https://doi.org/10.1016/j.ijnurstu.2020.103787.
35. Bonacaro A, Solfrizzo FG, Regano D, Negrello F, Domeniconi C, Volpon A, Taurchini S, Toselli P, Baesti C. Antimicrobial stewardship in healthcare: exploring the role of nurses in promoting change, identifying barrier elements and facilitators-a meta-synthesis. Healthcare (Basel). 2024;12(21):2122. https://doi.org/10.3390/healthcare12212122.
36. Pegues DA. The infection control committee. In: Lautenbach E, Malani PN, Woeltje KF, Han JH, Shuman EK, Marschall J, editors. Practical healthcare epidemiology. 4th ed. Cambridge: Cambridge University Press; 2018. p. 10–7.
37. Hamilton RA, Williams N, Ashton C, Gilani SAD, Hussain S, Jamieson C, et al. Nurses' attitudes, behaviours, and enablers of intravenous to oral switching (IVOS) of antibiotics: a mixed-methods survey of nursing staff in secondary care hospitals across the Midlands region of England. J Hosp Infect. 2024;131:174–81. https://doi.org/10.1016/j.jhin.2023.09.005.
38. Monsees E, Goldman J, Vogelsmeier A, Popejoy L. Nurses as antimicrobial stewards: Recognition, confidence, and organizational factors across nine hospitals. Am J Infect Control. 2020;48(3):239–45. https://doi.org/10.1016/j.ajic.2019.12.002.
39. Tang JW, Holmes A. Changing the culture of antimicrobial prescribing: embracing the butterfly effect. J Hosp Infect. 2019;101(1):1–2. https://doi.org/10.1016/j.jhin.2018.11.008.
40. Wood C. Leadership and management for nurses working at an advanced level. Br J Nurs. 2021;30(5):282–6. https://doi.org/10.12968/bjon.2021.30.5.282.
41. Rout J, Brysiewicz P. Perceived barriers to the development of the antimicrobial stewardship role of the nurse in intensive care: views of healthcare professionals. South Afr J Crit Care. 2020;36(1) https://doi.org/10.7196/SAJCC.2020.v36i1.410.
42. Kostas-Polston EA, Thanavaro JL, Arvidson C, Taub L. Advancing nurse practitioner knowledge of health policy and the policy process. J Nurse Pract. 2015;11(3):335–41. https://doi.org/10.1016/j.nurpra.2014.11.017.
43. Cappelli E, Zaghini F, Fiorini J, Sili A. Healthcare-associated infections and nursing leadership: a systematic review. J Infect Prev. 2024;27:17571774241287467. https://doi.org/10.1177/17571774241287467.
44. World Health Organization. Guidelines on core components of infection prevention and control programmes at the national and acute health care facility level. Geneva: WHO; 2016. https://www.ncbi.nlm.nih.gov/books/NBK401782/
45. Centers for Disease Control and Prevention. Core infection prevention and control practices for safe healthcare delivery in all settings – recommendations of the healthcare infection control practices advisory committee. Atlanta: CDC; 2022. https://www.cdc.gov/infection-control/hcp/core-practices/index.html
46. European Specialist Nurses Organisation. Empowering nurses through education, recognition, and autonomy: a strategic contribution to health workforce stability in the EU [Internet]. Brussels: ESNO; 2024. https://www.esno.org/assets/files/Empowering_Nurses_through_Education_Recognition_Autonomy.pdf
47. Bridey C, Le Dref G, Bocquier A, Bonnay S, Pulcini C, Thilly N. Nurses' perceptions of the potential evolution of their role in antibiotic stewardship in nursing homes: a French qualitative study. JAC Antimicrob Resist. 2023;5(1):dlad008. https://doi.org/10.1093/jacamr/dlad008.
48. Scheepers LN, Niesing CM, Bester P. Facilitators and barriers to implementing antimicrobial stewardship programs in public South African hospitals. Antimicrob Steward Healthc Epidemiol. 2023;3(1):e34. https://doi.org/10.1017/ash.2022.355.

49. Castro-Sánchez E, Gilchrist M, Ahmad R, Courtenay M, Grimshaw JM, Holmes AH. Nurse roles in antimicrobial stewardship: lessons from public sectors models of acute care service delivery in the United Kingdom. Antimicrob Resist Infect Control. 2019;8:162. https://doi.org/10.1186/s13756-019-0621-4.

50. Castro-Sánchez E, Drumright LN, Gharbi M, Farrell S, Holmes AH. Mapping antimicrobial stewardship in undergraduate medical, dental, pharmacy, nursing and veterinary education in the United Kingdom. PLoS One. 2016;11(2):e0150056. https://doi.org/10.1371/journal.pone.0150056.

51. Bos M, Schouten J, De Bot C, Vermeulen H, Hulscher M. A hidden gem in multidisciplinary antimicrobial stewardship: a systematic review on bedside nurses' activities in daily practice regarding antibiotic use. JAC Antimicrob Resist. 2023;5(6):dlad123. https://doi.org/10.1093/jacamr/dlad123.

52. Durrant RJ, Doig AK, Buxton RL, Fenn JP. Microbiology education in nursing practice. J Microbiol Biol Educ. 2017;18(2):18.2.43. https://doi.org/10.1128/jmbe.v18i2.1224.

53. Yano R, Okubo T, Shimoda T, Matsuo J, Yamaguchi H. A simple and short microbiology practical improves undergraduate nursing students' awareness of bacterial traits and ability to avoid spreading infections. BMC Med Educ. 2019;19(1):53. https://doi.org/10.1186/s12909-019-1483-4.

54. Nie H, Yue L, Peng H, Zhou J, Li B, Cao Z. Nurses' engagement in antimicrobial stewardship and its influencing factors: a cross-sectional study. Int J Nurs Sci. 2023;11(1):91–8. https://doi.org/10.1016/j.ijnss.2023.12.002.

55. Olufunke O, et al. The challenges of implementing infection prevention and antimicrobial stewardship programs in resource-constrained settings. Antimicrob Resist Infect Control. 2022;11(1):108. https://doi.org/10.1186/s13756-022-01124-9.

56. Pierce J, Apisarnthanarak A, Schellack N, Cornistein W, Maani AA, Adnan S, Stevens MP. Global antimicrobial stewardship with a focus on low- and middle-income countries. Int J Infect Dis. 2020;96:621–9. https://doi.org/10.1016/j.ijid.2020.05.126.

57. Kwon CY, Lee B. Effects of stress on burnout among infection control nurses during the COVID-19 pandemic in South Korea: a cross-sectional study. BMC Nurs. 2023;22(1):54. https://doi.org/10.1186/s12912-024-02209-z.

58. Courtenay M, Gillespie D, Lim R. Patterns of GP and nurse independent prescriber prescriptions for antibiotics dispensed in the community in England: a retrospective analysis. J Antimicrob Chemother. 2023;78(10):2544–53. https://doi.org/10.1093/jac/dkad267.

59. van Knippenberg-Gordebeke G. Screen and clean to beat MRSA: success story from The Netherlands. Healthc Infect. 2010;15(1):3–9. https://doi.org/10.1071/HI10002.

60. Redefining the antibiotic stewardship team: recommendations from the American Nurses Association/Centers for Disease Control and Prevention Workgroup on the role of registered nurses in hospital antibiotic stewardship practices. JAC Antimicrob Resist. 2019;1(2):dlz037. https://doi.org/10.1093/jacamr/dlz037.

61. Greendyke WG, Carter EJ, Salsgiver E, Bernstein D, Simon MS, Saiman L, Calfee DP, Furuya EY. Exploring the role of the bedside nurse in antimicrobial stewardship: survey results from five acute-care hospitals. Infect Control Hosp Epidemiol. 2018;39(3):360–2. https://doi.org/10.1017/ice.2017.255.

62. Rout J, Brysiewicz P. Exploring the role of the ICU nurse in the antimicrobial stewardship team at a private hospital in KwaZulu-Natal, South Africa. South Afr J Crit Care. 2017;33(2):46–50. https://www.ajol.info/index.php/sajcc/article/view/162183

63. Kibira J, Kihungi L, Ndinda M, Wesangula E, Mwangi C, Muthoni F, Augusto O, Owiso G, Ndegwa L, Luvsansharav UO, Bancroft E, Rabinowitz P, Lynch J, Njoroge A. Improving hand hygiene practices in two regional hospitals in Kenya using a continuous quality improvement (CQI) approach. Antimicrob Resist Infect Control. 2022;11(1):56. https://doi.org/10.1186/s13756-022-01093-z.

64. Mehta V, Ajmera P, Kalra S, Miraj M, Gallani R, Shaik RA, Serhan HA, Sah R. Human resource shortage in India's health sector: a scoping review of the current landscape. BMC Public Health. 2024;24(1):1368. https://doi.org/10.1186/s12889-024-18850-x.

65. Lowe H, Woodd S, Lange IL, Janjanin S, Barnet J, Graham W. Challenges and opportunities for infection prevention and control in hospitals in conflict-affected settings: a qualitative study. Confl Heal. 2021;15(1):94. https://doi.org/10.1186/s13031-021-00428-8. Erratum in: Confl Health. 2022;16(1):2. 10.1186/s13031-022-00433-5
66. USAID. Strengthening antimicrobial stewardship in Nigeria. Technical Brief. Washington, DC: USAID; 2023. https://www.mtapsprogram.org/wp-content/uploads/2023/06/MTaPS-Nigeria-Technical-Brief-AMS-December-2022.pdf.
67. The Joint Commission. Antibiotic stewardship – understanding the updated requirements – effective January 1, 2023. What are the expectations for a hospital's antibiotic stewardship program.   https://www.jointcommission.org/standards/standard-faqs/critical-access-hospital/medication-management-mm/000002449/

Antimicrobial Stewardship

12

Enrique Castro-Sánchez

Abstract

Antimicrobial resistance (AMR) is a critical global health threat that requires multifaceted strategies, with antimicrobial stewardship (AMS) playing a central role. Historically, AMS has been physician- and pharmacist-led, overlooking the significant potential of nursing. This chapter highlights the crucial need for and benefits of integrating nurses into AMS programs, addressing misconceptions about their roles, and enhancing their education. Nurses, who comprise the largest healthcare workforce, possess unique patient insights and are crucial for medication administration, patient education, and infection prevention. However, evidence suggests a knowledge gap and a perceived peripheral role in AMS among nurses. To address this gap, educational initiatives, clear role definitions, and institutional support are essential. European and international examples demonstrate successful nurse integration, emphasising the need for collaborative networks and leadership development in the nursing profession. Overcoming professional hierarchies and socioeconomic barriers is vital. Integrating nurses into AMS enhances patient-centred care, optimises antimicrobial use, and strengthens the global fight against AMR, aligning with nursing's core values of quality and safety.

Keywords

Antimicrobial stewardship · Antimicrobial resistance · Nursing roles · Interprofessional collaboration · Healthcare education

E. Castro-Sánchez (✉)
Department of Infectious Diseases, Imperial College London, London, UK

Global Health Research Group, University of Balearic Islands, Palma de Mallorca, Spain
e-mail: e.castro-sanchez@imperial.ac.uk

12.1   Introduction

The complexity and ubiquity of drug-resistant infections, which are difficult and
sometimes impossible to treat and threaten the ecosphere, demand comprehensive,
multidisciplinary, and sustained international interventions because of their substantial clinical, economic, and societal impact [1]. The emergence and spread of
drug-resistant organisms have rendered many routinely used antimicrobial treatments ineffective, leading to prolonged illness, unnecessary suffering, increased
mortality, and escalating healthcare costs [2]. Many other interventions in modern
healthcare, such as surgery or oncotherapy, will be collateral victims of antimicrobial resistance (AMR), as antimicrobial prophylaxis is crucial in these areas.

12.2   Transdisciplinary Cooperation, Key to Address
         Antimicrobial Resistance

The complexity of AMR demands a multifaceted approach that integrates efforts from
various sectors, including healthcare, agriculture, environmental management and
policymaking. International collaboration and cooperation are paramount, as resistant
microorganisms do not respect geographical boundaries or national economic might.
Addressing AMR requires coordinated strategies for surveillance, research and development of new antimicrobials, implementation of stewardship programs, and public
awareness campaigns [3]. Moreover, the economic implications of AMR are profound
and will only increase, with projections suggesting significant reductions in the global
gross domestic product if AMR is left substantially unchecked [4]. This underscores
the urgency of sustained investment and action to mitigate the spread of AMR and
preserve the efficacy of existing antimicrobials for future generations.

12.2.1 Antimicrobial Stewardship, a Formidable Collaborative
         Against Antimicrobial Resistance

Antimicrobial stewardship (AMS) is central to combating AMR and comprises strategic interventions that promote the rational and prudent use of antimicrobials to
preserve their effectiveness and limit the emergence of resistance [5]. These objectives are achieved through multidisciplinary collaboration among infectious disease
specialists, clinical pharmacists, microbiologists, and other health care professionals. AMS initiatives encompass a wide range of activities, including the development of evidence-based guidelines for prescribing practices, implementation of
surveillance systems to monitor antimicrobial use and resistance patterns, and education of healthcare professionals and the public on the importance of responsible
antimicrobial use [6]. AMS programs also focus on improving diagnostic accuracy
to ensure that antimicrobials are prescribed only when necessary and that the most
appropriate agent is selected based on the specific pathogen and its susceptibility
profile [7].

12.2.2 Why Include Nurses in AMS Programs?

Historically, AMS programs have been physician-led or pharmacist-driven, with nurses frequently perceived as peripheral contributors [8]. The scale of the challenge presented by drug-resistant infections, the worldwide shortages of personnel such as physicians or pharmacists traditionally in charge of AMS programs, and the recognition that involving other healthcare professionals in these programs would benefit health systems while affording professional growth and expanding competencies. However, it is important to remember that healthcare workers are an extremely scarce asset worldwide. The World Health Organization warns that, in the next 15 years, the world will require approximately 13 million additional healthcare workers to maintain and increase health systems and services worldwide [9].

Nurses are not only the largest health professional group worldwide, but in many low- and middle-income settings, they represent a high proportion of healthcare professionals in relation to other clinicians, such as physicians or pharmacists, encouraging calls for their increased involvement and leadership in AMS programs [10]. These calls highlight many features of the nursing profession, work, and expertise which would be valuable in AMS. Nurses, with their continuous presence at the bedside and intimate knowledge of patient conditions, are uniquely positioned to play a crucial role in AMS. Their responsibilities in medication administration, patient education, and monitoring of treatment responses place them at the forefront of antimicrobial use and its consequences for patients. Furthermore, nurses plug gaps in communication between different healthcare team members, potentially compromising the coordinated approach necessary for successful AMS implementation [11].

12.3 Enhancing the Participation and Leadership of Nurses in AMS

Despite their numerical strength and extensive patient interactions, nursing involvement in AMS has traditionally been limited, characterised by intermittent and informal engagement rather than structured integration into AMS decision-making [12]. By effectively excluding or minimising nursing within and about AMS, healthcare systems and leaders miss out on valuable assets that could significantly improve antimicrobial and broader health outcomes. Early nurse participation in AMS was often narrowly focused on specific clinical tasks, such as ensuring the timely collection of microbiological specimens, accurate antimicrobial administration, educating patients and families regarding antimicrobial treatments and adherence, and infection prevention [13]. Although critical and necessary, these contributions were traditionally perceived as supplementary rather than core stewardship roles.

This wide range of clinical roles has been supplemented by others in areas such as education, leadership, and research related to AMS for nursing. For example, the surge in nurse prescribing worldwide has greatly leveraged the normalisation of nurse participation in AMS programmes [14], although prescribing powers are not yet the norm internationally. Evidence suggests that whenever nurses engage in antimicrobial prescribing, their performance in terms of adherence to clinical guidelines and resolution of clinical cases is of high quality [15], a recurring theme when examining how nurses perform in different spheres of AMS.

12.3.1 Barriers to the Participation of Nurses in AMS

Historically, nurses' involvement in AMS activities may have reflected prevailing views about stewardship as a medical responsibility focused on diagnostic decision-making and prescribing choices [16]. Stewardship was a matter of prescribing antibiotics and prescribing them well, a notion further entrenched by hierarchical professional dynamics within healthcare, where prescribing autonomy has typically rested on physicians and, to a lesser extent, other healthcare professionals, including nurses in very specific contexts and health systems [17]. As a result of these ideas, there may have been a significant gap in the integration of nursing expertise and perspectives in comprehensive AMS programs, potentially constraining the effectiveness and reach of these initiatives across healthcare settings, and also creating barriers to their further implementation and normalisation (Fig. 12.1).

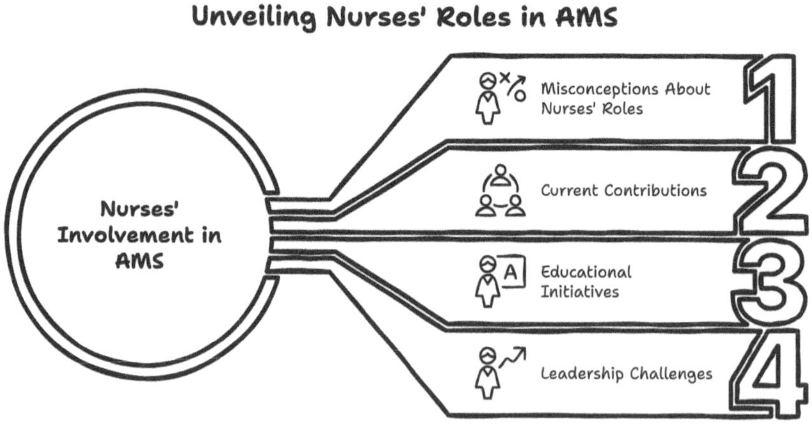

Fig. 12.1 Unveiling the involvement of nurses in AMS. (Author's own)

12.3.1.1 Stewardship Is not What Nurses Think They Should Do...

Integrating nurses into AMS programs requires a comprehensive approach that addresses multiple aspects of healthcare practice and education. It is clearly not a matter of just thinking that they should 'do' more AMS work. This integration should begin with challenging and correcting widespread internal and external misconceptions about the role of nurses in AMS, which often undervalue their potential contributions [12]. For example, studies conducted among healthcare workers worldwide have consistently highlighted the chasm in the familiarity and willingness of nurses to engage with AMS activities and programs relative to other professional groups [18], leading many nurses to believe that their role in AMS is and should remain peripheral or absent from AMS.

Such responses and hesitance to participate in stewardship programs may also simply reflect a frequent and perhaps unattractive narrative which allocates tasks such as reminding prescribers about the duration of antimicrobial courses or challenging inappropriate prescriptions [19]. These activities do not seem to be proposed in partnership or agreement with nurses, are not reflected in nurses' responsibilities in other clinical areas, and fail to recognise how they would expose nurses to uncomfortable experiences where gender, social status, education, professional tradition, and power imbalances may operate [20].

There may be a need to further consolidate the concept of AMS among nurses, tailored to their understanding and meaning of infection and infection management, and their expectations of contribution [21]. For now, at least, the AMS nomenclature may not contribute or help encourage nurses to participate in AMS activities. While nurses may understand that they ought to participate in the optimal management of antimicrobials, there could be benefit in promoting that AMS is way more than just offering the right antibiotic prescription (at the right time, dose, etc.), which is unlikely to be relevant to the broad corpus of nurses, and connect to contemporary views on, for example, infection prevention and control, where nurses have traditionally led interventions and programs, and where they have respect and recognition from other professions [22], promotion of vaccinations (which would prevent infection and thus reduce the need for antimicrobials), and the kind of socially conscious interventions highlighted in Chapters 15 and 16 in this volume. It may also be much more beneficial for AMS programs to stress how optimal nursing care is, by definition, the optimal use of antimicrobials, and how optimal use of antimicrobials is closely related to optimal nursing care [11].

12.3.1.2 Stewardship for Nurses: Do Not Do What I Say, but What I Do

The idea that more work is needed before nurses widely 'speak stewardship' is coupled, paradoxically, with the realisation that nurses already do much stewardship work, albeit this may be invisible to them and others or be embedded in much of the 'invisible nursing work' reported in other areas [23]. In addition to pivotal roles in activities fundamental to AMS objectives, including timely collection and management of microbiological specimens, accurate and timely antimicrobial administration, and patient education on antimicrobial therapies, or others such as advocating for the discontinuation of antimicrobial therapies when appropriate, studies worldwide have made clear how nurses can be seen leading AMS committees, developing and delivering education and continuous professional education and resources in AMS and infection, and contributing to point prevalence studies as well as other forms of research and quality improvement related to AMS [24].

It is encouraging to see that there is a growing body of literature reporting on nurse-specific and nurse-focused AMS interventions, which highlight how these infections can be highly impactful and effective by targeting classic nursing behaviours, such as improving hydration among long-term care residents and older patients [25], or improving the request for urinalysis or the performance of urine dipsticks which often results in prescribing behaviours driven by a misunderstanding about what a urinary tract infection is among nurses [26]. Overall, these interventions, which are often of low cost and complexity, achieve important results which are well sustained over time. These results should also encourage clinicians and researchers interested in engaging with nurses in AMS to start from what nurses routinely do and improve such performance before considering adding additional roles and actions, such as those mentioned before challenging prescriptions or reminding subscribers.

12.3.1.3 Nursing Education in AMS: More Content, Better Quality, and Increased Purpose

Educational initiatives targeting pre-registration and continuing professional education play a crucial role in bridging conceptual and operational gaps and reinforcing the alignment between nursing activities and AMS objectives [27]. Comprehensive education programs encompassing core AMS competencies —such as microbiology fundamentals, antimicrobial pharmacology, principles of infection prevention, and stewardship-specific interventions— have been developed gradually and increasingly, and once in place, they significantly enhance nurses' knowledge, self-efficacy, and active participation in AMS roles [28]. Initiatives such as interprofessional simulation training, interactive online modules, and serious games have been effective in improving nurses' competencies and confidence [29]. These innovations bolster clinical knowledge and cultivate essential communication and collaborative skills for effective nursing participation and leadership within interprofessional AMS teams [30].

The globalisation of nursing education and the increasing opportunities for collaboration and networking available for nurses worldwide may help mitigate the existing fragmentation and lack of cohesion within AMS nursing educational resources [31]. Additionally, the increasing number of conferences focused on AMS in nursing, including sessions relevant to AMS nursing, offers exciting opportunities to promote optimal interprofessional learning.

Furthermore, embedding AMS within nursing education, clinical practice standards, and institutional frameworks confers additional strategic benefits beyond improved stewardship. The formal recognition and integration of AMS competencies within professional standards empower nurses, enhancing their autonomy, clinical decision-making capabilities, and job satisfaction [32]. Institutional support for nurse-led stewardship encourages nurses' active involvement in policy formulation, clinical guideline development, and continuous quality improvement initiatives. Such structural embedding ensures the sustainability and scalability of AMS interventions, fostering resilient healthcare responses to AMR [30].

12.3.1.4 Leadership in AMS Nursing Across the World

In addition to this understanding of AMS issues with labels and concepts and educational gaps, a final challenge for the involvement of nurses in AMS is the lack of support from institutional and professional leaders for this nurse involvement. Perhaps due to the many other issues and problems affecting the nursing profession worldwide, from frustration about working conditions and burnout to workloads [33], it may simply be that developing competencies and roles related to AMS is not an opportunity and has not been prioritised by nursing leadership. It may also be too ambitious for a common view across health systems, countries, and traditions of the nursing profession regarding nurses' participation in AMS.

Successful European AMS nursing implementations demonstrate the benefits of both highly visible nurse consultant roles and broader educational initiatives that integrate AMS competencies across nursing cadres [34]. While nurse consultant roles significantly enhance AMS visibility and organisational commitment, broader professional role strategies yield sustained improvements in AMS practices and nursing capacity, highlighting the complementary nature of these approaches [35]. However, to implement these roles, it may be necessary to examine the status of vital determinants such as legal frameworks, codes of professional practice, and the views of other professional groups, who at times lobby for different depths or timings of implementation of nursing roles [36].

Furthermore, barriers to nursing AMS engagement reflect deeper structural issues, including professional hierarchies, interprofessional dynamics, and nurses' socioeconomic positioning within healthcare settings. To address these challenges, international collaborative networks have emerged as powerful tools for empowering nurses in AMS. The Brazilian Nurses Network Tackling Antimicrobial Resistance (REBRAN) [37] and the Nursing AMS Forum hosted by the British Society for Antimicrobial Chemotherapy (BSAC) exemplify successful initiatives that have bolstered nurse participation and leadership in antimicrobial stewardship.

Within Europe, numerous initiatives exemplify the successful integration of nursing roles within AMS frameworks. The UK's 'Start Smart then Focus' AMS toolkit illustrates core stewardship actions intrinsically linked to routine nursing care, such as the timely administration of antimicrobials, diligent specimen management, patient education, and infection prevention [38]. Additionally, educational programs, such as the Erasmus+ Intensive Programme on AMS, illustrate success-ful models for integrating AMS competencies across diverse European nursing cur-ricula. Organisations such as the European Specialist Nurses Organisation (ESNO) have pioneered nurse-focused AMS resources, significantly enhancing nurses' stewardship capacity and engagement [39].

These professional communities provide crucial platforms for nurses to share their experiences, best practices, and innovative strategies for AMS. By facilitating knowledge exchange, these networks enable nurses to develop expertise and confi-dence in their stewardship. Moreover, they serve as advocacy channels, amplifying nurses' voices in policy discussions and promoting the recognition of their vital contributions to AMS [40]. Through professional development opportunities, such as workshops, webinars, and mentorship programs, these communities equip nurses with the skills and knowledge necessary to overcome institutional barriers and assume leadership positions in stewardship programs.

12.3.2 Structural and Professional Enablers of Nursing Participation in AMS

Therefore, the successful integration of nurses into AMS depends heavily on culti-vating strong institutional and professional leadership, both within and outside the nursing profession. This involves creating supportive environments in which nurses are empowered to assume leadership roles in stewardship initiatives, leveraging their unique clinical expertise, patient advocacy skills, and leadership potential [41]. By recognising nurses as essential stakeholders rather than merely supportive per-sonnel, healthcare organisations can significantly enhance the effectiveness of their AMS programs. This approach not only aligns with nursing's fundamental values of patient-centred care, quality, and safety but also makes a substantial contribution to the global effort to combat AMR.

Nurses can also help address some of these challenges concerning support from leaders and decision makers. For example, many nursing leaders may have diffi-culty convincing policymakers and decision-makers of the need to develop and implement AMS nursing roles. This difficulty may stem from the fact that there is usually very limited, if any, available evidence about the return on investment of these emerging roles [42], particularly at a time when such role development may mean that generalist nursing cadres are further depleted. For example, the develop-ment of advanced practice in IPC and AMS, as highlighted in Chap. 11 of this vol-ume, may lead generalist nurses to lose some of their components, resulting in increased workloads and the risk of burnout. Therefore, it is vital that nurse research-ers and clinical academics ensure that data are available so that the evaluation of these roles in terms of impact and benefit does not just relate to their professional growth but includes hard outcomes which demonstrate value for money at the clini-cal, health system, and social levels.

It is encouraging to see how multiple nursing regulatory bodies and professional societies have embraced the participation of nurses in AMS, including national and international White Papers [43, 44] that not only highlight the need for nurses to engage in AMS but also indicate the expectations imposed by these regulatory bodies regarding such participation. For example, the Standards of Practice (2018) set by the Nursing and Midwifery Council in the UK provide a strong professional foundation for nursing involvement in AMS and infection management, even if not explicitly framed as such [45]. Key domains, such as pharmacology, evidence-based practice, and safe prescribing, underpin nurses' responsibilities in optimising antimicrobial use. Standards require nurses to understand the effects, contraindications, and adverse reactions of medicines (for example, 4.6) that directly support safe and rational antibiotic use. Moreover, the emphasis on person-centred care and health promotion (1.10) aligns with the broader goals of reducing infection risk and unnecessary antimicrobial exposure. Nurses are also expected to educate patients (4.8) and support self-management, which includes fostering adherence to and appropriate expectations about antibiotics. The standards also foreground interprofessional collaboration, leadership, and quality improvement (5.4, 6.5), which are essential for embedding AMS practices in health systems. Finally, the call to understand how providers work together (7.2) reinforces the multidisciplinary nature of the AMS. Collectively, these standards enable and arguably obligate nurses to play an active role in AMS. In essence, nurses should not have any difficulty justifying their participation in AMS efforts, at least from the perspective of regulatory bodies.

12.4   Recognising Context: Key Health System and Nursing Factors for Effective AMS Implementation

Calls to expand nursing roles in AMS must be grounded in a careful understanding of each health system's structural, professional, and cultural contexts. The success of AMS initiatives will depend not on the mere replication of idealised models but on the thoughtful adaptation of roles that align with local resources, regulatory frameworks, and the evolving identity of the nursing profession [16].

One possible model is the development of advanced practice nurses or nurse consultants specialising in AMS and IPC. Although these roles are likely to involve a small number of highly trained individuals per institution, they can have significant strategic visibility and catalyse institutional change through focused leadership, education, and clinical expertise. Their impact, though perhaps limited in scale, may signal a strong organisational commitment to stewardship and interprofessional collaboration. Alternatively, AMS principles can be embedded across the entire nursing workforce by integrating core competencies into daily clinical practice. This approach, while less visible externally, may have a broader systemic impact by transforming AMS into a routine element of nursing care. However, without formal recognition, these contributions risk being overlooked [35] (Fig. 12.2). Ultimately, tailoring stewardship roles to fit each context is not optional—it is essential for effectiveness, sustainability, and professional legitimacy.

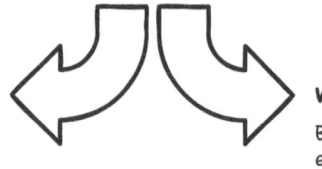

Potential approaches for deployment of AMS nursing roles

Advanced Practice Nurses
High visibility and strategic impact through specialized roles.

Workforce Integration
Broad systemic impact by embedding AMS into routine practice.

Fig. 12.2 Potential approaches for the deployment of AMS nursing roles. (Author's own)

12.5   Conclusion

Antimicrobial resistance is a defining challenge of our time that demands inclusive and contextually grounded responses. Antimicrobial stewardship remains central to this effort; however, its traditional frameworks have marginalised the profession that constitutes the largest share of the global health workforce: nursing. This oversight is not just a missed opportunity; it is a structural weakness in stewardship systems.

Nurses already contribute meaningfully to AMS through patient education, infection prevention, timely therapy administration, and care coordination. However, these contributions often remain invisible, unsupported, or unrecognised because of professional hierarchies, narrow definitions of stewardship, and conceptual disconnects. Integrating nurses into AMS must go beyond expanding tasks; it requires reframing stewardship to reflect nursing's values, expertise, and leadership. Implementation must be sensitive to the realities of each health system, avoiding prescriptive models in favour of flexible, scalable frameworks. Embedding AMS within routine nursing care and investing in visible leadership roles are not mutually exclusive; both are necessary and complementary.

Future research must evaluate the clinical and systemic impact of nursing roles in AMS, identifying not only cost-effectiveness but also cultural and professional facilitators. Without meaningful nursing participation, AMS will remain limited in scope and reach, and ultimately in its potential to mitigate drug-resistant infections.

References

1. O'Neill J. Tackling drug-resistant infections globally: final report and recommendations. Review on Antimicrobial Resistance. London: Wellcome Trust & HM Government; 2016.
2. Antimicrobial Resistance Collaborators. Global burden of bacterial antimicrobial resistance in 2019: a systematic analysis. Lancet. 2022;399(10325):629–55. https://doi.org/10.1016/S0140-6736(21)02724-0.
3. World Health Organization. Global action plan on antimicrobial resistance. Geneva: WHO; 2015.

4. Jonas O, Irwin A, Berthe FCJ, Le Gall FG, Marquez PV. Drug-resistant infections: a threat to our economic future. Washington, DC: World Bank; 2017.
5. Dyar OJ, Huttner B, Schouten J, Pulcini C. What is antimicrobial stewardship? Clin Microbiol Infect. 2017;23(11):793–8. https://doi.org/10.1016/j.cmi.2017.08.026.
6. Howard P, Pulcini C, Hara GL, West RM, Gould IM, Harbarth S, et al. An international cross-sectional survey of antimicrobial stewardship programmes in hospitals. J Antimicrob Chemother. 2015;70(4):1245–55. https://doi.org/10.1093/jac/dku497.
7. Barlam TF, Cosgrove SE, Abbo LM, MacDougall C, Schuetz AN, Septimus EJ, et al. Implementing an antibiotic stewardship program: guidelines by the Infectious Diseases Society of America and the Society for Healthcare Epidemiology of America. Clin Infect Dis. 2016;62(10):e51–77. https://doi.org/10.1093/cid/ciw118.
8. Charani E, Ahmad R, Tarrant C, Birgand G, Leather A, Møller MH, et al. Opportunities for system-level improvement in antibiotic decision making: a qualitative study of the experiences of junior doctors across 3 hospitals in England. BMJ Open. 2021;11(4):e041303. https://doi.org/10.1136/bmjopen-2020-041303.
9. World Health Organization. Global strategy on human resources for health: workforce 2030. Geneva: WHO; 2016.
10. International Council of Nurses. The role of nurses in tackling antimicrobial resistance. Geneva: ICN; 2019.
11. Olans RN, Olans RD, DeMaria A Jr. The critical role of the staff nurse in antimicrobial stewardship – unrecognized, but already there. Clin Infect Dis. 2016;62(1):84–9. https://doi.org/10.1093/cid/civ697.
12. Reeves S, Bader J, Fournier K, Kent F, Wagner SJ. Antimicrobial stewardship: a qualitative study of the perspectives of nurses and infection prevention staff. Am J Infect Control. 2020;48(5):492–7. https://doi.org/10.1016/j.ajic.2019.09.007.
13. Fowler T, Conway S, Zarb P, Roca I, Hernández-Santiago V, Monnet DL, et al. Driving forward antimicrobial stewardship: the role of nurses and the midwifery community. J Antimicrob Chemother. 2016;71(11):3225–6. https://doi.org/10.1093/jac/dkw361.
14. Kleinpell R, Scanlon A, Hibbert D, Ganz F, East L, Fraser D, et al. Addressing issues impacting advanced nursing practice worldwide. Online J Issues Nurs. 2014;19(2):5. https://doi.org/10.3912/OJIN.Vol19No02Man05.
15. Brett J, Fitzpatrick R, Waring J. The role of advanced nurse practitioners in antimicrobial stewardship: a scoping review. J Hosp Infect. 2022;119:52–61. https://doi.org/10.1016/j.jhin.2021.10.015.
16. Charani E, Smith I, Skodvin B, Perozziello A, Lucet JC, Arnoldo L, et al. Investigating the cultural and contextual determinants of antimicrobial stewardship programmes across low-, middle- and high-income countries – a qualitative study. PLoS One. 2019;14(1):e0209847. https://doi.org/10.1371/journal.pone.0209847.
17. Tarrant C, Krockow EM, Nakkawita WMID, Colman AM. Moral and contextual dimensions of "inappropriate" antibiotic prescribing in secondary care: a three-country interview study. Front Sociol. 2020;5:7. https://doi.org/10.3389/fsoc.2020.00007.
18. Kpokiri EE, Bowles T, Allan L, Mohomed I, Bal AM, Cumpston M, et al. Perceptions and attitudes of healthcare workers towards antimicrobial stewardship: a systematic review and thematic analysis. JAC Antimicrob Resist. 2020;2(3):dlaa092. https://doi.org/10.1093/jacamr/dlaa092.
19. Castro-Sánchez E, Bennasar-Veny M, Smith M, Singleton S, Bennett E, Appleton J, et al. European Commission guidelines for the prudent use of antimicrobials in human health: a missed opportunity to embrace nursing participation in stewardship. Clin Microbiol Infect. 2018;24(8):914–5. https://doi.org/10.1016/j.cmi.2018.02.030.
20. Broom A, Broom J, Kirby E, Scambler G. Antimicrobials and the social: an interdisciplinary analysis of the problem of antimicrobial resistance. Glob Public Health. 2017;12(4):512–26. https://doi.org/10.1080/17441692.2016.1185319.
21. Blackburn J, et al. What is the knowledge, perceptions, and experiences of nurses regarding antimicrobial stewardship? A systematic review. Wound Pract Res. 2025;33(1)

22. Naughton C, Ellis J, Kearney P, Healy P, Doody O. Nurses' views of their role in antimicrobial stewardship within an acute healthcare setting. J Clin Nurs. 2020;29(1–2):138–50. https://doi.org/10.1111/jocn.15070.

23. Bos M, Schouten J, De Bot C, Vermeulen H, Hulscher M. A hidden gem in multidisciplinary antimicrobial stewardship: a systematic review on bedside nurses' activities in daily practice regarding antibiotic use. JAC Antimicrob Resist. 2023;5(6):dlad123. https://doi.org/10.1093/jacamr/dlad123.

24. Bulabula ANH, Jenkins A, Mehtar S, Namahoro D, Mshana SE, Jentsch U, et al. Practical implementation of antimicrobial stewardship programmes in Africa: a systematic review. JAC Antimicrob Resist. 2020;2(3):dlaa070. https://doi.org/10.1093/jacamr/dlaa070.

25. Crayton E, Richardson M, Fuller C, Smith G, Liu S, Forbes G, et al. Interventions to improve appropriate antibiotic prescribing in long-term care facilities: a systematic review. BMC Geriatr. 2020;20(1):1–19. https://doi.org/10.1186/s12877-020-01803-5.

26. van Buul LW, van der Steen JT, Doncker SM, Achterberg WP, Schellevis FG, Veenhuizen RB, et al. Factors influencing antibiotic prescribing in long-term care facilities: a qualitative in-depth study. BMC Geriatr. 2014;14:136. https://doi.org/10.1186/1471-2318-14-136.

27. Courtenay M, Castro-Sánchez E, Fitzpatrick M, Gallagher R, Lim R, Weiss M. Developing consensus-based antimicrobial stewardship competencies for UK undergraduate health-care professional education. J Hosp Infect. 2019;103(3):244–50. https://doi.org/10.1016/j.jhin.2019.06.021.

28. Timen A, van de Sande-Bruinsma N, van der Hoek W, Voeten HA, Lie-A-Huen L, van Dissel JT. Educational programs to enhance nursing staff's knowledge and attitudes regarding anti-biotic use and resistance: a systematic review. J Hosp Infect. 2020;105(3):355–64. https://doi.org/10.1016/j.jhin.2020.04.014.

29. Seo M, Park H. Effects of simulation-based education for nursing students: a systematic review and meta-analysis. Nurse Educ Today. 2022;112:105327. https://doi.org/10.1016/j.nedt.2022.105327.

30. Monsees E, Goldman J, Popejoy L. Staff nurses as antimicrobial stewards: an integra-tive literature review. Am J Infect Control. 2017;45(8):917–22. https://doi.org/10.1016/j.ajic.2017.04.004.

31. Pulcini C, Binda F, Lamkang AS, Trett A, Charani E, Goff DA, et al. Developing core ele-ments and checklist items for global hospital antimicrobial stewardship programmes: a consensus approach. Clin Microbiol Infect. 2021;27(5):692–8. https://doi.org/10.1016/j.cmi.2020.11.024.

32. Naughton C, Prior M, McLaughlin E, O'Donnell C, Chambers D, Killen M, et al. Antimicrobial stewardship: the role of the nurse and the nurse prescriber in the UK. Br J Community Nurs. 2021;26(6):278–84. https://doi.org/10.12968/bjcn.2021.26.6.278.

33. Shah MK, Gandrakota N, Cimiotti JP, Ghose N, Moore M, Ali MK. Prevalence of and factors associated with nurse burnout in the US. JAMA Health Forum. 2021;2(10):e212395. https://doi.org/10.1001/jamahealthforum.2021.2395.

34. Sneddon J, Gilchrist M, Wickens HJ, Brennan L, Chaves RL, Gil-Navarro MV, et al. Development and impact of a competency framework for educational development in antimi-crobial stewardship. J Antimicrob Chemother. 2016;71(10):2978–89. https://doi.org/10.1093/jac/dkw301.

35. Castro-Sánchez E, Gilchrist M, Ahmad R, Courtenay M, Bosanquet J, Holmes AH. Nurse roles in antimicrobial stewardship: lessons from public sectors models of acute care service delivery in the United Kingdom. Antimicrob Resist Infect Control. 2019;8:162. https://doi.org/10.1186/s13756-019-0621-4.

36. Turale S, Klopper HC, Coetzee SK. Global nursing: what the COVID-19 pandemic has revealed. Int J Nurs Stud. 2022;128:104324. https://doi.org/10.1016/j.ijnurstu.2022.104324.

37. da Silva RMC, Monteiro CCF, Moura ML, da Costa BA, Tavares CMM, Secoli SR. The role of the Brazilian Network of Nurses and Patient Safety Researchers and the Brazilian Nurses Network Tackling Antimicrobial Resistance (REBRAN) in promoting antimicrobial steward-ship. Rev Lat Am Enfermagem. 2023;31:e3952. https://doi.org/10.1590/1518-8345.6021.3952.

38. Public Health England. Start smart – then focus: Antimicrobial stewardship toolkit for English hospitals. London: PHE; 2015. https://www.gov.uk/government/publications/antimicrobial-stewardship-start-smart-then-focus

39. European Specialist Nurses Organisation (ESNO). The role of specialist nurses in antimicrobial resistance and prevention of infection: a guide for nurses and stakeholders. Brussels: ESNO; 2021. https://www.esno.org/assets/files/AMR/AMR-booklet-ESNO-2021.pdf

40. Ritchie H, McIntyre L, Rotter T, MacDonald MB. Interprofessional collaboration and nurses' involvement in antimicrobial stewardship: a scoping review. J Clin Nurs. 2022;31(7–8):823–34. https://doi.org/10.1111/jocn.16057.

41. Broom J, Broom A, Kirby E. Cultivating hospital antibiotic prescribing: the role of interprofessional relationships and team dynamics. Qual Health Res. 2019;29(4):504–16. https://doi.org/10.1177/1049732318806201.

42. Monsees EA, Popejoy L, Jackson MA, Lee B. Integrating staff nurses in antimicrobial stewardship: opportunities, barriers, and a call to action. Jt Comm J Qual Patient Saf. 2020;46(7):381–7. https://doi.org/10.1016/j.jcjq.2020.02.003.

43. Royal College of Nursing (RCN). Antimicrobial resistance: RCN position on the essential role of nursing staff in antimicrobial stewardship. London: RCN; 2017. https://www.rcn.org.uk/professional-development/publications/rcn-antimicrobial-resistance-uk-position-001-268

44. American Nurses Association (ANA). Redefining the Antibiotic Stewardship Team: Recommendations from the American Nurses Association/Centers for Disease Control and Prevention Workgroup on the Role of Registered Nurses in Hospital Antibiotic Stewardship Practices. Silver Spring: ANA; 2017. https://www.nursingworld.org/practice-policy/advocacy/state/nurses-role-in-antimicrobial-stewardship/

45. Nursing and Midwifery Council. Future nurse: Standards of proficiency for registered nurses. London: NMC; 2018. https://www.nmc.org.uk/standards/standards-for-nurses/standards-of-proficiency-for-registered-nurses/

Nurses Leadership in IPC, AMS, and Vaccination Programmes

13

Tihana Gašpert and Julie Storr ⓘ

Abstract

Effective leadership is a cornerstone of high-quality healthcare, particularly evident in infection prevention and control (IPC), antimicrobial stewardship (AMS), and vaccination programmes. Nurses play a pivotal role in these areas, leveraging their expertise in patient education, advocacy, and interdisciplinary collaboration. Strong nursing leadership supports the implementation of evidence-based IPC practices, improves vaccine uptake, and addresses community-specific needs to combat the challenges posed by antimicrobial resistance and healthcare-associated infections. This chapter explores the integral role of nursing leadership in IPC, AMS, and vaccination efforts, emphasizing its impact on safeguarding public health.

Keywords

Nurses · Leadership · Infection prevention and control · Antimicrobial stewardship · Vaccination programmes

T. Gašpert (✉)
University Hospital Rijeka, Rijeka, Croatia

Faculty of Health Sciences, University of Maribor, Maribor, Slovenia

J. Storr
CEO & Cofounder KS Healthcare Consulting Past President Infection Prevention Society, UK & Ireland, London, UK

13.1   Introduction

Good leadership has been described as one of the prerequisites for the achievement of high-quality healthcare [1]. As each of the chapters in this book attest, infection prevention and control (IPC) plays a crucial contribution to the overall quality of healthcare delivery. To optimize this contribution, the ability to influence and persuade—to lead, is fundamental for all aspects of IPC, from the establishment of IPC programmes themselves, through to the implementation of guidelines at the point of care. Leadership is a key determinant of healthcare quality. In infection prevention and control (IPC), antimicrobial stewardship (AMS), and vaccination efforts, nurses act as central figures, applying their expertise to guide best practices and improve patient outcomes. The International Council of Nurses succinctly summarized this in their statement to the World Health Assembly in 2022 [2]: "Nurses play a crucial role in educating patients and their families, leading IPC teams and initiatives, and supporting the multidisciplinary team to apply IPC principles and best practices across health care settings, including efforts to combat antimicrobial resistance." This chapter will explore leadership in the context of IPC, antimicrobial stewardship (AMS) and vaccination programmes. It will reflect on what good leadership is and why it is important, with a focus on nurses' leadership.

Nursing leadership plays a pivotal role in the success of vaccination programmes, serving as a cornerstone for public health initiatives. As trusted healthcare providers, nurses bring unique skills in education, advocacy, and community engagement, which are essential for improving vaccine uptake and addressing vaccine hesitancy. Effective nursing leadership ensures the seamless coordination of resources, fosters interdisciplinary collaboration, and adapts strategies to meet diverse community needs. By leveraging their clinical expertise and leadership capabilities, nurses can drive the implementation of equitable and efficient vaccination programmes that safeguard public health.

13.2   Nurses Leadership in IPC and AMS

When considering the relationship between leadership, nursing, and IPC it is important not to overlook patient-related factors, which undoubtedly play a role in whether or not a healthcare-associated infection (HAI) occurs and its severity. However, HAIs are also influenced by a complex combination of many additional factors, and this is where leadership, particularly nurse leadership, comes into play [3]. These factors include (not exclusively):

- Policies and guidelines and their implementation.
- The infrastructure and systems that enable the right practices at the right time.
- Organizational culture including values.
- Knowledge, attitude, and skill of the health workforce.
- Effective measurement and feedback.

- Advocacy and communications for IPC as a force for good.
- Health worker behaviour (influenced by all of the preceding factors).

With these factors in mind, the available competency frameworks, discussed in more detail in the next section, make reference to the importance of role models and champions as this relates to implementation. The potential role of nurses as champions and influencers of best practice has been described, particularly in relation to hand hygiene improvement [4].

Effective IPC leadership transforms efforts to prevent and control infection from a theoretical solution to an evidence-based strategy for reducing HAIs. Nurse leaders, through advocacy, education, and implementation of best practices, play a key role in ensuring IPC measures lead to tangible patient safety improvements. Those who influence IPC at every level of the health system, including nurse leaders, therefore play an important role in changing behaviours, influencing practice, and improving health care. Nurses therefore play a central role in the prevention of infection, including efforts to tackle antimicrobial resistance, influenced not least by their constant presence and interaction in the lives of those who access care [5]. Building on this premise, the International Council of Nurses highlighted the leadership role of nurses in activities to combat AMR, including leading IPC teams and initiatives, and supporting the multidisciplinary team to apply IPC principles and best practices [6]. When considering antimicrobial stewardship (AMS), the nursing workforce has been described as a "potential AMS powerhouse" [7]. However, Castro-Sanchez goes on to highlight ongoing concerns that nurses remain underutilized in AMS efforts and face multiple barriers to greater AMS engagement, including lack of role clarity, inadequate education, hierarchical cultures limiting their autonomy, and failure to meaningfully involve them in stewardship leadership and decision-making [8].

Drilling deeper into the precise contribution warrants an exploration of the different elements of IPC programmes as they relate to nurse's leadership. This is important due to the ubiquity of the nursing workforce and indeed some authors have referred to nurses and those who lead them as the last layer in the Swiss Cheese Model [9].

13.2.1 Leadership and the Building Blocks of IPC Programmes

The World Health Organization (WHO) outlines the building blocks or core components that are required for effective IPC within their evidence-based guidelines [10]. Occupying a central role is an IPC programme itself, a programme that is integrated and aligned with other relevant programmes including those focused on AMS. In parallel, there should be an environment that supports health workers to do the right thing, including addressing workforce capacity, overcrowding, and a hygienic environment, infrastructure, and materials that facilitate IPC practices. These components are complemented by evidence-based guidelines and policies, training and education including simulation, surveillance systems locally and nationally, monitoring of IPC practices and timely feedback. Surrounding all of this, the WHO recommends a multimodal strategy to support behaviour at the point of care. As a minimum, the WHO guidance states that at the level of secondary and tertiary health care facilities chief nurses, together with other professionals, have a critical role in the decision to establish the minimum requirements of an IPC programme [11]. A recent global report highlights the ongoing challenges and gaps in achieving these IPC core components in all regions, with lack of leadership emphasized as a specific gap [12].

13.2.2 Leadership and IPC Competence

As Storr previously articulated, both the published literature and international guidance in relation to IPC reveals a number of relevant and interesting insights on leadership, including on what is meant by "good leadership" [13]. Factors such as effective communication and persuasion were highlighted as critical skills together with instilling respect and trust. In many instances in healthcare IPC decision-making and guidance falls under the purview of the nursing profession, since nurses continue to form the largest group fulfilling these roles, although this is changing. In addition, given that nurses form the largest percentage of the overall health workforce, nurses play a central role in the implementation of IPC practices at the point of care [14]. It is clear that nurses provide professional leadership of IPC programmes and are uniquely positioned with the knowledge, skills, and attributes to direct effective infection control practices and policies within their healthcare settings [15]. Competence is therefore an important leadership consideration.

Across the globe, a number of entities have developed IPC competences. The WHO's core competences were informed by a number of regional, national, and professional society competences [16]. Their target audience are those in charge of (or participating in) IPC programmes at the national, sub-national, or facility level and explicitly are targeted at IPC and AMR focal points, IPC officers, link persons, and diverse professionals participating in IPC programme activities. In light of the fact that since its origins in the 1960s, IPC in almost all countries saw the role of infection preventionists filled by nurses, these competences tend to be of significant relevance to the nursing profession, although more recently there has been an expansion to other disciplines [17]. IPC programme management and leadership is one of 16 core competencies described by the WHO. Within this domain, the use of management strategies and leadership for planning and operationalizing of an IPC programme and/or teams is addressed. It includes the need to develop competence in relation to cost-benefit and feasibility considerations, the development or adaptation and implementation of evidence-based IPC guidelines, standard operating protocols (SOPs), training resources, and monitoring/audit tools; the organization and provision of training and education for health workers; and the undertaking of monitoring and feedback activities of adherence with guideline recommendations. Furthermore, the use of data and evidence for decision-making is highlighted together with the use of leadership and communication skills to interact with teams, senior management, health workers, patients and families, and other audiences. The WHO suggests that leaders empower others to develop, implement, and evaluate their own solutions to problems [16].

The European Centre for Disease Prevention and Control (ECDC) published their IPC competences in 2013 [18] in which the importance of leadership is articulated for both the junior and more experienced infection preventionists, in relation to the formulation of IPC indicators, leadership towards a shared vision of IPC and a cohesive work ethos, the organization and leadership of regular reviews of policies and procedures in collaboration with multidisciplinary experts and leadership and support for other stakeholders, such as health care workers, consumers, and consumer groups to establish and evaluate the infection control aspects of quality and patient safety programmes.

13.2.3 What the Literature Has to Say on leadership, Nursing, and IPC

Historically, there has been a dearth of literature specifically focused on leadership and IPC through a nursing lens; however, this is changing. There is some merit to be had in looking at the influence of leaders per se on the implementation of efforts related to improving the quality of health service delivery, acknowledging that IPC is one part of this jigsaw puzzle [19–21]. The wider literature will be briefly touched upon before turning attention to available publications on leadership, nurse leaders, and IPC.

A report in 2018 by the WHO, OECD, and the World Bank [1] emphasized that the key ingredient in influencing a culture of continuous quality improvement is consistency of leadership from governments, policy makers, clinical leaders, health system managers and civil society "this does not require a high level of resources – it rather requires investment in a culture shift towards transparency for continuing improvement." Frenk suggests that one of the most complex challenges in health systems is to nurture people (leaders) who can develop the strategic vision, technical knowledge, political skills, and ethical orientation to lead the complex processes of policy formulation and implementation and goes on to state that "without leaders, even the best designed systems will fail" [22]. Fillingham et al. emphasized that effective leadership in complex systems is not solely an attribute of "top bosses", but can be best understood as "a shared process of many 'small' (and great) leaders working together with empowered followers to get things done in the context of a shared understanding of local needs". Using such a lens—these authors state that if the problem exists at the level of the system, then logically the solutions will not be exclusively at the level of the individual. This is an important consideration for IPC, IPC leadership, and nursing leadership therein. In other words, leadership development must focus on systems, including incentives and organizational relationships, as well as individuals [23].

In their multisite study, Saint et al. explored the importance of leadership in preventing HAI and found that successful IPC leaders cultivated a culture of clinical excellence and were focused on overcoming barriers, including effective strategies for tackling resistance to change and improvement [24]. Furthermore, effective leaders were found to be inspirational. They thought strategically while acting locally and were political - leveraging their personal prestige to move initiatives forward and form partnerships across disciplines. Strong leadership from IPC professionals was emphasized by participants in a UK Health Foundation study as a prerequisite for effective organizational IPC [25]. Furthermore, significant emphasis was placed on the necessity for frontline clinicians to assume ownership and leadership of IPC initiatives. A critical insight was that IPC leadership must be distributed across the organization, with clinical champions identified in all departments. This approach was deemed particularly important due to the constant tension at the point of care between addressing immediate priorities and adhering to routine best practices. The report highlights the necessity for IPC practitioners—who predominantly remain nurses—to demonstrate both robust and influential leadership. Additionally, they must serve as effective mentors, fostering empowerment among others to take ownership of IPC practices. Gould et al. [26] further highlight the importance of distributed leadership [26]. The authors review some the available literature on leadership and IPC and highlight how IPC leadership can be provided by staff at the front line of patient care as well as across other levels of healthcare, but that IPC expertise is important to legitimize this leadership. It reflects on the notion of formal and informal or spontaneous leadership.

Gould et al. [26] also emphasize the significance of distributed leadership in IPC. The authors review existing literature on leadership within the context of IPC and underscore that leadership can be effectively exercised by frontline staff as well as individuals operating at various levels of the healthcare system. However, they note that IPC expertise is essential for legitimizing such leadership roles. Additionally, the discussion highlights the distinction between formal leadership roles and informal or spontaneous leadership initiatives.

Mugomeri identified weak leadership and inadequate IPC governance as significant barriers to the effectiveness of IPC committees [27]. The findings emphasize a strong association between leadership competence and the success of IPC programmes, reinforcing the critical role of leadership in achieving effective IPC. Effective leadership is recognized as essential for capacity building, enhancing decision-making processes, and fostering positive interpersonal relationships among healthcare workers. Additionally, leadership is highlighted as crucial at the policy level, ensuring the establishment of robust policies and guidelines to support the implementation of national IPC programmes and the strengthening of national surveillance systems. Landerfelt et al. have also emphasized that effective nurse leaders play a pivotal role in fostering work environments that promote a culture of safety [28]. Their findings indicated that enhancements in leadership were associated with a reduction in catheter-associated urinary tract infections (CAUTIs), thereby reinforcing prior research suggesting that effective nurse leaders establish environments that provide nurses with the necessary resources to support IPC practices.

13.3   Nurses Leadership in Vaccination Programmes

Nurses are perpetually regarded with trust by the public [29]; interactions between nurses and patients have been demonstrated to impact patients' decision-making and care experiences, while nurses' perspectives and endorsements regarding vaccination can significantly affect patients' vaccination rates [30, 31]. Nurses are at the forefront of healthcare, engaging closely with patients daily, and are essential in educating, administering, monitoring, managing, and occasionally prescribing vaccinations, possessing practical insights and experiences regarding vaccination hesitancy. Nurses have a vital role in advocating for and facilitating immunizations, significantly impacting the increase in vaccine uptake for diseases such as human papillomavirus, measles, mumps, rubella, and influenza [32]. Nursing professionals leverage their community positioning and daily interactions with users and patients across various settings to educate vaccine recipients, enhance public awareness, and directly administer vaccines, a significant endeavor to achieve extensive coverage swiftly [33, 34]. Similar to previous vaccination initiatives, nurses are responsible for ensuring the proper handling, storage, and safe administration of vaccines, while also playing a pivotal role in promoting vaccination and assisting in the design and execution of effective campaigns [33, 34].

Nurses have been uniquely positioned during the COVID-19 pandemic to utilize various scientific knowledge essential for accessing vulnerable populations, particularly those encountering obstacles to vaccine reception [35].

Nurses are essential stakeholders in mass vaccination campaigns, and their insights are crucial for success. Their evidence-informed knowledge is unique among healthcare professionals, stemming from their diverse roles as providers, care team members, care coordinators, primary patient contacts, health promotion communicators, and educators [36]. Incorporating their evidence-informed knowledge, insights, and perspectives is vital for guiding policy discussions during critical healthcare decision-making processes [37].

In 2018, the International Council of Nursing, supported by Pfizer, conducted a survey to assess nursing participation in immunization initiatives across 15 OECD countries [31]. The results revealed that only 3 of the 15 countries (20%) demonstrated exemplary nurse engagement in immunization roles, 8 (53%) were categorized as expanding, and 4 (27%) were classified as emerging [31]. There are numerous obstacles to the engagement of nursing and nursing leadership in the mass immunization initiatives. The findings can be classified into four primary themes: (1) absence of voice, acknowledgement, and valuation, (2) employment-related obstacles, (3) dispersal of responsibility and authority, (4) supply and accessibility challenges [37]. Therefore, it is imperative to conduct education to enhance nurses' understanding and attitudes regarding immunizations [38].

Nurses are essential leaders in vaccination programmes, with responsibilities that include administration, strategic planning, education, and fostering public trust. Their leadership comprises of the following:

- Storage: Nurses guarantee vaccinations are maintained under ideal settings to preserve efficacy, consistently monitoring equipment and rectifying temperature fluctuations.
- Education and Advocacy: They disseminate precise vaccine information to mitigate hesitation and enhance public confidence. Nurses, as trusted experts, are optimally situated to combat disinformation and facilitate informed decision-making.
- Policy: Nurses frequently participate in committees to influence immunization policies, promoting equity and efficacy. Their observations inform national policy regarding training, resource distribution, and immunization timelines.
- Programme Implementation: Nurses spearhead immunization campaigns, formulate protocols, evaluate hazards, oversee administration, and guarantee follow-up care. Their participation in data analysis and community engagement has been associated with increased vaccination rates.

By consolidating these roles, nurses not only augment vaccine administration but also strengthen the health system's ability to oversee extensive vaccination initiatives [34, 39].

13.4   Conclusion

Considering the future, on behalf of the Crystal Ball Initiative, published the findings of a survey of international IPC experts who considered the various desirable skills that might be required among IPC personnel in the future [40]. The following were highlighted: first-hand clinical experience (nursing, medicine), epidemiology, microbiology, data science, implementation and behaviour science, leadership, project management, organizational management, and complexity science to communication and marketing skills. The authors reflected on this long list of skills that would be required to future-proof IPC for the 2030s and beyond and highlighted the challenge that healthcare institutions would face to integrate all of this required expertise. Although leadership was listed as just one of the range of skills, based on the literature explored in this chapter leadership will be pivotal for effective IPC, AMS, and vaccination programmes that will contribute to high-quality healthcare and the sustainability of these programmes and their associated interventions in the future.

Nursing leadership is indispensable in achieving the goals of vaccination programmes. Through their commitment to patient care and health promotion, nurse leaders advocate for evidence-based practices, address vaccine access disparities, and build community trust. Their leadership not only enhances programme effectiveness but also reinforces the role of nursing as a central pillar of public health. As vaccination programs continue to evolve, empowering nurse leaders will remain critical to achieving a healthier and more resilient society.

Literature

1. World Health Organization. Delivering Quality health services: a global imperative. OECD; 2018.
2. International Council of Nurses. Statement to the eventy-fifth World Health Assembly: Provisional agenda item 14.6. 2022. Infection Prevention and control https://www.icn.ch/sites/default/files/2023-05/WHA75_item%2014.6_ICN%20statement%20IPC.pdf Accessed January 15 2025. ICoNSttS-fWHAPaiIpac.
3. Storr J. New Zealand Phoenix Rising National Conference (invited international keynote speaker). 2019.
4. Sopirala MM, Yahle-Dunbar L, Smyer J, Wellington L, Dickman J, Zikri N, et al. Infection control link nurse program: an interdisciplinary approach in targeting health care-acquired infection. Am J Infect Control. 2014;42(4):353–9.
5. Edwards R, Drumright L, Kiernan M, Holmes A. Covering more territory to fight resistance: considering nurses' role in antimicrobial stewardship. J Infect Prev. 2011;12(1):6–10.
6. International Council of Nurses. Position statement: antimicrobial resistance. 2017. https://www.icn.ch/sites/default/files/inline-files/ICN_PS_Antimicrobial_resistance.pdf. Accessed 11 Feb 2025.
7. Sartelli M, Coccolini F, Catena F, Pagani L. Global Infection prevention and management in healthcare. 2024.
8. Castro-Sánchez E, Bosanquet J, Courtenay M, Gallagher R, Gotterson F, Manias E, et al. Nurse: an underused vital asset against drug-resistant infections. Lancet. 2022;400:10354.
9. Perneger TV. The Swiss cheese model of safety incidents: are there holes in the metaphor? BMC Health Serv Res. 2005;5:1–7.
10. Storr J, Twyman A, Zingg W, Damani N, Kilpatrick C, Reilly J, et al. Core components for effective infection prevention and control programmes: new WHO evidence-based recommendations. Antimicrob Resist Infect Control. 2017;6:1–18.
11. Minimum requirements for infection prevention and control programmes. Geneva: World Health Organization; 2019. https://apps.who.int/iris/handle/10665/330080. Accessed 11 Feb 2025.
12. World Health Organization. Strategic framework for enhancing prevention and control of mpox 2024–2027. World Health Organization; 2024.
13. Elliott P, Storr J, Jeanes A. Infection prevention and control: a social science perspective. CRC Press; 2023.
14. Storr J, Kilpatrick C, Seale H. The relevance of nursing to the achievement of person-centered infection prevention and control. J Res Nurs. 2024;17449871241281437
15. Macbeth D, Viengkham C, Shaban RZ. Credentialling in Australia for infection prevention and control: Philosophy, principles and practice. Infect Dis Health. 2025;30(1):61–73.
16. Core competencies for infection prevention and control professionals. Geneva: World Health Organization; 2020. https://apps.who.int/iris/handle/10665/335821. Accessed 11 Feb 2025.
17. Billings C, Bernard H, Caffery L, Dolan SA, Donaldson J, Kalp E, et al. Advancing the profession: an updated future-oriented competency model for professional development in infection prevention and control. Am J Infect Control. 2019;47(6):602–14.
18. Brusaferro S, Cookson B, Kalenic S, Cooper T, Fabry J, Gallagher R, et al. Training infection control and hospital hygiene professionals in Europe, 2010: agreed core competencies among 33 European countries. Eurosurveillance. 2014;19(49)
19. Amelung V, Stein V, Goodwin N, Balicer R, Nolte E, Suter E. Handbook integrated care. Springer; 2021.
20. Aarons GA, Green AE, Trott E, Willging CE, Torres EM, Ehrhart MG, et al. The roles of system and organizational leadership in system-wide evidence-based intervention sustainment: a mixed-method study. Admin Pol Ment Health. 2016;43:991–1008.

21. Peterson E, Dwyer J, Howze-Shiplett M, Davison C, Wilson K, Noykhovich E. Presence of leadership and management in global health programs: compendium of case studies. Washington DC: The George Washington University; 2011.
22. Frenk J. The global health system: strengthening national health systems as the next step for global progress. PLoS Med. 2010;7(1):e1000089.
23. Fillingham D, Weir B. System leadership: lessons and learning from AQuA's integrated care discovery communities. 2014.
24. Saint S, Kowalski CP, Banaszak-Holl J, Forman J, Damschroder L, Krein SL. The importance of leadership in preventing healthcare-associated infection: results of a multisite qualitative study. Infect Control Hosp Epidemiol. 2010;31(9):901–7.
25. Health Foundation. Infection prevention and control: lessons from acute care in England: towards a whole health economy approach. Health Foundation; 2015.
26. Gould D, Gallagher R, Allen D. Leadership and management for infection prevention and control: what do we have and what do we need? Elsevier; 2016. p. 165–8.
27. Mugomeri E. The efficacy of infection prevention and control committees in Lesotho: a qualitative study. Am J Infect Control. 2018;46(3):e13–e7.
28. Landerfelt PE, Lewis A, Li Y, Cimiotti JP. Nursing leadership and the reduction of catheter-associated urinary tract infection. Am J Infect Control. 2020;48(12):1546–8.
29. Kieft RA, de Brouwer BB, Francke AL, Delnoij DM. How nurses and their work environment affect patient experiences of the quality of care: a qualitative study. BMC Health Serv Res. 2014;14:1–10.
30. Hill MC, Salmon D, Chudleigh J, Aitken LM. Practice nurses' perceptions of their immunization role and strategies used to promote measles, mumps, and rubella vaccine uptake in 2014–2018: a qualitative study. J Adv Nurs. 2021;77(2):948–56.
31. Bajnok I, Shamian J, Catton H, Hons E, Skinner T, Pavlovic T. The role of nurses in immunisation. International Council of Nurses; 2018.
32. World Health Organization. Ottawa charter for health promotion. World Health Organization. Regional Office for Europe; 1986.
33. Barría PRM. Nursing and its essential role in the vaccination against COVID-19: New challenge in a pandemic scenario. Investigación y Educación en Enfermería. 2021;39(3)
34. de Graaf Y, Oomen B, Castro-Sanchéz E, Geelhoed J, Maria Vrijhoef HJ. Nurses' roles, views and knowledge regarding vaccines and vaccination: a pan-European survey. Int J Care Coord. 2023;26(3–4):129–36.
35. Johnson KE, Lin L-C, Horton SEB, Todd A, Guillet N, Morgan S. Vamos-Vaxnow: a nurse-led interdisciplinary disaster response to address vaccine equity in central Texas during the COVID-19 pandemic. Health Emerg Disaster Nurs. 2022;9(1):23–30.
36. Wang E, Clymer J, Davis-Hayes C, Buttenheim A. Nonmedical exemptions from school immunization requirements: a systematic review. Am J Public Health. 2014;104(11):e62–84.
37. Perlman S, Shamian J, Catton H, Ellen M. Assessing the country-level involvement of nurses in COVID-19 vaccination campaigns: a qualitative study. Int J Nurs Stud. 2023;146:104569.
38. Hunsaker S, Garrett L, Merrill K, Rhodes R. Meeting patients where they are: a nurse-driven quality improvement project to provide influenza vaccinations in the emergency department. J Emerg Nurs. 2023;49(4):553–63. e3
39. Burden S, Henshall C, Oshikanlu R. Harnessing the nursing contribution to COVID-19 mass vaccination programmes: addressing hesitancy and promoting confidence. Wiley Online Library; 2021. p. e16–20.
40. Sax H, Marschall J. Infection prevention and control in 2030: a first qualitative survey by the crystal ball initiative. Antimicrob Resist Infect Control. 2024;13(1):88.

Quality Approach in IPC

14

Joséphine Declaye

Abstract

Infection prevention and control (IPC) is a fundamental pillar of patient safety and healthcare quality. Its effectiveness depends on a structured, evidence-based quality management approach that ensures consistency, adaptability, and measurable impact.

The integration of continuous quality improvement (CQI) methods—such as the Plan-Do-Check-Act (PDCA) cycle—enables healthcare institutions to systematically identify gaps, implement targeted interventions, and monitor progress. Key components of a high-performing IPC program include tailored application of guidelines, robust surveillance systems, multimodal implementation strategies, ongoing staff education, and clearly defined roles and responsibilities. Nurses, as frontline actors, play a critical role in antimicrobial stewardship and protocol adherence.

Root Cause Analysis (RCA), using tools like the Ishikawa diagram and Failure Modes and Effects Analysis (FMEA), provides a structured framework for identifying systemic failures and prioritizing high-risk vulnerabilities. Importantly, patient education enhances adherence to IPC measures, yet remains underutilized. Simulation-based training reinforces practical competencies and decision-making under pressure, contributing to organizational resilience. Embedding these quality management principles into IPC fosters a culture of safety, improves clinical outcomes, and supports sustainable reductions in healthcare-associated infections and antimicrobial resistance.

J. Declaye (✉)
ESNO, Siz Nursing and University of Liège, Liège, Belgium
e-mail: jdeclaye@uliege.be

© The Author(s), under exclusive license to Springer Nature Switzerland AG 2025
B. Oomen, S. Gastaldi (eds.), *Principles of Nursing Infection Prevention Control*,
Principles of Specialty Nursing, https://doi.org/10.1007/978-3-032-01446-7_14

Keywords

Infection control · Quality improvement · Antimicrobial resistance · Stewardship · Surveillance

14.1   Introduction

Effective infection prevention and control (IPC) is essential not only for safeguarding patients and healthcare workers but also for reducing healthcare-associated infections (HAIs) and antimicrobial resistance (AMR). However, successfully implementing IPC measures is a complex endeavor that demands consistency, accountability, and adaptability. This is where a quality management approach becomes indispensable.

Quality management offers a structured framework that enables healthcare organizations to systematically assess, implement, and continuously refine IPC practices. By integrating evidence-based methodologies, data-driven decision-making, and continuous quality improvement (CQI) cycles—such as the Plan-Do-Check-Act (PDCA) model—organizations can identify process gaps and apply targeted interventions. For instance, rigorous quality management practices have been shown to reduce HAIs by up to 70% [1], yet HAIs continue to affect approximately 7% of patients in high-income countries and 15% in low- and middle-income countries [2, 3].

A key element in this quality-driven framework is the pivotal role of nurses in antimicrobial stewardship. Nurses are often at the frontline of patient care and infection control. Their active involvement in monitoring, education, and the implementation of IPC protocols ensures that antimicrobial use is optimized and that best practices are consistently applied. Embedding quality management principles into IPC not only enhances compliance and optimizes resource allocation but also empowers nurses to lead antimicrobial stewardship initiatives—ultimately reducing infection rates and improving patient outcomes on a global scale.

14.2   Quality in Heathcare

Quality in healthcare is defined as the degree to which health services increase the likelihood of desired health outcomes and conform to current professional standards [4]. A Quality Management System (QMS) provides a structured framework that documents an organization's processes, procedures, and responsibilities to achieve specific quality objectives and ensure compliance with established standards.

Key dimensions of quality in healthcare include:

Effectiveness: Delivering care that reliably produces the intended health outcomes.
Safety: Minimizing risks and preventing harm to both patients and healthcare staff.
Timeliness: Providing care promptly to avoid unnecessary delays in treatment.

Efficiency: Optimizing the use of resources and reducing waste without compromising quality.
Equity: Ensuring that care is accessible and delivered fairly to all patients.
Patient-Centeredness: Focusing on patients' needs, values, and preferences, and engaging them in decision-making processes.

A quality management approach in healthcare involves continuous monitoring, rigorous evaluation, and ongoing process adaptation to improve outcomes and enhance patient safety [5]. Through systematic quality improvement initiatives, healthcare organizations can ensure that care remains safe, effective, and patient-centered, thereby fostering an environment of sustained excellence in healthcare delivery.

14.3   Specificity of Quality Management in IPC

Quality management in infection prevention and control (IPC) requires adapting general quality improvement principles to address the unique challenges of preventing infections in healthcare settings. This requires a tailored approach with key aspects including the following:

14.3.1 Adapting Guidelines to Local Conditions

IPC programs must be aligned with the specific healthcare environment in which they operate. This involves tailoring guidelines to match available resources, workforce capacity, and institutional infrastructure, ensuring that protocols are both feasible and relevant [6].

14.3.2 Targeted Surveillance and Monitoring

Implementing surveillance systems that capture local epidemiological data is essential. Continuous tracking of HAIs, antimicrobial resistance (AMR), and compliance with IPC protocols allows healthcare workers to detect trends, intervene in a timely manner, and drive continuous improvement.

14.3.3 Integration of Multimodal Strategies (MMIS)

IPC interventions are most effective when they combine system changes, staff education, robust monitoring, and cultural reinforcement. This multimodal approach ensures long-term adherence to best practices and enhances the overall effectiveness of infection control measures [7].

14.3.4 Customization of Interventions

While standardization is important, IPC measures must also be customized to address the specific needs and priorities of each healthcare setting. This balance between uniformity and flexibility ensures that clinical decision support systems and infection prevention strategies are aligned with local institutional priorities and workforce dynamics [8].

14.3.5 Interdisciplinary Collaboration

Effective IPC requires coordination among diverse sectors, including patient safety, AMR programs, emergency preparedness, and quality management. Strong interdepartmental relationships foster a culture of shared responsibility and accountability, ensuring that interventions are well-integrated and sustainable [6].

By incorporating these tailored approaches, healthcare facilities can optimize their IPC measures, ensuring that improvements are both patient-centered and sustainable. This specificity in quality management not only reduces HAIs and AMR but also strengthens the overall resilience of the healthcare system.

14.4 Key Components of a Quality Approach in IPC

A quality approach in IPC relies on key principles that ensure infection prevention is effective, sustainable, and integrated into healthcare settings:

- **Systematic improvement:** A structured methodology like the **Plan-Do-Study-Act (PDSA) cycle** ensures continuous assessment and refinement of IPC practices [7].
- **Data-driven decisions:** Monitoring, audits, and feedback allow for targeted interventions, improving IPC effectiveness [2, 9].
- **Multidisciplinary collaboration:** Teamwork across IPC, patient safety, and quality management fosters a coordinated approach [10].
- **Standardization:** Applying evidence-based guidelines ensures consistent training, implementation, and assessment of IPC measures.
- **Staff training and education:** Ongoing professional development strengthens IPC knowledge and skills.
- **Defined roles and responsibilities:** Ensuring clear objectives and action plans with dedicated resources supports IPC sustainability [11].
- **Regulatory compliance:** Aligning IPC with national and international regulations enhances accountability and patient safety [3].

By integrating these elements, IPC programs can establish a strong foundation for preventing infections, reducing AMR, and enhancing overall patient care quality.

14.4.1 Patient Education as a Key Component of a Quality Approach in IPC

In addition to the core elements outlined above, patient education is increasingly recognized as an essential component of a robust IPC strategy. Educating patients and their families on infection control measures empowers them to actively participate in their own care, serving as a vital adjunct to traditional healthcare practices. When patients are informed about the importance of hand hygiene, isolation precautions, and the rationale behind infection control protocols. They are more likely to adhere to these practices and even prompt healthcare workers to maintain compliance. Current evidence is limited on effective strategies for involving patients in IPC. The review highlights the need for targeted approaches to clarify patient roles and address power imbalances between patients and healthcare professionals [12, 13].

This active engagement not only enhances patient safety but also reinforces other quality management components—such as systematic improvement and data-driven decision-making—by creating an additional layer of vigilance against healthcare-associated infections (HAIs) and antimicrobial resistance (AMR). Despite its proven benefits, patient education on infection control remains underutilized in many hospital settings. Strengthening this component by integrating structured education programs can help bridge the existing gap, ultimately leading to more sustainable and effective IPC outcomes.

14.4.2 Staff Training and Education in IPC

Ongoing professional development is a critical pillar in maintaining and advancing infection prevention and control (IPC) practices. Continuous education not only reinforces core IPC protocols—such as hand hygiene, proper use of personal protective equipment (PPE), and environmental cleaning—but also supports the evolution of antimicrobial stewardship strategies. For instance, simulation-based training offers a risk-free environment for healthcare workers, enabling them to practice realistic scenarios that mirror high-pressure clinical situations. This method not only improves technical competency but also enhances critical decision-making skills under stress, preparing staff to respond swiftly and effectively during infectious outbreaks.

Moreover, integrating simulation exercises with antimicrobial stewardship initiatives helps cultivate leadership among nurses. These training sessions enable nurses to develop expertise in optimizing antimicrobial use, understanding diagnostic stewardship, and implementing de-escalation strategies. As a result, they become key players in reducing healthcare-associated infections (HAIs) and combating antimicrobial resistance (AMR) [14, 15].

This comprehensive approach to staff education ensures that IPC strategies remain dynamic, evidence-based, and adaptable to evolving clinical challenges. It fosters a culture of continuous improvement and interprofessional collaboration, ultimately leading to improved patient outcomes and enhanced safety across healthcare settings.

Robust, ongoing education and support are key drivers of improved prescribing behavior among healthcare professionals. As demonstrated in a comprehensive study by Lutters et al. (2004), clinicians who receive targeted, multidisciplinary training—including evidence-based guidelines, expert lectures, regular ward rounds, and personalized counseling—are better equipped to adopt best practices in antimicrobial use. This underscores the critical role of structured education in sustaining high standards in IPC and antimicrobial stewardship [16].

14.4.3 Defined Roles and Responsibilities

Clearly defined roles and responsibilities are vital for the long-term sustainability of IPC programs. When objectives are explicit, action plans are well-documented, and dedicated resources are allocated, every team member—from frontline healthcare workers to administrators—knows precisely what is expected of them. This clarity fosters accountability and streamlines interdepartmental collaboration, ensuring that infection control measures are consistently and effectively implemented. Ultimately, such structured organization underpins the integration of IPC practices into routine care, enhancing patient safety and reducing infection rates [11].

14.5 Key Performance Indicators (KPIs)

In quality management, Key Performance Indicators (KPIs) are vital tools for assessing performance and guiding improvement efforts. KPIs are quantifiable measures that demonstrate how effectively an organization is achieving its key objectives. In the context of infection prevention and control (IPC), KPIs are essential for evaluating the success of interventions and driving continuous quality improvement. Unlike general quality management KPIs—which may focus broadly on patient outcomes, resource efficiency, or overall safety—IPC-specific KPIs are designed to capture the nuances of infection control practices. They focus on measurable aspects such as hand hygiene compliance, adherence to personal protective equipment (PPE) protocols, and reductions in healthcare-associated infections (HAIs).

A well-structured IPC KPI framework is built on several key characteristics:

- **Specific:** KPIs must be clearly defined and directly linked to strategic IPC objectives. For example, tracking the reduction in HAIs per 10,000 patient days provides a focused measure of infection control success.
- **Measurable:** Reliable data collection methods are necessary to establish baselines and set targets, enabling meaningful comparisons over time.
- **Actionable:** The insights derived from KPI data should inform targeted interventions, such as corrective feedback or additional staff training.

- **Relevant:** KPIs should align with both organizational goals and the specific challenges of IPC, ensuring that they address critical areas like antimicrobial resistance (AMR) and outbreak prevention.
- **Time-Bound:** Establishing a clear timeframe for achieving targets facilitates regular monitoring and timely adjustments.

For example, WHO recommends using electronic monitoring systems, direct observation audits, and feedback-driven interventions to improve hand hygiene compliance [3]. Additionally, surveillance data—such as infection rates per 1000 patient days—provide insights into the effectiveness of IPC strategies and help prioritize areas for improvement.

By contrasting these IPC-specific KPIs with those in general quality management, it becomes clear that while the principles remain similar, the focus in IPC is on the rapid detection and mitigation of infection risks. This targeted approach ensures that improvement efforts are not only data-driven but also finely tuned to the challenges of preventing infections in diverse healthcare settings.

14.6 Plan-Do-Check-Act (PDCA) Cycle for IPC Improvement

The Plan-Do-Check-Act (PDCA) cycle—often referred to as the Deming Wheel 1986 [17]—serves as a cornerstone for driving continuous improvement in infection prevention and control (IPC). It offers a clear, iterative framework for pinpointing and resolving gaps in IPC practices. By following PDCA's structured steps and aligning them with Root Cause Analysis (RCA), healthcare teams can refine solutions, maintain high standards of patient safety, and build a culture of sustained quality.

Below, we will explore each phase of the PDCA cycle in more detail, illustrating how its systematic approach can be practically applied to enhance IPC outcomes.

Plan
In this initial phase, healthcare teams assess current IPC performance by identifying gaps—such as low hand hygiene compliance or high HAI rates—through baseline assessments and root cause analysis. Based on this information, they set clear, SMART (Specific, Measurable, Achievable, Relevant, Time-Bound) objectives and select evidence-based interventions tailored to their specific needs.

Do
During the Do phase, the planned interventions are implemented on a pilot scale. These may include revised protocols, competency-based training for staff, enhanced environmental cleaning, and initiatives related to antimicrobial stewardship. This phase allows for the practical testing of changes in a controlled environment.

Check

The Check phase focuses on evaluating the effectiveness of the implemented interventions. Teams monitor key performance indicators (KPIs), conduct regular audits, and use statistical tools such as statistical process control (SPC) to measure improvements and identify any shortcomings. This evaluation provides critical feedback for further adjustments.

Act

In the final phase, successful interventions are standardized and integrated into routine practice. Lessons learned are used to refine the process further, and resources are allocated to sustain improvements over the long term. This phase ensures that effective strategies become part of the organizational culture, leading to sustained reductions in HAIs and antimicrobial resistance (AMR).

By incorporating the PDCA cycle into IPC quality management, healthcare organizations can continuously refine their infection control strategies in a systematic, iterative manner. This approach ensures that interventions are both evidence-based and adaptable to evolving challenges in healthcare settings.

14.7   Root Cause Analysis in IPC

Root Cause Analysis (RCA) is a systematic method used to identify the underlying factors that contribute to failures or adverse events. In the world of quality management, RCA serves as a critical tool to go deeper than superficial symptoms and pinpoint critical issues.

When applied to infection prevention and control (IPC), RCA enables healthcare organizations to identify why infection control measures fail, leading to healthcare-associated infections (HAIs) and increased antimicrobial resistance (AMR).

Moreover, RCA can also help to identify what works effectively by revealing successful processes and interventions. These can be replicate and scale up. By distinguishing both the gaps and the strengths within IPC practices, organizations can optimize their strategies, reinforcing effective measures while addressing areas that require improvement. This holistic approach ultimately contributes to safer and more efficient healthcare environments.

14.7.1 Ishikawa Diagram

In IPC, RCA is particularly valuable because the challenges are often multifactorial. A widely used RCA tool is the fishbone diagram—also known as the Ishikawa (1982) diagram—which organizes potential causes into key categories. Traditionally, these categories are represented by the 5M framework (Man, Machine, Material, Method, Measurement) or its expanded version, the 8M framework (adding Mother Nature, Management, and Maintenance). This structured visualization helps teams systematically explore how human factors, equipment, materials, processes, measurement systems, environmental conditions, managerial practices, and maintenance issues interact to impact infection control.

Man (People)
In the context of IPC, human factors—such as the adequacy of staff training, compliance with protocols, and communication—are often at the heart of infection control challenges. Addressing "Man" helps organizations understand if errors stem from gaps in knowledge or behavioral issues, which are critical for designing effective training and engagement strategies.

Machine
Equipment plays a pivotal role in IPC, from ensuring that PPE is available and functional to maintaining proper sterilization tools. Focusing on "Machine" allows organizations to evaluate whether equipment malfunctions or outdated technologies are contributing to increased infection risks.

Material
The quality and appropriateness of the materials used—such as disinfectants, hand rubs, and cleaning supplies—directly impact IPC outcomes. Analyzing "Material" highlights whether suboptimal supplies or inconsistent products may be undermining infection control efforts.

Method
The processes and protocols (or "Method") underlying IPC practices determine consistency and reliability. By scrutinizing these methods, organizations can identify if the procedures in place are too complex, not standardized, or misaligned with best practices, leading to variability in outcomes.

Measurement
Effective monitoring is essential for IPC. "Measurement" assesses the tools and metrics used to track compliance and infection rates. Reliable measurement systems ensure that data reflects true performance and that any deviations are promptly dctcctcd.

Extending to the 8M framework to enrich the analysis:

Mother Nature (Environment)
The physical environment, including factors like ventilation and cleanliness, is critical in preventing pathogen spread. Evaluating environmental conditions helps identify external factors that may compromise IPC.

Management
Leadership and organizational support are key determinants of IPC success. Assessing "Management" clarifies whether sufficient resources, clear policies, and active oversight are in place.

Maintenance

Regular upkeep of equipment and facilities ensures that IPC measures remain effective over time. Focusing on "Maintenance" emphasizes the need for ongoing support to avoid degradation of critical IPC infrastructure.

14.7.2 Risk Prioritization

Risk prioritization is a critical component of Root Cause Analysis (RCA) that enables healthcare organizations to identify which factors most significantly impact infection control outcomes. By employing tools such as risk assessment matrices and Failure Modes and Effects Analysis (FMEA), teams can systematically evaluate each potential root cause based on its impact on patient safety and its likelihood of occurrence.

A risk assessment matrix provides a visual framework for plotting potential failure points. Each identified issue is assigned scores for severity (impact) and probability (likelihood), allowing teams to quickly pinpoint high-risk areas that require immediate attention. For instance, a frequent lapse in hand hygiene—if both highly likely and severe in impact on HAI rates—would be prioritized over less critical issues.

FMEA further enhances this approach by quantifying risks and analyzing the effects of each failure mode on the overall system. By breaking down complex processes into discrete components, FMEA enables teams to assess root causes and estimate potential consequences, resulting in a risk priority number (RPN) for each issue. This numerical value guides resource allocation and intervention prioritization, ensuring that improvement efforts are both focused and sustainable.

Integrating these risk prioritization tools into RCA reinforces effective IPC practices and mitigates high-risk vulnerabilities, aligning improvement efforts with critical insights from recent research in infectious disease management [18, 19].

14.7.3 Other Tools

Beyond this structured categorization, several complementary approaches can deepen the RCA process, ensuring a more holistic, data-driven, and sustainable strategy in infection prevention and control:

- **Integrating Systems Thinking:** Examine how different components of the healthcare system interact, emphasizing the interplay between human, technical, and organizational factors.
- **Leveraging Data Analytics Tools:** Incorporate trend analysis, statistical process control, and digital dashboards to identify patterns over time and quantify deviations.

- **Stakeholder Involvement:** Engage multidisciplinary teams and front-line staff in brainstorming and validating potential root causes to ensure a comprehensive understanding.
- **Iterative Action Plans:** Develop structured action plans that include corrective measures, verification of implementation, and follow-up assessments to ensure sustainability.
- **Documentation and Continuous Learning:** Maintain detailed records of RCA findings, interventions, and outcomes to build a knowledge base for future training and process refinement.

14.8 Conclusion

Building a culture of quality in infection prevention and control is a dynamic, human-centered journey, anchored in good practice and guided by rigorous data. Evidence-based guidelines and hands-on education empower both staff and patients to translate knowledge into routine actions that prevent infections. Continuous monitoring and timely feedback foster a collective sense of ownership, while Plan-Do-Check-Act cycles and Root Cause Analysis ensure that interventions remain focused and adaptable. As new research emerges and local conditions shift, leaders at every level must champion actions that reduce antimicrobial resistance and keep patient safety at the core.

Ultimately, this integrated and evolving approach delivers fewer infections, healthier outcomes, greater workplace satisfaction, and a higher standard of care for all.

References

1. World Health Organization. Implementation of post-market surveillance in cervical cancer programmes [Internet]. 2021 [cited 2025 Feb 22]. https://www.who.int/publications/i/item/9789240020207
2. Sonpar A, Hundal CO, Totté JEE, Wang J, Klein SD, Twyman A, et al. Multimodal strategies for the implementation of infection prevention and control (IPC) interventions – update of a systematic review for the WHO guidelines on core components of IPC programmes at the facility level. Clin Microbiol Infect [Internet]. 2025 [cited 2025 Feb 22]. https://www.sciencedirect.com/science/article/pii/S1198743X25000163
3. World Health Organization. Guidelines on core components of infection prevention and control programmes at the national and acute health care facility level [Internet]. World Health Organization; 2016 [cited 2025 Feb 22]. https://iris.who.int/handle/10665/251730
4. Guyatt GH, Oxman AD, Vist GE, Kunz R, Falck-Ytter Y, Alonso-Coello P, et al. GRADE: an emerging consensus on rating quality of evidence and strength of recommendations. BMJ. 2008;336(7650):924–6.
5. Page MJ, McKenzie JE, Bossuyt PM, Boutron I, Hoffmann TC, Mulrow CD, et al. The PRISMA 2020 statement: an updated guideline for reporting systematic reviews. BMJ. 2021;372:n71.
6. World Health Organization. Global report on infection prevention and control 2024: executive summary [Internet]. World Health Organization; 2024 [cited 2025 Feb 26]. https://iris.who.int/handle/10665/379863

7. Storr J, Twyman A, Zingg W, Damani N, Kilpatrick C, Reilly J, et al. Core components for effective infection prevention and control programmes: new WHO evidence-based recommendations. Antimicrob Resist Infect Control. 2017;6(1):6.

8. Mitchell BG, Gardner A, Stone PW, Hall L, Pogorzelska-Maziarz M. Hospital staffing and health care-associated infections: a systematic review of the literature. Jt Comm J Qual Patient Saf. 2018;44(10):613–22.

9. Baines R, Regan de Bere S, Stevens S, Read J, Marshall M, Lalani M, et al. The impact of patient feedback on the medical performance of qualified doctors: a systematic review. BMC Med Educ. 2018;18(1):173.

10. Mitchell BG, Shaban RZ, MacBeth D, Russo P. Organisation and governance of infection prevention and control in Australian residential aged care facilities: a national survey. Infect Dis Health. 2019;24(4):187–93.

11. Organization WH. Global strategy on human resources for health: workforce 2030 [Internet]. World Health Organization; 2016 [cited 2025 Mar 5]. https://iris.who.int/handle/10665/250368

12. Hammoud S, Amer F, Lohner S, Kocsis B. Patient education on infection control: a systematic review. Am J Infect Control. 2020;48(12):1506–15.

13. Fernandes Agreli H, Murphy M, Creedon S, Ni Bhuachalla C, O'Brien D, Gould D, et al. Patient involvement in the implementation of infection prevention and control guidelines and associated interventions: a scoping review. BMJ Open. 2019;9(3):e025824.

14. Dellit TH, Owens RC, McGowan JE, Gerding DN, Weinstein RA, Burke JP, et al. Infectious Diseases Society of America and the Society for Healthcare Epidemiology of America guidelines for developing an institutional program to enhance antimicrobial stewardship. Clin Infect Dis. 2007;44(2):159–77.

15. McGaghie WC, Issenberg SB, Cohen ER, Barsuk JH, Wayne DB. Does simulation-based medical education with deliberate practice yield better results than traditional clinical education? A meta-analytic comparative review of the evidence. Acad Med J Assoc Am Med Coll. 2011;86(6):706–11.

16. Lutters M, Harbarth S, Janssens JP, Freudiger H, Herrmann F, Michel JP, et al. Effect of a comprehensive, multidisciplinary, educational program on the use of antibiotics in a geriatric university hospital. J Am Geriatr Soc. 2004;52(1):112–6.

17. Deming WE. Out of the crisis [Internet]. MIT Press; 2018 [cited 2025 Mar 31]. https://direct.mit.edu/books/monograph/4192/Out-of-the-Crisis

18. Failure Modes and Effects Analysis (FMEA) Tool | Institute for Healthcare Improvement [Internet]. [cited 2025 Feb 26]. https://www.ihi.org/resources/tools/failure-modes-and-effects-analysis-fmea-tool

19. Vecchia M, Sacchi P, Marvulli LN, Ragazzoni L, Muzzi A, Polo L, et al. Healthcare Application of failure mode and effect analysis (FMEA): is there room in the infectious disease setting? A scoping review. Healthcare. 2025;13(1):82.

Social Determinants of Healthcare-Associated Infections and Antimicrobial Resistance

15

Enrique Castro-Sánchez

Abstract

This chapter examines the impact of social determinants of health (SDOH) on healthcare-associated infections (HAIs) and antimicrobial resistance (AMR). This highlights how factors such as socioeconomic position, education, living conditions, and access to healthcare significantly influence infection risks and the spread of AMR. This chapter illustrates how poverty, inadequate sanitation, overcrowding, and low health literacy contribute to increased vulnerability to infection and the misuse of antibiotics. It also explores how gender and discrimination exacerbate these problems. There is further discussion on the substantial socioeconomic costs of infections and AMR, including direct healthcare expenses, lost productivity, and strain on healthcare systems. Finally, this chapter advocates for health systems to address the SDOH by developing effective public health interventions and achieving health equity, tackling both individual behaviours and broader societal factors.

Keywords

Social determinants of health · Healthcare-associated infections · Antimicrobial resistance · Health equity · Infection prevention and control

E. Castro-Sánchez (✉)
Department of Infectious Diseases, Imperial College London, London, UK

Global Health Research Group, University of Balearic Islands, Palma de Mallorca, Spain
e-mail: e.castro-sanchez@imperial.ac.uk

15.1   Introduction

Healthcare-associated infections (HAIs) and antimicrobial resistance (AMR) are significant public health challenges that disproportionately affect vulnerable populations globally [1]. Interventions to address these clinical and public health issues frequently emphasise the contribution of individual behaviours, such as hand hygiene, vaccination, and optimal adherence to antibiotic courses. These behaviours are undoubtedly important and useful. However, the capacity and ability to carry them out effectively depend on broader determinants which shape and modulate individual behaviours and outcomes [2].

Social determinants of health (SDOH) are increasingly recognised as critical factors influencing the incidence and spread of HAIs and AMR, the availability of interventions, and their success [3]. This chapter explores the close and complex relationship between the SDOH and infection-related healthcare challenges, highlighting the need for comprehensive approaches that address both individual and societal factors.

15.2   What Are the Social Determinants of Health?

The World Health Organization (WHO) defines social determinants of health (SDOH) as "the conditions in which people are born, grow, live, work, and age" [4]. These conditions encompass a wide range of characteristics, including socioeconomic position, education and educational attainment, neighbourhood and physical environment, employment, and social support networks, as well as access to healthcare, to name a few (Box 15.1).

These broad categories and their relationships have been recently refined by models such as the social ecological model [5], which recognises the reciprocity and interdependence of health outcomes with intrapersonal, interpersonal, institutional, and public policies. Ultimately, these factors are shaped by the distribution of money, power, and resources at the global, national, and local levels [6].

Box 15.1 Selected Social Determinants of Health of Relevance to Infections and Resistance

Socio-economic Status: Gender, income, education, employment, and occupation.

Physical Environment: Housing, neighbourhood safety, and environmental exposures.

Social and Community Context: Social support, discrimination, and access to healthcare.

Health Behaviours: Diet, physical activity, and substance use.

The effects of SDOH are broad and interconnected, fostering health inequities by affecting access to healthcare, quality of care, and health behaviours. Citizens living in poverty face numerous barriers to maintaining good health, which extend beyond limited access to healthcare services [7]. Financial constraints often force them to make difficult choices regarding essential needs, such as food, housing, and medical care. This can lead to inadequate nutrition, as affordable food options are often less nutritious and more calorie-dense, contributing to obesity and related health issues [8], which are frequently associated with infections [9] or contact with health and social care services, thus placing them at risk for HCAIs. Substandard housing conditions may expose them to environmental hazards, such as mould or pest infestations, further compromising their health with infectious risks [10]. Additionally, chronic stress associated with financial instability can have long-term negative effects on both physical and mental well-being [11].

Education level also plays a crucial role in infection-related health outcomes, influencing not only health literacy but also overall life choices and opportunities [12]. Those with lower levels of education may struggle to understand complex clinical information relevant to support preventive behaviours, such as vaccination [13], follow antimicrobial treatment plans [14], navigate the healthcare system effectively, or adequately manage chronic conditions. Furthermore, education often correlates with employment opportunities and income levels, creating a cycle in which limited education leads to lower-paying jobs, which, in turn, restricts access to quality healthcare and health-promoting resources [15]. These factors contribute to persistent health disparities across socio-economic groups, highlighting the need for comprehensive approaches that address both healthcare access and the broader social determinants of health.

The inequities generated by SDOH, that is, the systematic, unjust, and avoidable differences by these determinants, are also spread unevenly among individuals, with groups of people such as migrants or women typically more likely to be marginalised and left behind not only because of the determinants but also due to the ineffectiveness of mitigating interventions or policies [16]. These disparities are further exacerbated by intersectionality, where multiple social identities and systems of oppression interact to create compounded disadvantages [17]. For instance, migrant women may face unique challenges arising from the intersection of their gender and immigration status, leading to greater barriers in accessing healthcare, education, and employment opportunities [18].

15.2.1 The Impact of SDOH on Infections

As briefly illustrated before, SDOH can influence the risk of infection, including healthcare-associated infections (HAIs, broadly, infections that patients acquire while receiving care in a healthcare facility or in contact with the healthcare system) in multiple ways (Fig. 15.1).

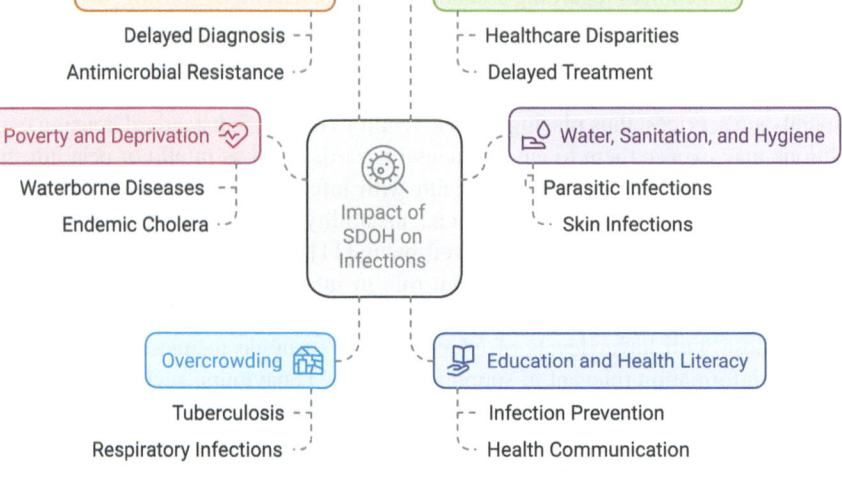

Fig. 15.1 Selected impacts of social determinants on infections. (Author's own)

15.2.1.1 Poverty and Deprivation

People living in poverty often lack access to basic necessities, such as clean water and proper sanitation. This increases their vulnerability to a wide range of infections, as contaminated water and inadequate sanitation can easily spread pathogens [19]. For example, waterborne diseases, such as cholera and typhoid fever, are particularly prevalent in impoverished communities with poor sanitation infrastructure [20]. Furthermore, if sanitation remains inadequate, the faeces of infected individuals can further contaminate the environment, perpetuating the cycle of disease transmission. Globally, there have been numerous cholera outbreaks in impoverished regions. For instance, Nigeria has grappled with endemic cholera for decades and has experienced significant outbreaks over the years. Even in mid-2024, reports indicate ongoing cholera transmission in Nigeria [21]. The humanitarian crisis in Yemen provides another compelling example of the link between disrupted WASH infrastructure and cholera outbreaks. The ongoing conflict has severely damaged or destroyed essential water and sanitation systems, leaving 16 million Yemenis –a significant proportion of the population– without access to these basic necessities, and resulting in 2016 in Yemen's worst cholera outbreak in history, affecting more than one million people [22].

Another study conducted in Vellore, southern India, provided valuable insights into the specific risk factors associated with typhoid fever in an urban setting [23]. The study revealed that mothers consuming food from street vendors in the week preceding the illness were independently associated with an increased risk of typhoid in their children. Conversely, treating household drinking water was found to be protective against the disease.

15.2.1.2 Water, Sanitation, and Hygiene

Additionally, inadequate hygiene practices due to limited access to clean water, sanitation, and hygiene (WASH) can lead to the rapid spread of skin infections and parasitic diseases [19]. Soil-transmitted helminth (STH) infections are a group of common parasitic infections directly linked to poor sanitation [24]. The main species that infect humans include roundworms (*Ascaris lumbricoides*), whipworms (*Trichuris trichiura*), and hookworms (*Necator americanus* and *Ancylostoma duodenale*). These infections are transmitted through contact with soil contaminated with human faeces containing parasitic eggs. In communities with inadequate sanitation, individuals often defaecate outdoors, leading to widespread soil contamination. These parasitic infections can have significant health consequences, particularly for vulnerable populations, such as children, including anaemia and malnutrition [25]. These health challenges not only impact individuals but also strain the already limited healthcare resources in low-income areas, creating a cycle of poverty and illness that is difficult to break.

15.2.1.3 Overcrowding and Accommodations

Overcrowded living conditions, which are common in poor communities, can also create an environment where infectious diseases can be rapidly harboured and disseminated. The proximity and shared spaces in overcrowded settings facilitate pathogen transmission through airborne droplets, direct contact, and contaminated surfaces [26]. Tuberculosis (TB) serves as a classic and excellent example of a respiratory infection strongly associated with poverty and overcrowding. Research has consistently shown an inverse relationship between TB incidence and per-capita gross domestic product, highlighting poverty as a significant underlying factor [27]. Studies have also found a positive association between household crowding and TB incidence. For instance, a study in Harare, Zimbabwe, identified living in a home with two or more people per room as a significant risk factor for TB [28].

15.2.1.4 Education and Health Literacy

Health literacy, the ability to access and understand health information and make effective decisions about health and care, is directly linked to education and has gained much attention recently because of its role in the transmission of infections [13]. Low health literacy can hinder a person's ability to understand and follow infection prevention practices, such as hand hygiene with soap and water for a sufficient duration, or they may not grasp the concept of cross-contamination and the need to avoid touching their eyes, nose, and mouth with unwashed hands [29, 30]. Similarly, they may struggle to follow instructions for cleaning and dressing wounds, leading to improper wound care and a heightened risk of infection [31].

Additionally, they may have difficulty understanding medication labels and instructions, leading to incorrect dosages or missed doses [32]. These lapses in infection prevention due to low health literacy can increase the risk of HCAIs and the development of AMR.

15.2.1.5 Access to Healthcare

Limited access to healthcare can delay the diagnosis and treatment of infections, leading to several adverse outcomes for the patient, including disease progression, the development of complications, and increased morbidity [33], as well as the risk of HCAIs. Moreover, delayed treatment may force the use of broader-spectrum antimicrobials or prolonged therapy [34], which can contribute to the development of antimicrobial resistance. This, in turn, can further limit treatment options for both individual patients and the wider population.

15.2.1.6 Racism and Other Forms of Institutionalised Discrimination

Racial and ethnic minorities, along with other marginalised groups, including those based on socio-economic position, gender, sexual orientation, disability, and language preference, may face discrimination in healthcare settings and care, including IPC [35]. Discrimination can manifest in various ways, leading to inadequate infection prevention practices such as improper hand hygiene, delayed isolation precautions, and substandard environmental cleaning. For example, studies have indicated that minorities might experience implicit bias from healthcare providers, resulting in less comprehensive explanations of hygiene protocols [36]. This can lead to a lack of understanding and adherence to crucial preventive measures. Additionally, marginalised groups may receive less education and counselling on infection prevention due to communication barriers or cultural insensitivity, leading to lower compliance with preventive measures [37]. For instance, language barriers or limited health literacy (as seen above, a product of limited education, which, in turn, can be the result of limited economic means) can prevent people from receiving adequate instructions on proper wound care or medication usage.

Furthermore, discrimination can result in the delayed or inappropriate treatment of infections, contributing to the development and spread of AMR. A lack of trust in the healthcare system, stemming from past experiences of discrimination, might cause individuals from marginalised groups to delay seeking treatment for infections. For example, research has shown that all minorities report experiencing discrimination when accessing healthcare, and in the United States, Spanish-speaking Hispanics specifically face difficulties in accessing care [38, 39]. This delay can lead to more severe illness and the need for broader-spectrum antibiotic therapy.

Income disparities also contribute to this issue, as historically underrepresented racial and ethnic groups and other marginalised groups often experience poorer healthcare experiences and are more likely to delay or forgo medical care due to cost [40], or be offered therapeutic options, including antimicrobials, based on the assumptions made by the clinical teams regarding both the financial capacity of marginalised communities –for example, with cheaper antibiotics which may not be optimal, in health systems where patients must pay the full cost of the medicine out of pocket [41]– or their assumed understanding of the treatment plan.

15.2.2 The Impact of Social Determinants of Health on Antimicrobial Resistance

Socio-economic status plays a significant role in the development of AMR through multiple interconnected pathways. In LMICs, limited access to healthcare, inadequate sanitation, and overcrowding contribute to the spread of infectious diseases, leading to increased antibiotic use and potential misuse. Additionally, individuals with a lower socio-economic position may face barriers to obtaining proper clinical care, resulting in self-medication or incomplete antibiotic courses, which can promote the emergence of resistant bacteria.

Conversely, in higher-income environments, the overuse of antibiotics in healthcare settings and agriculture can drive AMR development. Affluent populations may have greater access to antibiotics, potentially leading to unnecessary prescriptions and overconsumption [42]. Furthermore, socio-economic factors influence dietary patterns and exposure to environmental contaminants, which can affect the human microbiome and its susceptibility to antibiotic-resistant organisms [43]. The complex interplay between socio-economic status and AMR underscores the need for targeted interventions that address both the social determinants of health and responsible antimicrobial use across all socio-economic strata.

15.2.2.1 Poverty and Deprivation

Poverty and economic hardship can limit access to healthcare services, resulting in delayed diagnosis, inappropriate self-medication, and misuse of over-the-counter antibiotics [44]. People in resource-constrained settings may be compelled to seek care outside formal healthcare facilities, exacerbating the risk of suboptimal antibiotic use. Furthermore, economic barriers can force patients to prematurely discontinue treatments or rely on cheaper, possibly counterfeit, or substandard antibiotics, thus enhancing the risk of resistance emergence and transmission [45].

15.2.2.2 Water, Sanitation, and Hygiene

Environmental conditions, particularly water, sanitation, and hygiene (WASH), critically influence the dynamics of AMR. Poor sanitation infrastructure, often prevalent in LMICs, fosters the rapid dissemination of resistant microorganisms through environmental contamination and human-to-human transmission. The lack of clean water and effective waste management exacerbates microbial exposure, contributing to higher infection rates and subsequently increased antibiotic use, thus fuelling resistance [46]. Improvements in WASH infrastructure and hygiene practices have been associated with a reduced incidence of resistant infections, highlighting a pivotal area for public health interventions [47].

15.2.2.3 Education and Health Literacy

As with infections, education and health literacy significantly shape individuals' antibiotic usage behaviour. Populations with limited health literacy may possess inadequate knowledge regarding the appropriate use of antibiotics, frequently using these medications for viral infections, such as influenza and common colds, conditions against which antibiotics are ineffective [48]. Misunderstandings about the need for or benefits of completing prescribed antibiotic courses further compound this misuse, accelerating the development of resistance. Educational interventions aimed at improving public understanding of AMR and appropriate antimicrobial use have been effective in mitigating resistance, underscoring the crucial role of education and health literacy in AMR prevention [49].

15.2.2.4 Occupational Environments

Occupational factors also significantly impact AMR, particularly in sectors characterised by frequent and close human-animal-environment interactions, such as agriculture and healthcare. Agricultural practices involving extensive antibiotic use for growth promotion or prophylaxis in livestock considerably amplify the selective pressure, promoting the emergence of resistance in animal populations [50]. Resistant organisms can then be transmitted to humans via direct contact, food consumption, or environmental pathways. Similarly, healthcare workers, particularly in LMICs, may experience increased exposure to resistant organisms due to inadequate or lacking infection prevention measures, limited availability of protective equipment, and high patient turnover rates, which heighten the risk of occupationally acquired infections and their further spread to communities [51].

Although not a social determinant of health, globalisation fosters the movement of people and products worldwide and plays a pivotal role in propagating resistant organisms [52]. Whether these movements are driven by the desire (or need) of workers to migrate seeking better employment or conditions under the current economic system, or whether globalisation fosters food production systems that enhance intensive livestock or farming practices which result in increased use of antibiotics, enhanced connectivity, and increased global mobility, enabling rapid cross-border dissemination of AMR pathogens, challenging the effectiveness of national and regional containment strategies [53]. Travellers can also act as vectors, introducing resistant strains into new geographic areas, where these microorganisms can become established and further transmitted within local populations [54].

15.3   Gender and Sex

Gender, encompassing both biological (sex) and sociocultural factors, significantly influences susceptibility, exposure, and outcomes related to infectious diseases and AMR [55]. Understanding these sex-specific dynamics is crucial for effective public health interventions, including those addressing infections. Biologically, females generally exhibit stronger innate and adaptive immune responses than males, potentially offering greater protection against infection. This is partly attributed to hormonal influences; oestradiol appears to provide protective immunity, whereas testosterone may suppress anti-infectious responses.

Sociocultural factors also play vital roles. Gendered occupational roles lead to varying exposure risks [56]. For instance, men may face higher exposure in certain work environments, whereas women, often overrepresented in healthcare and care-giving, have increased exposure to pathogens. Healthcare access is also influenced by gender norms and power differentials, impacting prevention and treatment. Infection patterns reveal gender differences. For example, in sub-Saharan Africa, men generally showed higher COVID-19 incidence and case fatality rates [57] while women are significantly more prone to urinary tract infections due to ana-tomical differences [58]. Tuberculosis and Hepatitis C infection also show higher incidence and severity in men [59, 60], but clinicians and researchers ought to care-fully disentangle the effect of behaviours and cultural traditions from the biology whenever hypothesising about the chain of infection.

AMR is also affected by sex and gender. Inequity impacts access to healthcare and treatment-seeking behaviour [61, 62]. Women are often prescribed more antibi-otics, and their roles in household management and childcare can influence the use of antimicrobials. Gender norms influence health outcomes by affecting knowledge of health problems and preventive measures. They also shape health-seeking behav-iours and adherence to treatment [63].

Addressing gender-specific aspects of infection and AMR requires more gender-sensitive research, policymaking, and healthcare delivery. There is a need for com-prehensive gender-disaggregated data and policies that promote equitable access to health care and treatment.

15.4   The Significant and Multifaceted Socio-economic Impacts of IPC and AMR

Infectious diseases represent a substantial global health challenge, extending their impact far beyond individual well-being to exert considerable pressure on societies, economies, and political structures worldwide [64, 65]. Compounding this issue is the escalating threat of AMR, making infections more difficult and thus costly to treat, thereby amplifying the already significant socio-economic consequences of infectious diseases [66].

The interconnectedness of these challenges demands a comprehensive under-standing of their multifaceted impacts across various societal levels. At the indi-vidual and household levels, the economic burden of infection and AMR manifests through both direct and indirect costs. Direct costs encompass out-of-pocket expen-ditures for healthcare services, including consultations with healthcare profession-als, the purchase of prescribed medications, and potential hospitalisation [67]. For instance, a study on COVID-19 revealed that the mean out-of-pocket spending after hospital discharge ranged from $534 for privately insured patients to $680 for Medicare Advantage beneficiaries, illustrating the immediate financial strain on individuals [68]. These expenses can be particularly devastating for households already burdened by non-communicable diseases, increasing their risk of cata-strophic health expenditures. The emergence of AMR further exacerbates these direct costs, as treatment failures necessitate the use of more expensive second-line antimicrobial drugs, placing an even greater financial burden on patients and their families. This situation is particularly critical in low-income countries, where a sig-nificant portion of healthcare spending is through direct out-of-pocket payments, potentially pushing vulnerable populations into debt and poverty [66].

Beyond direct healthcare costs, individuals and households face substantial indi-rect economic burdens. The challenge of AMR amplifies these indirect costs, as prolonged illnesses and premature deaths due to treatment failures result in extended periods of lost income and diminished economic well-being for affected households [69]. For individuals in precarious employment or lacking adequate sick leave pro-visions, these indirect costs can have long-lasting and severe financial repercussions for them.

The health system also experiences significant economic strain due to infection and AMR. Infectious diseases lead to increased hospital admissions, extended lengths of stay, and higher overall treatment costs. For example, patients with healthcare-associated infections tend to have significantly longer hospital stays, driving up healthcare expenditures [70]. Surges in infectious disease cases can also overwhelm healthcare systems, leading to capacity strain, treatment delays, and potentially compromised quality of care, as observed during the recent COVID-19 pandemic. Moreover, combating AMR requires the use of more sophisticated and potentially costly diagnostic tools to accurately identify resistant pathogens.

At the societal level, the economic consequences of infection and AMR are extensive. Infectious diseases diminish the labour supply and negatively impact overall economic output. Long-term epidemics like HIV/AIDS and malaria have significantly hindered economic growth in several low-income nations by reducing productivity and discouraging foreign investment [71]. Projections indicate that AMR could lead to substantial global GDP losses in the coming decades, posing a significant threat to long-term economic stability. The burden of infectious diseases can exacerbate economic instability, social fragmentation, and political unrest, par-ticularly in developing countries with fragile healthcare infrastructure. Childhood infections can negatively affect development and educational attainment, with long-term consequences for human capital and future economic productivity. Moreover, antibiotic resistance in animals can significantly impact the agricultural sector through increased livestock illness and mortality, affecting food security and caus-ing economic losses to farmers.

Interestingly, the relationship between socio-economic status and AMR can manifest in unexpected ways. Some authors have reported elevated resistance rates among wealthier populations within specific contexts, possibly due to greater access to antibiotics and increased healthcare-seeking behaviours, leading to antibiotic overuse and consequent resistance development [72]. Similarly, pregnant women with high health literacy were reportedly more likely to avoid some recommended immunisations due to concerns about uncommon or extremely uncommon adverse events for their babies, without adequately contextualising the impact that such missed vaccinations would have on their babies' risk associated with the infection the very same vaccines successfully prevent [73]. These paradoxical scenarios underscore the complexity of addressing AMR, requiring nuanced, culturally sensitive, and context-specific strategies.

15.5   Conclusion

Social determinants of health play a significant role in the incidence and spread of healthcare-associated infections and antimicrobial resistance. Addressing these social factors is essential for achieving equitable and sustainable public health improvements. By recognising the complex interplay between social, economic, and environmental factors and health outcomes, healthcare providers, policymakers, and communities can work together to create a healthier and more equitable world.

References

1. World Health Organization. Global report on infection prevention and control. Geneva: WHO; 2022. https://www.who.int/publications/i/item/9789240051164
2. Chandler CI. Current accounts of antimicrobial resistance: stabilisation, individualisation and antibiotics as infrastructure. Palgrave Commun. 2019;5:53. https://doi.org/10.1057/s41599-019-0263-4.
3. Khalid F, Yang GL, McGuire JL, Robson J, Ashraf S, Muneer I, et al. Social determinants of health and antimicrobial resistance: a systematic review. Antibiotics (Basel). 2022;11(6):767. https://doi.org/10.3390/antibiotics11060767.   https://www.ncbi.nlm.nih.gov/pmc/articles/PMC9221393/
4. World Health Organization. Social determinants of health. Geneva: WHO; 2023. https://www.who.int/health-topics/social-determinants-of-health
5. McLeroy KR, Bibeau D, Steckler A, Glanz K. An ecological perspective on health promotion programs. Health Educ Q. 1988;15(4):351–77. https://doi.org/10.1177/109019818801500401.
6. Marmot M, Allen JJ. Social determinants of health equity. Am J Public Health. 2014;104(Suppl 4):S517–9. https://doi.org/10.2105/AJPH.2014.302200.
7. Braveman P, Gottlieb L. The social determinants of health: it's time to consider the causes of the causes. Public Health Rep 2014;129(Suppl 2):19–31. https://doi.org/10.1177/00333549141291S206.
8. Drewnowski A, Darmon N. The economics of obesity: dietary energy density and energy cost. Am J Clin Nutr. 2005;82(1 Suppl):265S–73S. https://doi.org/10.1093/ajcn/82.1.265S.
9. Huttunen R, Syrjänen J. Obesity and the risk and outcome of infection. Int J Obes. 2013;37(3):333–40. https://doi.org/10.1038/ijo.2012.62.
10. Krieger J, Higgins DL. Housing and health: time again for public health action. Am J Public Health. 2002;92(5):758–68. https://doi.org/10.2105/ajph.92.5.758.
11. Braveman P, Egerter S, Barclay C. Stress and health. Exploring the social determinants of health. Issue Brief No. 3. Princeton: Robert Wood Johnson Foundation; 2011. https://www.rwjf.org/en/library/research/2011/03/stress-and-health.html
12. Nutbeam D, Lloyd JE. Understanding and responding to health literacy as a social determinant of health. Annu Rev Public Health. 2021;42:159–73. https://doi.org/10.1146/annurev-publhealth-090419-102529.

13. Castro-Sánchez E, Chang PWS, Vila-Candel R, Escobedo AA, Holmes AH. Health literacy and infectious diseases: why does it matter? Int J Infect Dis. 2016;43:103–10. https://doi.org/10.1016/j.ijid.2015.12.019.

14. Salm F, Ernsting C, Kuhlmey A, Kanzler M, Gastmeier P, Gellert P. Antibiotic use, knowledge and health literacy among the general population in Berlin, Germany, and its impact on adherence. PLoS One. 2018;13(2):e0193336. https://doi.org/10.1371/journal.pone.0193336.

15. Zimmerman EB, Woolf SH, Haley A. Understanding the relationship between education and health: a review of the evidence and an examination of community perspectives. In: Kaplan RM, Spittel ML, David DH, editors. Population health: behavioral and social science insights. AHRQ Publication No. 15–0002. Rockville: Agency for Healthcare Research and Quality and Office of Behavioral and Social Sciences Research, National Institutes of Health; 2015. https://www.ahrq.gov/sites/default/files/publications/files/population-health.pdf.

16. World Health Organization. Health inequities and their causes. Geneva: WHO; 2018. https://www.who.int/news-room/facts-in-pictures/detail/health-inequities-and-their-causes

17. Bowleg L. The problem with the phrase women and minorities: intersectionality – an important theoretical framework for public health. Am J Public Health. 2012;102(7):1267–73. https://doi.org/10.2105/AJPH.2012.300750.

18. Keygnaert I, Guieu A, Ooms G, Vettenburg N, Temmerman M, Roelens K. Sexual and reproductive health of migrants: does the EU care? Health Policy. 2014;114(2–3):215–25. https://doi.org/10.1016/j.healthpol.2013.10.007.

19. Prüss-Ustün A, Bartram J, Clasen T, Colford JM Jr, Cumming O, Curtis V, et al. Burden of disease from inadequate water, sanitation and hygiene in low- and middle-income settings: a retrospective analysis of data from 145 countries. Trop Med Int Health. 2014;19(8):894–905. https://doi.org/10.1111/tmi.12329.

20. Rizzo C, Barchitta M, Cantarini L, Agodi A. The impact of water, sanitation, and hygiene on the health of vulnerable populations: a systematic review. Ann Ig. 2021;33(6):472–85. https://doi.org/10.7416/ai.2021.2495.

21. Eneh S, Onukansi F, Anokwuru C, Ikhuoria O, Edeh G, Obiekwe S, Dauda Z, Praise-God A, Okpara C. Cholera outbreak trends in Nigeria: policy recommendations and innovative approaches to prevention and treatment. Front Public Health. 2024;12:1464361. https://doi.org/10.3389/fpubh.2024.1464361. https://www.frontiersin.org/journals/public-health/articles/10.3389/fpubh.2024.1464361

22. Al-Mekhlafi HM. Yemen in a time of cholera: current situation and challenges. Am J Trop Med Hyg. 2018;98(6):1558–62. https://doi.org/10.4269/ajtmh.17-0811. Epub 2018 Mar 15. PMID: 29557331; PMCID: PMC6086153

23. Giri S, Kattula D, John J, et al. Case-control study of household and environmental transmission of typhoid fever in urban Vellore, India. J Infect Dis. 2021;224(Suppl 5):S584–91. https://doi.org/10.1093/infdis/jiab378. https://academic.oup.com/jid/article-pdf/224/Supplement_5/S584/41245690/jiab378.pdf

24. World Health Organization. Soil-transmitted helminthiasis. [Internet]. Geneva: WHO; [cited 2025 Mar 21]. https://espen.afro.who.int/diseases/soil-transmitted-helminthiasis

25. Echazú A, Bonanno D, Juarez M, Cajal SP, Heredia V, Caropresi S, et al. Effect of poor access to water and sanitation as risk factors for soil-transmitted helminth infection: selectiveness by the infective route. PLoS Negl Trop Dis. 2015;9(9):e0004111. https://doi.org/10.1371/journal.pntd.0004111.

26. Ali S, Islam MA, Rahman M, et al. Effect of in-house crowding on childhood hospital admissions for acute respiratory infections in Bangladesh. PLoS One. 2021;16(4):e0250801. https://doi.org/10.1371/journal.pone.0250801.

27. Liyew AM, Clements ACA, Akalu TY, Gilmour B, Alene KA. Ecological-level factors associated with tuberculosis incidence and mortality: a systematic review and meta-analysis. PLOS Glob Public Health. 2024;4(10):e0003425. https://journals.plos.org/globalpublichealth/article?id=10.1371/journal.pgph.0003425

28. Gomo E, Mungofa S, Chideme M, et al. Prevalent infectious tuberculosis in Harare, Zimbabwe: burden, risk factors, and implications for control. PLoS One. 2012;7(6):e39492. https://doi.org/10.1371/journal.pone.0039492.
29. Fitzpatrick T, Tenkorang EY. Health literacy and hand hygiene practices among older adults: implications for infection prevention. Am J Infect Control. 2019;47(10):1169–73.
30. González-Chica DA, Luque-Fernández MA, Buitrago-Garcia D, et al. Health literacy and preventive health behaviors during the COVID-19 pandemic. Int J Environ Res Public Health. 2021;18(4):1759.
31. Low Health Literacy Is Associated with Higher Rates of Postoperative Infection. Abstract 344.840041 presented at: 2020 ACS Quality and Safety Conference VIRTUAL; August 21–24, 2020.
32. Wolf MS, Davis TC, Bass PF, et al. Patients with low health literacy make more errors interpreting medication instructions and warning labels. J Health Commun. 2006;11(Suppl 1):1–12.
33. Suneja M, Beekmann SE, Dhaliwal G, Miller AC, Polgreen PM. Diagnostic delays in infectious diseases. Diagnosis (Berl). 2022;9(3):332–9. https://doi.org/10.1515/dx-2021-0092. PMID: 35073468; PMCID: PMC9424060
34. Berkowitz KA, et al. Delay of appropriate antibiotic treatment is associated with high mortality in patients with sepsis. J Hosp Med. 2019;14(8):488–94.
35. Nix CD, Bubb TN, Maddox VB. Recommendations from the association for professionals in infection control and epidemiology health inequalities & disparities task force. Am J Infect Control. 2023;51:107–9.
36. Cohen RA, Terlizzi EP, Villarroel MA. Experiences of racial and ethnic discrimination in health care – United States, 2019. MMWR Morb Mortal Wkly Rep. 2023;72(16):437–44.
37. Bayeh R, Yampolsky MA, Ryder AG. The social lives of infectious diseases: why culture matters to COVID-19. Front Psychol. 2021;12:648086. https://doi.org/10.3389/fpsyg.2021.648086. PMID: 34630195; PMCID: PMC8495420
38. Smedley BD, Stith AY, Nelson AR, editors. Unequal treatment: confronting racial and ethnic disparities in health care. National Academies Press; 2003.
39. González-Hernández G, et al. Barriers to healthcare access among hispanics in the United States: a literature review. J Immigr Minor Health. 2017;19(3):694–700.
40. Chen A, Escarce JJ. Quantifying income-related inequality in healthcare delivery in the United States. Med Care. 2004;42(1):38–47.
41. Vu HTL, Pham TTT, Duong YH, Truong QA, Nguyen HK, Nguyen TTC, Trinh LX, Nguyen TTH, Le MQ, Vu VH, Chau DM, Huynh NT, Vo ETHD, Le HNM, Pham TN, Pollack TM, Van Doorn HR. Antibiotic prescribing practices of medical doctors in a resource-limited setting and the influence of individual perceptions and stewardship support: a survey in three tertiary hospitals in Vietnam. JAC Antimicrob Resist. 2024;6(2):dlae064. https://doi.org/10.1093/jacamr/dlae064.
42. Boyd SE, Moore LSP, Gilchrist M, Costelloe C, Castro-Sánchez E, Dean Franklin B, Holmes AH. Obtaining antibiotics online from within the UK: a cross-sectional study. J Antimicrob Chemother. 2017;72(5):1521–8. https://doi.org/10.1093/jac/dkx003.
43. Björk JM, et al. Environmental Influences on the Human microbiome and implications for public health. Curr Environ Health Rep. 2021;8(4):365–75.
44. Sachdev C, Anjankar A, Agrawal J. Self-medication with antibiotics: an element increasing resistance. Cureus. 2022;14(10):e30844. https://doi.org/10.7759/cureus.30844. PMID: 36451647; PMCID: PMC9704507
45. Torres NF, Solomon VP, Middleton LE. Evidence of factors influencing self-medication with antibiotics in low and middle-income countries: a systematic scoping review. Public Health. 2019;168:92–101.
46. Fuhrmeister ER, Harvey AP, Nadimpalli ML, Gallandat K, Ambelu A, Arnold BF, Brown J, Cumming O, Earl AM, Kang G, Kariuki S, Levy K, Pinto Jimenez CE, Swarthout JM, Trueba G, Tsukayama P, Worby CJ, Pickering AJ. Evaluating the relationship between community water and sanitation access and the global burden of antibiotic resistance: an ecological study. Lancet Microbe. 2023;4(8):e591–600. https://doi.org/10.1016/S2666-5247(23)00137-4.

47. Sambaza SS, Naicker N. Contribution of wastewater to antimicrobial resistance: a review article. J Glob Antimicrob Resist. 2023;34:23–9. https://doi.org/10.1016/j.jgar.2023.05.010.
48. Mostafa A, Abdelzaher A, Rashed S, AlKhawaga SI, Afifi SK, AbdelAlim S, Mostafa SA, Zidan TA. Is health literacy associated with antibiotic use, knowledge and awareness of antimicrobial resistance among non-medical university students in Egypt? A cross-sectional study. BMJ Open. 2021;11(3):e046453. https://doi.org/10.1136/bmjopen-2020-046453.
49. King S, Exley J, Taylor J, Kruithof K, Larkin J, Pardal M. Antimicrobial stewardship: the effectiveness of educational interventions to change risk-related behaviours in the general population: a systematic review. Rand Health Q. 2016;5(3):2.
50. Marshall BM, Levy SB. Food animals and antimicrobials: impacts on human health. Clin Microbiol Rev. 2011;24(4):718–33.
51. Zong Z, Zhang Q, Li X, et al. Knowledge, awareness and practices of healthcare workers regarding antimicrobial use, antimicrobial resistance and antimicrobial stewardship in a tertiary hospital in China. J Glob Antimicrob Resist. 2023;6(3):dlae076. https://doi.org/10.1093/jacamr/dlae076. Available from: https://academic.oup.com/jacamr/article/6/3/dlae076/7675733
52. Laxminarayan R, Van Boeckel TP, Teillant A, et al. Global antibiotic consumption and resistance: a cross-sectional analysis. Lancet Infect Dis. 2014;14(8):742–50.
53. Berndtson AE. Increasing globalization and the movement of antimicrobial resistance between countries. Surg Infect. 2020;21(7):579–85. https://doi.org/10.1089/sur.2020.145.
54. D'Souza AW, van Schaik W, Penders J, et al. Destination shapes antibiotic resistance gene acquisitions, abundance increases, and diversity changes in Dutch travelers. Genome Med. 2021;13(1):43. https://doi.org/10.1186/s13073-021-00868-0. https://genomemedicine.biomedcentral.com/articles/10.1186/s13073-021-00868-0
55. Gay L, Melenotte C, Lakbar I, Mezouar S, Devaux C, Raoult D, Bendiane MK, Leone M, Mège JL. Sexual dimorphism and gender in infectious diseases. Front Immunol. 2021;12:698121. https://doi.org/10.3389/fimmu.2021.698121.
56. Biswas A, Tiong M, Irvin E, Zhai G, Sinkins M, Johnston H, Yassi A, Smith PM, Koehoorn M. Gender and sex differences in occupation-specific infectious diseases: a systematic review. Occup Environ Med. 2024;81(8):425–32. https://doi.org/10.1136/oemed-2024-109451.
57. Dalal J, Triulzi I, James A, Nguimbis B, Dri GG, Venkatasubramanian A, Noubi Tchoupopnou Royd L, Botero Mesa S, Somerville C, Turchetti G, Stoll B, Abbate JL, Mboussou F, Impouma B, Keiser O, Coelho FC. COVID-19 mortality in women and men in sub-Saharan Africa: a cross-sectional study. BMJ Glob Health. 2021;6(11):e007225. https://doi.org/10.1136/bmjgh-2021-007225.
58. Saif-Al-Islam M, Mohamed H, Younis M, Abdelhamid M, Ali M, Khalaf S. Impact of gender difference on characteristics and outcome of chronic hepatitis C. Open J Gastroenterol. 2020;10:281–94. https://doi.org/10.4236/ojgas.2020.1011027.
59. Wang AC, Geng JH, Wang CW, Wu DW, Chen SC. Sex difference in the associations among risk factors with hepatitis B and C infections in a large Taiwanese population study. Front Public Health. 2022;10:1068078. https://doi.org/10.3389/fpubh.2022.1068078. Available from: https://www.frontiersin.org/journals/public-health/articles/10.3389/fpubh.2022.1068078
60. Peer V, Schwartz N, Green MS. Gender differences in tuberculosis incidence rates-a pooled analysis of data from seven high-income countries by age group and time period. Front Public Health. 2023;10:997025. https://doi.org/10.3389/fpubh.2022.997025. Erratum in: Front Public Health. 2023;11:1157235. 10.3389/fpubh.2023.1157235
61. Batheja D, Goel S, Charani E. Understanding gender inequities in antimicrobial resistance: role of biology, behaviour and gender norms. BMJ Glob Health. 2025;10:e016711.
62. Adewusi OJ, Cassidy R, Aboderin A, Bailey S, Hotham S. Gender differences in antibiotic use behaviour and access to antibiotics in low- and middle-income countries: a scoping review protocol. BMJ Open. 2024;14(12):e081279. https://doi.org/10.1136/bmjopen-2023-081279.
63. Gautron JMC, Tu Thanh G, Barasa V, Voltolina G. Using intersectionality to study gender and antimicrobial resistance in low- and middle-income countries. Health Policy Plan. 2023;38(9):1017–32. https://doi.org/10.1093/heapol/czad054. PMID: 37599460; PMCID: PMC10566319

64. Fonkwo PN. Pricing infectious disease. The economic and health implications of infectious diseases. EMBO Rep. 2008;9(Suppl 1):S13–7. https://doi.org/10.1038/embor.2008.110. PMID: 18578017; PMCID: PMC3327542

65. Ferraz MP. Antimicrobial resistance: the impact from and on society according to one health approach. Societies. 2024;14:187. https://doi.org/10.3390/soc14090187.

66. Dadgostar P. Antimicrobial resistance: implications and costs. Infect Drug Resist. 2019;12:3903–10. https://doi.org/10.2147/IDR.S234610. PMID: 31908502; PMCID: PMC6929930

67. Yu H, Alfred T, Nguyen JL, Zhou J, Olsen MA. Incidence, attributable mortality, and healthcare and out-of-pocket costs of clostridioides difficile infection in US Medicare advantage enrollees. Clin Infect Dis. 2023;76(3):e1476–83. https://doi.org/10.1093/cid/ciac467.

68. Pike J, Kompaniyets L, Lindley MC, Saydah S, Miller G. Direct medical costs associated with post-COVID-19 conditions among privately insured children and adults. Prev Chronic Dis. 2023;20:E06. https://doi.org/10.5888/pcd20.220292.

69. Safdar N, Saleem S, Salman M, Tareq AH, Ishaq S, Ambreen S, Hameed A, Habib MB, Ali TM. Economic burden of antimicrobial resistance on patients in Pakistan. Front Public Health. 2025;13:1481212. https://doi.org/10.3389/fpubh.2025.1481212.

70. Gidey K, Gidey MT, Hailu BY, Gebreamlak ZB, Niriayo YL. Clinical and economic burden of healthcare-associated infections: a prospective cohort study. PLoS One. 2023;18(2):e0282141. https://doi.org/10.1371/journal.pone.0282141.

71. Smith KM, Machalaba CC, Seifman R, Feferholtz Y, Karesh WB. Infectious disease and economics: the case for considering multi-sectoral impacts. One Health. 2019;7:100080. https://doi.org/10.1016/j.onehlt.2018.100080.

72. Ljungqvist U, van Kessel R, Mossialos E, Saint V, Schmidt J, Mafi A, Shutt A, Chatterjee A, Charani E, Anderson M. Mapping socioeconomic factors driving antimicrobial resistance in humans: an umbrella review. One Health. 2025;20:100986. https://doi.org/10.1016/j.onehlt.2025.100986.

73. Castro-Sánchez E, Vila-Candel R, Soriano-Vidal FJ, et al. Influence of health literacy on acceptance of influenza and pertussis vaccinations: a cross-sectional study among Spanish pregnant women. BMJ Open. 2018;8:e022132. https://doi.org/10.1136/bmjopen-2018-022132.

Infection Prevention and Control and Antimicrobial Resistance from a Planetary Perspective

16

Enrique Castro-Sánchez

Abstract

Antimicrobial resistance (AMR) is a critical global health challenge with profound implications for human, animal, and environmental health. The emergence and spread of drug-resistant pathogens threaten the effectiveness of antimicrobial treatments, leading to increased morbidity, mortality, and healthcare costs. Infection prevention and control (IPC) measures play a crucial role in mitigating the impact of AMR by preventing infections and reducing the need for antimicrobial use in patients. This chapter explores the interconnectedness of AMR and IPC from a planetary health perspective, emphasising the need for a holistic approach that considers the interplay between human activities, animal health, and environmental factors. This chapter examines the impact of climate change on the spread of infectious diseases and AMR, highlights successful interventions and programs implemented to address these challenges, and discusses the role of healthcare workers in preventing and controlling infections and AMR.

Keywords

Antimicrobial resistance · Infection prevention and control · Planetary health · Climate change · One Health

E. Castro-Sánchez (✉)
Department of Infectious Diseases, Imperial College London, London, UK

Global Health Research Group, University of Balearic Islands, Palma de Mallorca, Spain
e-mail: e.castro-sanchez@imperial.ac.uk

16.1   Introduction

There is no doubt about the scale of the threat presented by infections, particularly those difficult to treat, to humans and the ecosphere—millions of people died from antibiotic-resistant bacterial infections in 2019 [1]. Although the misuse and overuse of antimicrobials in human and animal health, as well as in agriculture, are the main drivers of antimicrobial resistance (AMR) [2], resistance is a natural and ubiquitous evolutionary mechanism which is present everywhere on the planet. The World Health Organization (WHO) has rated antibiotic resistance as a 'global security threat' impacting a wide range of key areas such as global health, food security, and human development [3].

Infection prevention and control (IPC) practitioners carry out and lead essential activities to prevent infections and reduce the need for antimicrobials, thereby mitigating the impact of AMR. However, these activities are often solely focused on clinical tasks or interventions conducted in clinical settings. This clinical interest and focus are not wrong or inappropriate; however, to minimise the dissemination of infections in healthcare and community settings and across society, effective IPC programs should seek to influence and address the determinants of such infections and resistance. These determinants ultimately operate much more 'upstream' (that is, away from health and social care settings and clinical work) and can also be affected by multiple factors and policies unrelated to human and animal health [4, 5].

The increasing recognition that addressing social determinants of health and illness (i.e. the conditions in which people are born, live, work, and play) [6, 7] is vital to improve infection-related outcomes for citizens worldwide has recently been coupled with the awareness that those same social determinants are closely interrelated with ecological factors. This chapter examines the interconnectedness of AMR and IPC from a planetary health perspective, recognising not only the close links between human, animal, and environmental health, but also the synergies between the factors which drive infections and the different planetary crises (climate crisis, biodiversity loss, and environmental damage) [8].

The content explores the impact of the climate crisis on the emergence, re-emergence, and transmission of infectious diseases and AMR, and the effect of IPC and AMS activities on the environment, highlighting successful interventions and programs implemented to address these challenges and discussing the role of healthcare workers and IPC nursing practitioners.

16.2   What Is Planetary Health?

Planetary health is an emerging transdisciplinary field that examines the interconnectedness and interdependence of human health, environmental systems, and broader planetary ecosystems [9]. Planetary health recognises that human well-being is dependent on the health of the Earth's natural systems, such as climate, biodiversity, water, and soil quality [10]. Emerging as a response to the environmental degradation's impacts on human and animal health, the Lancet Commission on Planetary Health defined planetary health as 'the health of the human civilisation and the state of the natural systems on which this health depends'. [11]. This notion emphasises the fundamental principle that human health cannot be sustained without ecosystem integrity.

16.2.1 Where Does Planetary Health Originate?

Planetary health is deeply rooted in public and environmental health (Fig. 16.1). Traditional public health acknowledges environmental factors such as air pollution and water quality as health determinants [12], a vision expanded by the ecohealth paradigm which considers ecosystems as key determinants of health, focusing on human–animal–environment interactions [13]. The 'One Health' perspective, primarily used in infectious disease research and infection prevention, emphasises the links between humans, animals, and environmental health, particularly in relation to zoonotic diseases, and has gained relevance for infection control [14]. Although global health focuses on human populations, it may be seen as being expanded by planetary health to include environmental sustainability [15]. Planetary health differs from previous disciplines in that it takes a systems approach, embraces movement building and change, and firmly aims to resolve injustice and inequity [16].

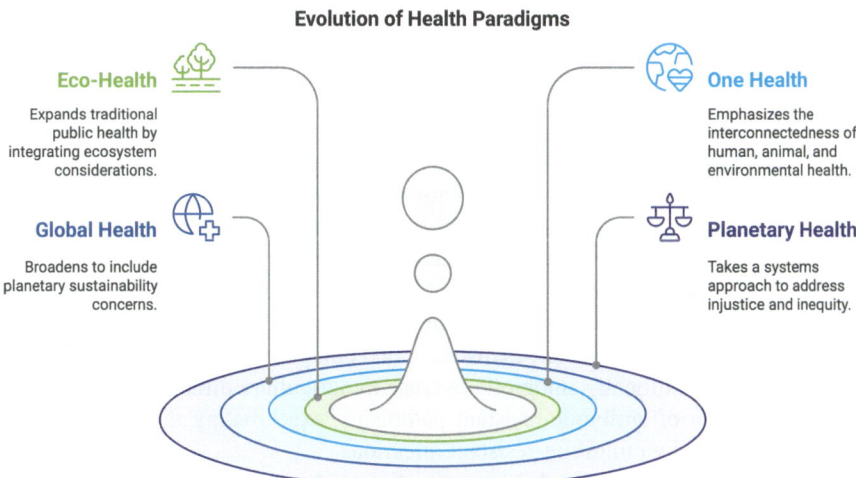

Fig. 16.1 The evolution of health paradigms. (Author's own)

16.3   The Impact of the Climate Crisis on Infectious Diseases and Antimicrobial Resistance

Globally, AMR and the climate crisis represent two critical and interconnected public health emergencies [17]. The climate crisis is profoundly altering environmental conditions, thereby influencing infectious disease dynamics and exacerbating the development of AMR. Rising temperatures have altered precipitation patterns, and the increasing frequency of extreme weather events has significantly affected disease ecology, influencing the spread, survival, and proliferation of pathogens [18].

For example, warmer temperatures can accelerate bacterial growth and enhance the horizontal transfer of antibiotic resistance genes, thereby increasing the risk of multidrug-resistant infections [19]. Additionally, climate-induced phenomena, such as flooding and drought, often drive increased antimicrobial usage across agriculture, livestock production, and healthcare settings, further intensifying the risk and spread of AMR [20].

Consequently, these environmental disruptions contribute to heightened transmission rates of infectious diseases, including vector-borne illnesses such as malaria and dengue fever, as well as waterborne diseases such as cholera [21]. The 2023 Lancet Countdown on Health and Climate Change highlighted this escalating threat, noting that changing climatic conditions, combined with increasing urbanisation and human mobility, significantly amplified global infection risks [22]. Indeed, global infection cases have doubled every decade since 1990, with nearly half of the world's population currently at risk of climate-sensitive infectious diseases [23].

Furthermore, extreme weather events caused by climate change exacerbate health risks by increasing mortality rates, displacement, and population vulnerability to infectious diseases. Biodiverse ecosystems play a crucial role in maintaining environmental resilience, providing essential services such as clean air, water, and food, and acting as natural barriers to emerging infectious diseases. Conversely, environmental degradation, including deforestation and pollution, undermines these protective effects, increases exposure to zoonotic pathogens, and contributes to respiratory, cardiovascular, and gastrointestinal conditions. These health impacts further escalate the use of antimicrobials, reinforcing the cycle of resistance.

Industrial agricultural practices exacerbate these problems by contributing to deforestation, greenhouse gas emissions, environmental degradation, and poor dietary outcomes [24]. These factors collectively impair immune system function, increase vulnerability to infectious diseases, and complicate effective antimicrobial management. Additionally, antibiotic overuse in agriculture directly contributes to the proliferation of antibiotic-resistant pathogens, exacerbating the public health challenges posed by multidrug-resistant infections.

Overall, the complex interplay between climate change, environmental degradation, increased antimicrobial use, and biodiversity loss demands integrated approaches to simultaneously address AMR and environmental sustainability and mitigate their impact on disproportionately affected vulnerable populations, including low-income individuals and Indigenous communities.

16.3.1 Balancing Infection Control, Antimicrobial Stewardship, and Environmental Sustainability in Healthcare

Infection prevention and, control and antimicrobial stewardship (AMS) are vital for patient safety and public health. However, they can also have unintended environmental consequences, such as greenhouse gas emissions, waste generation, and overall resource consumption [25]. It is important to frame the planetary footprint of IPC and AMS activities within the wider impact of healthcare systems, which contribute ~3–10% of national greenhouse gas emissions in high-resource settings [26]. For example, the National Health Service (NHS) in the UK is responsible for approximately 5.4% of the nation's carbon footprint [27], and the US healthcare sector accounts for approximately 8.5% of US annual emissions [28]. This impact has led the World Health Organization to advocate and encourage 'climate-resilient and environmentally sustainable health systems' [29].

Ensuring sustainability in IPC and AMS activities is not only about environmental stewardship but also about safeguarding health in the long term; the climate crisis and its effects, such as pollution and biodiversity loss, are projected to cause an additional ~14.5 million deaths by 2050 and can disrupt infectious disease risks, as highlighted [30]. Therefore, integrating sustainability into IPC and AMS practices is essential to protect both planetary and patient health.

16.3.2 The Environmental Impact of IPC Activities

IPC and AMS activities in healthcare directly and indirectly contribute to environmental degradation through carbon emissions, waste production, and high resource utilisation. For example, many IPC products and activities have a significant carbon footprint across their lifecycle (manufacture, transport, use, and disposal). The use of personal protective equipment (PPE) is a clear example of this impact. During the COVID-19 pandemic, the surge in disposable PPE led to a dramatic increase in the healthcare emissions. An estimated 3 billion PPE items used over 6 months in England (February–July 2020) had a carbon footprint of ~591 tonnes of CO_2 per day [31]. Perhaps unsurprisingly, gloves were the most-used item (1.8 billion gloves) and contributed the largest share of the PPE-related carbon footprint.

Beyond PPE, sterilisation and disinfection processes also contribute to emissions, as steam sterilisers (autoclaves) and sterilant production require energy. A study in a UK hospital sterilisation unit found that reprocessing a single surgical instrument can emit ~66–189 g of CO_2-equivalent, depending on how efficiently the loads are processed [32]. Likewise, the manufacture and use of antimicrobial agents leaves a considerable carbon and pollution footprint. Pharmaceutical production is energy-intensive, and the supply chain for antibiotics and other antimicrobials contributes to the overall emissions of healthcare. For instance, the carbon footprint of an antibiotic encompasses all greenhouse gases from production to disposal [33]. Although precise figures vary by drug, it is clear that unnecessary use of antimicrobials not only drives resistance but also generates avoidable emissions.

IPC and AMS practices produce large volumes of waste, much of which is plastic and is often classified as hazardous. The necessary reliance on single-use, disposable materials (e.g. gloves, gowns, and intravenous IV tubing) generates significant solid waste. In one study on a single general medical ward under contact precautions, 56 kg of disposable PPE waste were produced in just 24 h, over 1/3 of the ward's daily total solid waste [34]. Healthcare waste profiles differ among regions worldwide. High-resource settings generate approximately 0.5 kg of hazardous medical waste per hospital bed/day, whereas this figure is 0.2 kg per bed/day in low-resource settings [35]. However, due to poor segregation practices, the true amount of this waste in low-resource settings is likely to be higher.

Clinical waste disposal practices have environmental impacts. Infectious waste is often incinerated to eliminate biological risks; however, incineration at insufficient temperatures can release harmful pollutants such as dioxins and furans, and even well-controlled incineration produces greenhouse gases [36]. The improper disposal of antibiotics and other pharmaceuticals can further contaminate soil and water, fostering drug-resistant organisms in the environment [37, 38]. Single-use IPC materials also contribute to plastic pollution, as they mostly end up in landfills or require high-energy treatments.

The disposal of products crucial for IPC and AMS operations is not the sole resource-intensive stage of these activities. This process is inherently resource-intensive, consuming significant amounts of water and energy. Hand hygiene, a cornerstone of infection control, can be water-demanding when performed with soap and water. Each thorough hand wash, as recommended, uses clean water and often heated water, incurring energy costs for heating. In settings with inadequate infrastructure, water scarcity is frequent [39], prompting the use of alcohol-based hand rubs (ABHR) as an alternative (though ABHR production has its own carbon footprint due to ethanol distillation and packaging) [40]. Instrument reprocessing (cleaning, disinfection, and sterilisation of clinical instruments) requires both water and energy. Automated washers use large volumes of water and detergents, and steam sterilisers consume significant amounts of electricity or fuel to generate high-pressure steam [41]. If reprocessing is suboptimal (e.g. running sterilisers at partial loads), energy per instrument is wasted.

Furthermore, IPC-driven environmental controls in healthcare facilities contribute to energy consumption. Ventilation and air filtration systems are critical for IPC in operating theatres and isolation rooms; however, they are energy intensive. Hospital heating, ventilation, and air conditioning (HVAC) systems account for an estimated 57% of the total energy use in hospitals [42], largely because they must maintain strict air exchange rates, filtration, and climate parameters to control infection risks. Operating rooms, for instance, require high air exchange rates (15–20 air changes per hour with HEPA filtration) and maintained positive pressure, running 24/7, even when surgeries are not occurring. This makes surgical suites one of the most energy-demanding areas, consuming approximately 20–40% of a hospital's energy [43].

16.4   Sustainability Challenges and Barriers for IPC and AMS Activities

Implementing sustainable infection practices in healthcare settings faces numerous challenges. These barriers can be logistical, financial, regulatory, or cultural (Fig. 16.2).

Financial and economic barriers can hinder the good intentions to deploy 'greener' IPC and AMS. Environmentally friendly alternatives, such as reusable gowns and advanced waste treatment, require upfront investment or higher costs than disposable options. Reusable gowns incur laundry costs, whereas single-use items are immediately affordable (but have hidden long-term costs). There may be a perception that sustainability is expensive; however, hospitals that switched from disposable to reusable gowns reported a 50% reduction in gown expenditure without compromising safety [44].

In terms of logistical and infrastructure barriers, introducing reusable or lower-waste systems requires adequate infrastructure, such as sterile reprocessing facilities, trained staff, and space for onsite sterilisation. Many hospitals, especially smaller or low-resource hospitals, lack these resources. For example, hospitals need the capacity for high-temperature laundering or disinfection, quality control processes, and inventory management to circulate clean items. In low-income settings, basic requirements such as reliable electricity and water for sterilisation or hand hygiene may be lacking [39, 45]. Supply chain issues also pose barriers, and facilities might find it difficult to procure sustainable alternatives because of limited availability or higher cost per unit.

Infection control regulations and standards, although crucial for safety, may inadvertently favour disposable products and hinder sustainability. Medical device

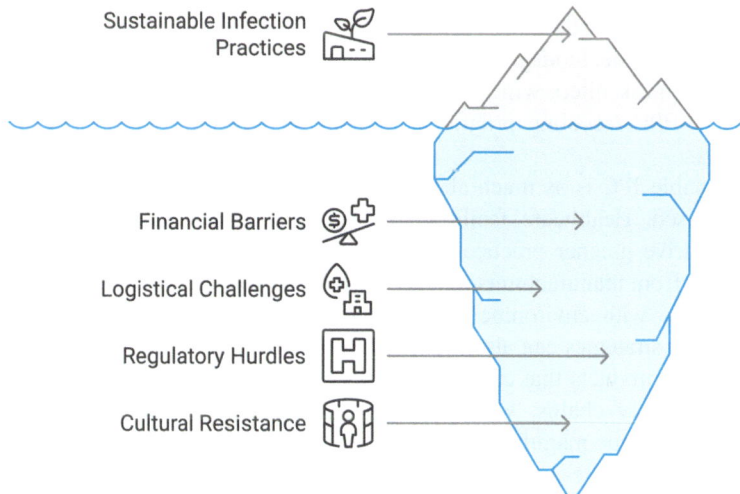

Fig. 16.2 Sustainability challenges for infection and AMS practices. (Author's own)

regulations often designate items as single use by default, particularly after high-profile IPC failures. This cautious approach can lead to the labelling of potentially reusable items as single use only, creating compliance challenges for hospitals. Health authorities' compliance audits often 'mark down' hospitals for lapses in disinfection practices, reinforcing the perception of disposable equipment as a simpler way to ensure compliance with infection control protocols.

Finally, behavioural and cultural challenges in healthcare include resistance to change due to decades of IPC practices, reinforcing the idea that disposable items are safe [46]. Educating healthcare workers and administrators about sustainable practices requires demonstrating safety, addressing concerns about compromising infection control, and overcoming convenience and habits. A lack of awareness and data on the environmental harm caused by IPC activities also hinders change [47]. At the leadership level, sustainability may not be a priority without strong institutional commitment or external pressure [48, 49].

16.5   Strategies for Sustainable IPC and AMS

Despite these challenges, various strategies and best practices can substantially reduce the environmental footprint of IPC and AMS without compromising their effectiveness. These strategies span technological solutions, process improvements, and policy initiatives and can be tailored to both high- and low-resource healthcare settings.

For example, adopting reusable and environmentally friendly materials could be a 'low-hanging fruit', and replacing single-use items with reusables would be impactful. Many PPE items and clinical instruments can be designed for reuse and safely reprocessed after use. For example, reusable isolation gowns made of durable fabric reduce greenhouse gas emissions, water usage, and solid waste compared to disposable paper/plastic gowns [50] without increasing infection rates. Where safe reuse is not feasible, biodegradable plastics may be considered; for example, gloves, gowns, and mask filters will break down faster after disposal [51]. Hospitals can implement PPE recycling programs for materials such as polypropylene masks and visors.

Sustainable IPC is as much about how products are sourced as it is about the products used. Healthcare facilities and systems can leverage their purchasing power to drive greener practices. Sustainable procurement policies may include purchasing from manufacturers that use recycled or low-carbon materials or choosing suppliers with environmentally responsible operations (e.g. ISO certified). Procurement strategies can also reduce waste, such as buying certain items in bulk or preferring products that are reusable or re-processable by design. Additionally, localising supply chains, where possible, can reduce transport emissions and encourage domestic manufacturing.

Healthcare facilities can reduce resource use through efficiency and innovation, aiming to eliminate unnecessary consumption and optimise processes. For example, autoclaves and washers should run with full loads of instruments in sterilisation departments to maximise utility per unit of energy and water. Better loading and packaging of surgical instrument sets can significantly reduce the per-instrument carbon footprint of sterilisation. HVAC settings in operating and isolation rooms should be adjusted to reduce energy when rooms are unoccupied. A hospital in Spain introduced a smart climate control system for its operating theatres, linking ventilation to the real-time surgical schedules. This initiative reduced energy consumption by 5.78 GWh over 4 years and avoided over 1200 tonnes of CO_2 emissions [52]. Water-saving measures include using no-touch faucet systems that cut off while hands are being lathered or promoting alcohol hand rub for routine decontamination when hands are not visibly soiled.

Diagnostic and antimicrobial stewardship can also be excellent sustainability strategies; avoiding unnecessary tests and treatments reduces waste. For example, reducing urine cultures and antibiotics for asymptomatic bacteriuria can improve patient care and save resources [53, 54]. Choosing an oral antibiotic over an intravenous one eliminates IV tubing, syringes, and single-use IV medications, reducing material waste and emissions and saving nurses' administration time [55, 56]. An even more preferable behaviour would be preventing infections in the community as much as in healthcare settings, avoiding the intensive resources required.

Behavioural and organisational hurdles may be gradually overcome by implementing strategies for education and awareness and shaping decision architecture to promote buy-in from healthcare workers. Incorporating sustainability into IPC and AMS training, guidelines, and institutional culture is a softer, yet important, approach. Infection prevention and control committees should consider the environmental impact when developing protocols. Health facilities may appoint sustainability champions or "green IPC/AMS" working groups to identify opportunities for improvement, at least until this perspective does not need to be seen as an add-on to others of safety and effectiveness [57]. Climate-smart healthcare delivers low-carbon, resilient, and safe care.

Unsurprisingly, support from institutional leaders and decision-makers is crucial for widespread changes in healthcare. These leaders can implement frameworks and incentives for sustainable IPC, such as setting waste or carbon reduction targets. National policies can also make a difference, including guidelines on environmentally sustainable healthcare practices and sustainability criteria for hospital accreditation. Some countries, such as the NHS in England, have committed to reaching net-zero emissions by 2045, which encourages hospitals to innovate in IPC [58]. Regulatory bodies can revise guidelines to incorporate evidence of what not to do and streamline approval processes for sustainable technologies. Collaboration with industry regulators is crucial to encourage the design of reusable devices and update labelling.

However, strategies need to be tailored to the context. Facilities in high-resource settings might focus on high-tech solutions (e.g. energy management systems or advanced reusables), whereas low-resource hospitals may focus on fundamental improvements (basic sanitation infrastructure, reuse of supplies when safe). However, the overarching principle remains: through thoughtful changes, IPC and AMS can maintain their core mission of patient safety while dramatically reducing their environmental footprint.

16.6   Recommendations

The way we prevent and manage infections today can inadvertently pose public health risks tomorrow through the climate crisis and its effects. The encouraging news is that many current strategies can mitigate these impacts without compromising the quality or safety.

1. Integrate sustainability and planetary perspective into IPC and AMS standards: Incorporate sustainability principles into infection control and antimicrobial prescribing guidelines. Encourage the use of reusable options, such as gowns and respirators, when safe, and discourage low-value, wasteful practices, such as routine contact precautions for low-risk pathogens. Regulatory bodies and accreditation programs should include environmental criteria and track IPC/AMS-related waste and emissions as quality metrics for sustainability. Embedding sustainability in good IPC and AMS practices will make it part of healthcare workers' mandates.
2. Invest in reusable systems and infrastructure: Target investments to overcome barriers to switching to reusable systems. Purchase reusable PPE/instrument sets and expand the sterile processing capacity to handle reprocessing loads. Improving infrastructure for cleaner waste treatment, such as on-site autoclave treatment for infectious waste, is necessary. Engage hospital leadership through successful case studies to secure funding.
3. Promote waste segregation and recycling: Staff should be trained on proper waste segregation, ensuring that only infectious waste is placed in biohazard bags. This reduces the incineration volume and cost. Initiate recycling of non-infectious waste (paper, cardboard, and clean plastic packaging). Partner with companies that recycle medical-grade plastics (where regulations allow) for used sterilisation wraps, mask plastics, etc. Set annual waste reduction targets to motivate improvements.
4. Optimise resource use through efficiency improvement. Review practices for waste reduction are also recommended. Adjust room air change frequency when rooms are unused, reduce excessive diagnostic testing, or use multi-dose vials instead of single-dose vials (when safe). Adopt energy-efficient technologies, such as motion-sensor faucets and energy-saving autoclave cycles. Prioritise resource-efficient options that achieve IPC goals with the least expenditure (e.g. alcohol hand rub over soap-and-water when appropriate). Checklists or toolkits should be developed for unit managers to assess and improve IPC/AMS resource efficiencies.
5. Strengthening education and awareness. Incorporate environmental impact into IPC training, hand hygiene campaigns, and antibiotic stewardship. For example, when training on PPE use, environmental cost and rational use should be included in the training. Celebrate and reward wards for reducing waste. Promote planetary health in infection control curricula for new healthcare professionals.
6. Encourage research and innovation. Support research on reconciling infection control with environmental sustainability issues. Key research needs include

biodegradable PPE, safer reprocessing methods for complex devices, and the impact of reduced-contact precautions on infection rates and resource use. Infection preventionists can collaborate with engineers, materials scientists, and environmental health experts to pilot solutions in hospitals. Findings should be shared widely to build evidence and coalitions of interested stakeholders.

7. Foster multidisciplinary and global collaborations to address sustainable IPC/AMS challenges. Infection control experts should collaborate with sustainability officers, hospital engineers, procurement officers, and policymakers. Form working groups or committees to combine perspectives and develop holistic solutions. Global health organisations and professional societies should prioritise sustainability in conferences and guidelines, facilitating the exchange of ideas across healthcare systems.

16.7 Conclusion

Sustainable infection prevention and control and optimal use of antimicrobials are attainable goals. This calls for rethinking entrenched practices and innovating on multiple fronts, but the benefits are manifold: reduced environmental harm, potential cost savings, and often improvements in the efficiency and resilience of healthcare delivery. IPC and AMS are poised to be allies in reducing the environmental footprint of healthcare if professionals lead and advocate for these changes. By aligning IPC and AMS with planetary health, we not only do no harm to our patients but also do less harm to the world in which they live. Future efforts should ensure that every advancement in infection prevention is evaluated not only for its immediate efficacy but also for its long-term sustainability. This integrated approach will help safeguard the health of current and future generations in an ever-changing global environment.

References

1. Murray CJL, Ikuta KS, Sharara F, Swetschinski L, Aguilar GR, Gray A, et al. Global burden of bacterial antimicrobial resistance in 2019: a systematic analysis. Lancet. 2022;399(10325):629–55. https://doi.org/10.1016/S0140-6736(21)02724-0.
2. Sakalauskienė GV, Radzevičienė A. Antimicrobial resistance: what lies beneath this complex phenomenon? Diagnostics (Basel, Switzerland). 2024;14:2319.
3. Ifedinezi OV, Nnaji ND, Anumudu CK, Ekwueme CT, Uhegwu CC, Ihenetu FC, Obioha P, Simon BO, Ezechukwu PS, Onyeaka H. Environmental antimicrobial resistance: implications for food safety and public health. Antibiotics (Basel, Switzerland). 2024;13:1087.
4. Lacotte Y, Ploy M-C, Årdal C. Infection prevention and control research priorities: what do we need to combat healthcare-associated infections and antimicrobial resistance? vol. 9. Results of a narrative literature review and survey analysis: Antimicrob Resist Infect Control; 2020. https://doi.org/10.1186/s13756-020-00801-x.
5. Stewardson AJ, Kramer A, Allegranzi B, et al. Updates and future directions regarding hand hygiene in the healthcare setting: insights from the 3rd ICPIC alcohol-based handrub

(ABHR) task force. Antimicrob Resist Infect Control. 2024;13:26. https://doi.org/10.1186/s13756-024-01374-9.

6. World Health Organization. Social determinants of health. Geneva: WHO; 2010. Available from: https://www.who.int/health-topics/social-determinants-of-health.

7. Macias-Konstantopoulos WL, Duber HC, Edwards CD, Sachs CJ, Riviello RJ, Diaz R, Collins KA, Wettstein ZS, Ranney ML, Hsu AP. Race, healthcare, and health disparities: a critical review and recommendations 6. For advancing health equity. West J Emerg Med. 2023;24:906. https://doi.org/10.5811/westjem.58408.

8. Myers SS, Frumkin H. Planetary health: protecting nature to protect ourselves. Washington, DC: Island Press; 2020.

9. Antó JM. Human health and the health of planet earth go together. J Intern Med. 2024;295:695–706.

10. Kopittke PM, Minasny B, Pendall E, Rumpel C, Mckenna BA. Healthy soil for healthy humans and a healthy planet. Crit Rev Environ Sci Technol. 2023;54:210–21.

11. Whitmee S, Haines A, Beyrer C, Boltz F, Capon AG, de Souza Dias BF, et al. Safeguarding human health in the Anthropocene epoch: report of The Rockefeller Foundation–Lancet Commission on planetary health. Lancet. 2015;386(10007):1973–2028. https://doi.org/10.1016/S0140-6736(15)60901-1.

12. Sundas A, Contreras I, Mujahid O, Beneyto A, Vehi J. The effects of environmental factors on general human health: a scoping review. Healthcare (Basel, Switzerland). 2024;12:2123.

13. Parkes MW, Bienen L, Breilh J, Hsu LN, McDonald M, Patz JA, et al. All hands on deck: transdisciplinary approaches to emerging infectious disease. EcoHealth. 2005;2(4):258–72. https://doi.org/10.1007/s10393-005-8385-3.

14. Murray MH, Buckley J, Byers KA, Stone C, Magle SB, Fake K, Schell CJ, Tuten H, Lehrer EW. One health for all: advancing human and ecosystem health in cities by integrating an environmental justice lens. Annu Rev Ecol Evol Syst. 2022;53:403–26.

15. Mago A, Kumar H, Maity R, Dhali A, Kumar B. Planetary health and its relevance in the modern era: a topical review. SAGE Open Med. 2024;12:20503121241254231. https://doi.org/10.1177/20503121241254231.

16. Iyer HS, Deville NV, Stoddard O, Cole J, Myers SS, Li H, Elliott EG, Jimenez MP, James P, Golden CD. Sustaining planetary health through systems thinking: public health's critical role. SSM Popul Health. 2021;15:100844.

17. Magnano San Lio R, Favara G, Maugeri A, Barchitta M, Agodi A. How antimicrobial resistance is linked to climate change: an overview of two intertwined global challenges. Int J Environ Res Public Health. 2023;20:1681.

18. Anikeeva O, Hansen A, Varghese B, Borg M, Zhang Y, Xiang J, Bi P. The impact of increasing temperatures due to climate change on infectious diseases. BMJ. 2024; https://doi.org/10.1136/bmj-2024-079343.

19. Baldrian P, López-Mondéjar R, Kohout P. Forest microbiome and global change. Nat Rev Microbiol. 2023;21:487–501.

20. Pepi M, Focardi S. Antibiotic-resistant bacteria in aquaculture and climate change: a challenge for health in the Mediterranean area. Int J Environ Res Public Health. 2021;18:5723.

21. Rocklöv J, Dubrow R. Climate change: an enduring challenge for vector-borne disease prevention and control. Nat Immunol. 2020;21(5):479–83. https://doi.org/10.1038/s41590-020-0648-y.

22. Romanello M, McGushin A, Di Napoli C, et al. The 2023 report of the lancet countdown on health and climate change: health at the mercy of fossil fuels. Lancet. 2023;402(10397):1610–54. https://doi.org/10.1016/S0140-6736(23)01859-7.

23. Watts N, Amann M, Arnell N, Ayeb-Karlsson S, Belesova K, Boykoff M, et al. The 2019 report of the lancet countdown on health and climate change: ensuring that the health of a child born today is not defined by a changing climate. Lancet. 2019;394(10211):1836–78. https://doi.org/10.1016/S0140-6736(19)32596-6.

24. Kwon H, Xu H, Liu X, Wang M. Greenhouse gas mitigation strategies and opportunities for agriculture. Agron J. 2021;113:4639–47.

25. Alruwaili RF, Alsadaan N, Alruwaili AN, Alrumayh AG. Unveiling the symbiosis of environmental sustainability and infection control in health care settings: a systematic review. Sustainability. 2023;15(22):15728. https://doi.org/10.3390/su152215728.
26. Lenzen M, Malik A, Li M, Fry J, Weisz H, Pichler PP, et al. The environmental footprint of health care: a global assessment. Lancet Planet Health. 2020;4(7):e271–9. https://doi.org/10.1016/S2542-5196(20)30121-2.
27. Tennison I, Roschnik S, Ashby B, Boyd R, Hamilton I, Oreszczyn T, et al. Health care's climate footprint: the NHS and climate change. Lancet Planet Health. 2021;5(2):e84–6. https://doi.org/10.1016/S2542-5196(20)30250-2.
28. Eckelman MJ, Huang K, Lagasse R, Senay E, Dubrow R, Sherman JD. Health care pollution and public health damage in the United States: an update. Health Aff (Millwood). 2020;39(12):2071–9. https://doi.org/10.1377/hlthaff.2020.01109.
29. World Health Organization. Operational framework for building climate resilient health systems. Geneva: World Health Organization; 2015. Available from: https://www.who.int/publications/i/item/9789241565073.
30. World Economic Forum. Quantifying the impact of climate change on human health. Geneva: World Economic Forum; 2024. Available from: https://www.weforum.org/publications/quantifying-the-impact-of-climate-change-on-human-health/.
31. Rizan C, Reed M, Bhutta MF. Environmental impact of personal protective equipment distributed for use by health and social care services in England in the first six months of the COVID-19 pandemic. J R Soc Med. 2021;114(5):250–63. https://doi.org/10.1177/01410768211001583.
32. Rizan C, Mortimer F, Stancliffe R, Bhutta MF. Plastics in healthcare: time for a re-evaluation. J R Soc Med. 2020;113(2):49–53. https://doi.org/10.1177/0141076819890554.
33. Andrzejewski A, Mascarenhas A, Mascarenhas J, Rosenbaum RK, Fantke P. A global life cycle assessment of 15 antibiotic drugs—impacts on climate change and freshwater ecotoxicity. Environ Int. 2021;156:106672. https://doi.org/10.1016/j.envint.2021.106672.
34. Thompson R, Nawaz M, MacEachern L, et al. The plastic pandemic: quantifying the waste generated by personal protective equipment (PPE) during the COVID-19 pandemic in a UK hospital. J Hosp Infect. 2023;129:144–51. https://doi.org/10.1016/j.jhin.2023.01.016.
35. World Health Organization. Health-care waste. Geneva: World Health Organization; 2018. Available from: https://www.who.int/news-room/fact-sheets/detail/health-care-waste.
36. World Health Organization. Safe management of wastes from health-care activities. 2nd ed. Geneva: WHO Press; 2014. Available from: https://www.who.int/publications/i/item/9789241548564.
37. Tell J, Caldwell DJ, Häner A, et al. Science-based targets for antibiotics in receiving waters from pharmaceutical manufacturing operations. Integr Environ Assess Manag. 2019;15(3):312–9. https://doi.org/10.1002/ieam.4141.
38. Larsson DGJ, Andremont A, Bengtsson-Palme J, et al. Critical knowledge gaps and research needs related to the environmental dimensions of antibiotic resistance. Environ Int. 2018;117:132–8. https://doi.org/10.1016/j.envint.2018.04.041.
39. World Health Organization, UNICEF. WASH in health care facilities: global baseline report 2019. Geneva: WHO and UNICEF; 2019. Available from: https://www.who.int/publications/i/item/9789241515504.
40. Trust C. Carbon footprinting alcohol-based hand rubs. London: Carbon Trust; 2021.
41. Rizan C, Bhutta MF. Sustainability in surgery: green operating theatres. Surgery (Oxford). 2022;40(1):9–15. https://doi.org/10.1016/j.mpsur.2021.10.004.
42. Short M, Al-Bazi A, Oughton EJ, Hanna RF, Chalabi Z. A systematic review of the energy demand of hospitals. Renew Sust Energ Rev. 2021;143:110903. https://doi.org/10.1016/j.rser.2021.110903.
43. Bolten A, Kringos DS, Spijkerman IJB, Sperna Weiland NH. The carbon footprint of the operating room related to infection prevention measures: a scoping review. J Hosp Infect. 2022;128:64–73.

44. Vozzola E, Overcash M, Griffing E. Environmental considerations in the selection of isolation gowns: a life cycle assessment of reusable and disposable alternatives. Am J Infect Control. 2020;48(5):529–36. https://doi.org/10.1016/j.ajic.2019.09.005.

45. Overcash M. A comparison of reusable and disposable perioperative textiles: sustainability state-of-the-art 2012. Anesth Analg. 2012;114(5):1055–66. https://doi.org/10.1213/ANE.0b013e318248f4c3.

46. MacNeill AJ, Hopf H, Khanuja A, Alizamir S, Bilec MM, Eckelman MJ, et al. Transforming the medical device industry: road map to a circular economy. Health Aff (Millwood). 2020;39(12):2088–97. https://doi.org/10.1377/hlthaff.2020.01118.

47. McGain F, Muret J, Lawson C, Sherman JD. Environmental sustainability in anaesthesia and critical care. Br J Anaesth. 2020;125(5):680–92. https://doi.org/10.1016/j.bja.2020.07.061.

48. Sherman JD, MacNeill A, Thiel C. Reducing pollution from the health care industry. JAMA. 2019;322(11):1043–4. https://doi.org/10.1001/jama.2019.11868.

49. Mortimer F, Isherwood J, Wilkinson A, Vaux E, Moghazy H. Sustainability in quality improvement: redefining value. Future Healthc J. 2018;5(2):88–93. https://doi.org/10.7861/futurehosp.5-2-88.

50. McGain F, Hendel SA, Story DA, et al. The environmental impact of reusable versus single-use perioperative textiles: a life cycle analysis. Anesth Analg. 2012;114(5):1055–66. https://doi.org/10.1213/ANE.0b013e31824f695f.

51. Kutralam-Muniasamy G, Pérez-Guevara F, Shruti VC, Elizalde-Martínez I, Roy PD. Bioplastics in the medical sector: a greener alternative? Sci Total Environ. 2022;807(Pt 3):150998. https://doi.org/10.1016/j.scitotenv.2021.150998.

52. Pujol M, Limón E, López-Contreras J, et al. The green surgical block 4.0: automation of the operating theatre's climate conditions using real-time patient flow data. J Hosp Infect. 2023;127:89–96. https://doi.org/10.1016/j.jhin.2023.05.004.

53. Morgan DJ, Malani P, Diekema DJ. Diagnostic stewardship—leveraging the laboratory to improve antimicrobial use. JAMA. 2017;318(7):607–8. https://doi.org/10.1001/jama.2017.8531.

54. Trautner BW, Grigoryan L. Approach to a positive urine culture in a patient without urinary symptoms. Infect Dis Clin N Am. 2014;28(1):15–31. https://doi.org/10.1016/j.idc.2013.10.002.

55. Wilkinson A, Wood P, Mortimer F, Low M. Sustainable prescribing: a multiprofessional consensus on environmentally sustainable prescribing practice. J Clean Prod. 2022;344:131069. https://doi.org/10.1016/j.jclepro.2022.131069.

56. Meddings J, Saint S, Krein SL, et al. Reducing unnecessary urinary catheter use and other strategies to prevent catheter-associated urinary tract infection: an integrative review. BMJ Qual Saf. 2014;23(4):277–89. https://doi.org/10.1136/bmjqs-2012-001774.

57. MacNeill AJ, McGain F, Sherman JD. Planetary health care: a framework for sustainable health systems. Lancet Planet Health. 2021;5(2):e66–8. https://doi.org/10.1016/S2542-5196(20)30281-4.

58. NHS England. Delivering a Net Zero National Health Service. London: NHS England; 2020. Available from: https://www.england.nhs.uk/greenernhs/a-net-zero-nhs/.

The ABC of Behavior Change in IPC and AMS and Social Marketing

17

Elisa Fabbri

Abstract

Infection control, which refers to the practical discipline of preventing healthcare-associated infections, is an essential process for any healthcare organization to control, reduce, and prevent infections in all care settings. These infection prevention and control (IPC) practices are all supported by scientific evidence and include hand hygiene, the use of personal protective equipment (PPE), patient screening, equipment decontamination, environmental sanitation, proper disposal/treatment of linens and waste, thorough risk assessment, and proper respiratory hygiene.

At the same time, the significant global increase in antimicrobial resistance (AMR) has led to a greater spread of microorganisms in all healthcare settings. This phenomenon is particularly impactful in countries with high antibiotic use.

Behavioral changes among healthcare workers are necessary to improve adherence to infection prevention and control guidelines. Despite significant investments in strategies to change behaviors, their effectiveness has not been adequately evaluated, which remains a crucial aspect, particularly in IPC and the fight against antimicrobial resistance (AMR).

Keywords

Behavior changes theory · IPC · AMR · Implementation · Change · Social marketing

E. Fabbri (✉)
IPC Nurse, Emilia-Romagna, Italy

© The Author(s), under exclusive license to Springer Nature Switzerland AG 2025
B. Oomen, S. Gastaldi (eds.), *Principles of Nursing Infection Prevention Control*,
Principles of Specialty Nursing, https://doi.org/10.1007/978-3-032-01446-7_17

17.1   Introduction

Preventing harm to patients, health workers (HWs), and visitors due to healthcare-associated infections (HAIs) is fundamental to achieve safe quality care and reduce antimicrobial resistance (AMR) [1, 2].

Similarly, preventing and reducing the transmission of infectious diseases that may pose global threats are equally crucial. Supported by many stakeholders in the field of infection prevention and control (IPC), the World Health Organization (WHO) has issued recommendations and specifications for effective IPC programmes, identified as core components of IPC programmes [1] and the approach for their implementation is presented in associated manuals for both national and facility level [3, 4].

By understanding the ABC of behavior change in IPC, AMS, and social marketing, interventions can be better designed to shift attitudes, influence behaviors, and work within the context of societal and environmental factors.

Behavior change is a crucial aspect in various areas of public health, particularly in infection prevention and control (IPC) and the fight against antimicrobial resistance (AMR) [5–10]. Through social marketing and other techniques, individual and collective behaviors can be influenced, reducing the risks of infection and the spread of antibiotic resistance. Here is how we can understand and apply the ABCs of behavior change, by defining:

1. Attitude: Focus on shaping the beliefs, perceptions, and values that individuals hold about infection control, antimicrobial use, or health behaviors.
2. Behavior: The core of behavior change, focusing on influencing actions such as washing hands, taking antibiotics as prescribed, or adopting healthier lifestyle choices.
3. Context: The environment that affects the ability to change, including healthcare infrastructure, policies, and socioeconomic conditions.

By integrating the ABC approach into IPC, AMS, and social marketing strategies, interventions can be more effectively tailored to drive sustainable behavior change.

Furthermore, continuing education is essential for staying updated on emerging scientific evidence and technological advancements. International collaboration plays a key role in developing innovative approaches that are adaptable to global health challenges. Emerging technologies, including artificial intelligence and the Internet of Things, are transforming nursing and healthcare practices, while implementation science facilitates the adoption of evidence-based best practices [11].

17.2 The ABC of Behavior Change

17.2.1 Attention: Raising Awareness

The first step in behavioral change is capturing the attention of the target audience (healthcare workers, users, etc.). Without awareness, effective intervention is impossible. In the context of Infection Prevention and Control (IPC) and Antimicrobial Resistance (AMR), this means educating individuals about the severity of infections, the risks of antibiotic resistance, and the importance of preventive measures.

Social marketing campaigns must leverage visible and accessible communication channels (e.g., social media, television ads, posters) to reach the public.

In the case of AMR, it is crucial to inform citizens about the risks of improper or excessive antibiotic use, for instance, raising awareness about the importance of completing a full prescribed course of antibiotics, avoiding self-medication, and preventing indiscriminate antibiotic use. Awareness remains a fundamental step in behavior change.

Modern technologies, such as health apps, social media, and instant messaging, have become powerful tools for increasing awareness and engaging people in real-time.

17.2.1.1 In IPC and AMS
- Early warning systems, mobile apps for infection monitoring, and hand hygiene reminders are innovative tools that enhance awareness of hospital-acquired infection risks and inappropriate antibiotic use.
- The use of real-time data to educate and raise awareness among healthcare professionals has proven to be a promising area.

17.2.1.2 Social Marketing
- Digital platforms (such as Facebook, Instagram, and TikTok) enable social marketing campaigns to reach a broad and diverse audience, promoting awareness of crucial topics such as mental health, healthy eating, and smoking prevention in an interactive way.

17.2.2 Understanding: Enhancing Behavioral Comprehension

Mere awareness is not enough; people need to understand why certain behaviors are harmful while others are beneficial. Information must be clear, scientifically grounded, and culturally adapted to the target population and professionals it is intended for.

For behavioral change in IPC, this involves educating both patients and healthcare professionals on the importance of daily hygiene practices, such as handwashing, proper management of medical devices, and mask use when necessary. Creating clear and easy-to-follow messages is essential to ensure that people not only understand the risks but also know how to act accordingly.

In the context of AMR, understanding how inappropriate antibiotic use leads to the selection of resistant bacteriais crucial. Scientific information must be communicated effectively, ensuring that the public recognizes individual responsibility in preventing antibiotic resistance.

Beliefs still play a significant role in shaping behavior, but advanced persuasion techniques from behavioral sciences, such as nudging ("gentle push") and framing (cognitive bias strategies), are becoming increasingly central. Recent research in behavioral psychology has demonstrated that small changes in how information is presented can significantly influence decision-making.

17.2.2.1 In IPC and AMS
- Promoting proper antimicrobial stewardship requires overcoming misconceptions. The use of visual evidence, such as infographics and simulations, is becoming a powerful strategy to change beliefs about AMR risks and infections.

17.2.2.2 Social Marketing
- Beliefs that hinder change, such as those related to smoking or unhealthy diets, can be more effectively modified through personalized messages and success stories, often reinforced by video testimonials or interviews on social media.

17.2.3 Behavior: Implementing and Sustaining Change

Real behavioral change occurs when people modify their habits. This is the most challenging part of the process: social marketing goes beyond raising awareness and focuses on encouraging the adoption of new behaviors, such as improving hygiene practices or using antibiotics responsibly.

For change to persist, it requires continuous reinforcement and motivation.

In IPC, this means promoting the adoption of daily hygiene routines in schools, hospitals, and communities. Implementing policies and incentives that encourage positive behaviors, such as frequent handwashing, is essential.

For AMR, promoting the responsible use of antibiotics is crucial. This involves educating people about preventive alternatives (such as vaccination and improved hygiene practices) and making it clear that both individual and collective health depend on adherence to these practices.

The focus is no longer solely on education and resources—modern strategies enhance self-efficacy, reinforcing digital skills and integrating technology into daily practice. Simulators and e-learning platforms represent a major advancement in improving healthcare professionals' competencies.

17.2.3.1 In IPC and AMS
- Digital platforms, online training courses, and clinical scenario simulations are innovative tools for enhancing skills and best practices adoption in IPC and AMS.
- Mobile apps that provide antibiotic prescribing guidelines have had a significant impact on responsible antimicrobial use.

17.2.3.2 Social Marketing

- Empowering consumers through accessible resources, such as online tutorials on health and nutrition, has enabled many individuals to develop fundamental skills for behavioral change independently.

Beyond these widely recognized strategies, which are supported by scientific evidence, additional approaches can further contribute to achieving sustainable behavior change.

17.2.4 Motivation

Motivation is viewed as a dynamic process that can be reinforced through immediate feedback and digital reward systems, such as apps that track progress and provide incentives (e.g., points, badges). These tools are reshaping how people are encouraged to adopt behavioral changes.

17.2.4.1 In IPC and AMS

- Healthcare professionals' motivation to adhere to IPC and AMS guidelines can be enhanced through real-time feedback systems, such as monitoring adherence rates and assigning digital recognitions for correct behaviors.
- Incentive-based approaches, including awards or recognition for best practices, are an emerging strategy for sustaining motivation.

17.2.4.2 Social Marketing

- Health-tracking apps and gamification platforms strengthen motivation through friendly competition, rewards, and visible progress tracking—a technique widely used in anti-obesity campaigns and smoking cessation programs.

17.2.5 Environment

The physical and social environment continues to shape behavior. However, the rise of digital and virtual environments is transforming how people interact with the world. Online platforms and virtual spaces provide new opportunities to modify social settings and promote healthy behaviors.

17.2.5.1 In IPC and AMS

- The hospital environment, now integrating advanced technologies such as automated hand hygiene monitoring systems, is improving compliance with IPC measures.
- Virtual work environments and digital meetings are also enhancing awareness and training for healthcare professionals, making education more efficient.

17.2.5.2 Social Marketing

- The creation of virtual social environments, such as online support groups and virtual communities, has revolutionized social marketing, enabling behavioral change through reinforced group dynamics and peer support.

17.2.6 Feedback and Reinforcement

In today's world, feedback is often provided in real-time through digital platforms, which play a crucial role in encouraging behavioral change. The use of apps and progress-tracking systems is becoming increasingly central to reinforcing positive behaviors.

17.2.6.1 In IPC and AMS

- Instant feedback systems, such as digital performance reports for individuals and teams, are advanced toolsthat support adherence to IPC and AMS measures.
- These systems provide immediate data on behaviors, allowing for timely corrections and continuous improvement.

17.2.6.2 Social Marketing

- Digital platforms offer immediate feedback to consumers, such as health scores or virtual badges, which incentivize sustained behavior change, encouraging actions like physical activity and improved nutrition.

17.3 Conclusion

Behavioral change is essential for the success of Infection Prevention and Control (IPC), optimal Antimicrobial Stewardship (AMS), and social marketing campaigns. Recent advancements in behavioral psychology, technology, and communication have enhanced our understanding of change processes and the most effective strategies to facilitate them. This chapter has explored an updated approach to the fundamentals of behavioral change in these fields, incorporating the latest innovations.

Implementing behavioral change in IPC and AMS is challenging, yet it is crucial to reduce infection risks and prevent the spread of antibiotic resistance. Leveraging marketing strategies as a tool for awareness and motivation is essential in transforming knowledge into daily actions. Only through collective commitment and strong collaboration between institutions, healthcare professionals, and communities can we achieve long-term public health improvements.

Behavioral change in IPC, AMS, and social marketing has significantly advanced due to modern technologies and new psychological insights. The integration of digital tools, advanced persuasion techniques, and virtual environments has improved intervention effectiveness, facilitating behavioral change at both individual and collective levels. Emerging technologies and theories provide powerful opportunities to address global health challenges more efficiently, but their implementation must be consistent and adapted to local organizational settings.

Marketing is a powerful tool for promoting behavioral change. Its principles are based on the use of traditional marketing techniques to influence positive public health behaviors [12, 13]. Effective social marketing campaigns should be:

- Culturally Adapted: Every community has values, beliefs, and behaviors that influence health decisions. Therefore, communication must be personalized.
- Motivational: Creating incentives (even psychological ones) that encourage change, such as rewards for adherence to good hygiene practices or proper antibiotic use.
- Sustainable: Campaigns must have sufficient duration to ensure lasting behavioral change. Positive reinforcement, such as public recognition or rewards, can help sustain behaviors over time.

An essential factor in facilitating behavioral change is strong leadership, which plays a key role in shaping social relationships within organizations. A recent review [14] analyzed leadership during the pandemic, highlighting how human traits, behavior, and emotional intelligence are critical elements in building trust—both institutionally (with citizens) and within professional teams.

Key leadership attributes such as empathy, compassion, attention to well-being, and honesty have been reaffirmed as fundamental qualities for establishing credibility and trust, which are necessary for implementing policies, behavioral changes, and interventions. These elements are closely linked to leaders' communication skills, particularly when operating within complex systems that require systemic and inclusive approaches. Leadership capacity is indispensable for driving behavioral change among all healthcare professionals.

Policymakers and organizational leaders must make informed decisions that facilitate the application of innovative strategies—this can no longer be delayed. Synergy between decision-makers and professionals must be continuous and consistent, extending across all healthcare settings. This is critical to achieving real behavioral changes in infection prevention and control measures as well as responsible antibiotic use.

The use of advanced informational and training technologies can help disseminate a culture of change, ensuring that dynamic, widespread actions are implemented across all healthcare contexts, including hospitals and community-based care settings.

References

1. World Health Organization. Guidelines on core components of infection prevention and control programmes at the national and acute health care facility level. Geneva: World Health Organization; 2016. http://www.who.int/infection-prevention/publications/ipc-componentsguidelines/en/.

2. World Health Organization. Global action plan on antimicrobial resistance. Geneva: World Health Organization; 2015. https://www.who.int/antimicrobial-resistance/publications/global-action-lan/en/.

3. World Health Organization. Interim practical manual supporting national implementation of the WHO guidelines on core components of infection prevention and control programmes. Geneva: World Health Organization; 2017. http://www.who.int/infection-prevention/tools/core-components/cc-implementationguideline.

4. World Health Organization. Improving infection prevention and control at the health facility: interim practical manual supporting implementation of the WHO guidelines on core components of infection prevention and control programmes. Geneva: World Health Organization; 2018. http://www.who.int/infectionprevention/tools/core-components/facility-manual.pdf.

5. Global strategy on infection prevention and control. World Health Organization 2023, ISBN 978-92-4-008051-5.

6. Infection prevention and control in-service education and training curriculum. World Health Organization 2024, ISBN 978-92-4-009412-3

7. WHO. Minimum requirements for infection prevention and control programmes. https://www.who.int/publications/i/item/9789241516945. Accessed Jan 2025.

8. WHO. Guidelines on core components of infection prevention and control programmes at the national and acute health care facility level. Geneva: World Health Organization; 2016.

9. WHO. Global report on infection prevention and control. Geneva: World Health Organization; 2022.

10. WHO. My 5 moments for hand hygiene. https://5mgame.lxp.academy.who.int/. Accessed Jan 2025.

11. Gastaldi S. L'infermiere specializzato nella prevenzione del rischio infettivo nell'era della globalizzazione: innovazione ed eccellenza professionale. GImPIOS. 2024;14(1):27.

12. Fattori G., Vanoli M., Il marketing sociale: opportunità e prospettive. In Cucco E., Pagani R., Pasquali M., Soggia A, Secondo rapporto sulla comunicazione sociale in Italia, Carocci Editore, Roma, 2011.

13. Caruso M, Gagliardi A. Tecnologie digitali nel cambiamento comportamentale in salute pubblica. J Public Health. 2021;29(4):565–76.

14. Osti T, Valz Gris A, Corona VF, Villani L, D'Ambrosio F, Lomazzi M, Favaretti C, Cascini F, Gualano MR, Ricciardi W. Public health leadership in the COVID-19 era: how does it fit? A scoping review. BMJ Leader. 2024;8:174–82.

NANDA

Tihana Gašpert

Abstract

This chapter explores nurses' systematic roles in intervention and outcomes through the lens of the NANDA International (NANDA-I) taxonomy, Nursing Interventions Classification (NIC), and Nursing Outcomes Classification (NOC) frameworks. The integration of these three essential tools enables nurses to deliver patient-centered care with precision, evidence-based rationale, and measurable outcomes.

NANDA-I provides standardized nursing diagnoses that identify patients' actual or potential health issues. These diagnoses guide the selection of appropriate interventions classified under NIC, which organizes nursing activities into a structured taxonomy. Meanwhile, NOC complements this process by defining expected outcomes that allow nurses to evaluate the effectiveness of their interventions. This chapter emphasizes the synergistic application of these frameworks in enhancing clinical decision-making, improving communication among healthcare teams, and fostering better patient outcomes. By adopting NANDA-I, NIC, and NOC, nurses not only meet the demands of contemporary healthcare but also contribute to advancing nursing as a science.

T. Gašpert (✉)
University Hospital Rijeka, Rijeka, Croatia

Faculty of Health Sciences, University of Maribor, Maribor, Slovenia

Keywords

NANDA International · Nursing Diagnoses · Nursing Interventions Classification (NIC) · Nursing Outcomes Classification (NOC) · Systematic nursing care · Patient-centered care · Evidence-based nursing · Clinical decision-making · Healthcare outcomes · Nursing documentation

18.1   Introduction

The Nursing Interventions Classification (NIC) constitutes one element of a tripartite framework, which includes NANDA International (NANDA-I) nursing diagnoses and the Nursing Outcomes Classification (NOC). Collectively, these three systems establish a thorough framework for nursing care planning, execution, and assessment. This cohesive strategy enables nurses to examine patients systematically, execute interventions efficiently, and review care outcomes impartially.

NANDA International (NANDA-I) offers standardized nursing diagnoses, facilitating nurses' recognition of health issues, dangers, and wellness states. Every diagnostic function is a foundation for devising interventions and is articulated in a clear, uniform language comprehensible worldwide. The NANDA-I taxonomy organizes these diagnoses into domains and classes, providing a comprehensive, evidence-based framework for clinical decision-making [1].

The Nursing Intervention Classification (NIC) expands on NANDA-I diagnoses by providing a defined terminology for detailing the precise actions nurses implement to meet patient requirements. The NIC comprises a taxonomy of more than 550 interventions categorized into areas and classes, encompassing physiological, behavioral, safety, family, health system, and community care aspects. Every intervention is meticulously delineated, accompanied by activities that facilitate its execution. The focus on evidence-based approaches guarantees that NIC interventions are both effective and adaptive in diverse clinical situations [2].

The Nursing Outcomes Classification (NOC) finalizes this triad by offering quantifiable patient outcomes that indicate the efficacy of nursing treatments. NOC results are precise, patient-centered, and linked to metrics that measure advancement. This method enables nurses to assess the efficacy of care plans, ensuring that interventions result in significant enhancements in patient health [3].

This synergistic framework—NANDA-I, NIC, and NOC—standardizes nursing practice, promotes interdisciplinary collaboration, and improves the quality and safety of patient care. This document offers a comprehensive examination of NIC about its integration with NANDA-I and NOC, highlighting its framework, applications, and critical significance in the advancement of the nursing profession [4].

18.2   NANDA-I

The publication of Nursing Diagnoses: Definitions and Classification by NANDA International represents a significant advancement in nursing science. This text standardizes nursing diagnoses by including the NANDA-I taxonomy, so ensuring clarity and consistency in clinical, academic, and research environments [5].

The NANDA-I Taxonomy II provides a structured framework for understanding nursing diagnoses, classifying them into 13 domains and other categories. This systematic approach allows nurses to accurately assess, diagnose, and formulate interventions tailored to the individual needs of each patient.

18.2.1 NANDA-I Taxonomy: Structure and Purpose

18.2.1.1 Domains and Classifications
The taxonomy has 13 domains, each representing a distinct area of patient care, which are subsequently divided into classes to emphasize specific aspects of health and well-being. The domains include:

- Domain 1: Health Promotion: Focuses on diagnoses intended to augment health and wellness.
- Domain 2: Nutrition encompasses diagnoses like "Imbalanced nutrition: less than body requirements" and "Ineffective breastfeeding patterns."
- Domain 3: Abolition and Substitution: Addresses diagnoses related to urinary and bowel function.
- Domain 4: Activity and Rest: Encompasses disorders related to sleep, mobility, and physical activity.
- Domain 5: Perception and Cognition.
- Domain 6: Self-Perception.
- Domain 7: Interpersonal Relationships: Focuses on caregiving obligations and family dynamics.
- Domain 8: Sexuality.
- Domain 9: Resilience and Stress Management: Addresses emotional responses.
- Domain 10: Essential Principles of Existence.
- Domain 11: Safety and Security: Recognizes hazards and injuries.
- Domain 12: Comfort.
- Domain 13: Advancement/Progression: Includes developmental impairments and related conditions.

Each section includes lectures that focus on specific patient scenarios, ensuring a comprehensive and cohesive approach to nursing care [5].

18.2.1.2 Specification of Attributes and Related Factors
Each diagnosis is related to certain qualities (observable signs or symptoms) and relevant circumstances (causal factors leading to the diagnosis). These qualities

provide a thorough framework for assessing patient circumstances and tailoring therapeutic procedures [5].

18.2.1.3 Evidence-Based Improvement

Over 70 diagnoses were revised following current evidence. The improvements included the standardization of diagnostic terminology, enhancement of clarity, and alignment with international best practices. The integration of evidence ensures that the taxonomy corresponds with advancements in medical knowledge and nursing practice [5].

18.2.1.4 Global Contributions and Translation Efforts

The development of the taxonomy is becoming a global endeavor. Nurses from more than 40 countries contribute to its advancement, ensuring applicability in diverse healthcare settings. The translation into about 20 languages enhances accessibility; nonetheless, challenges remain in preserving conceptual clarity across various cultures and languages.

The standardization of diagnostic terminology to enhance translation and application is a notable accomplishment. The term "lack" was clarified to distinguish between "absence" and "insufficiency," so reducing uncertainty for non-native English speakers. This program emphasizes the commitment to making taxonomy a universally applicable tool.

International cooperation improves cultural awareness in nursing diagnosis, ensuring their pertinence and respect across various healthcare systems and practices. The involvement of multinational committees ensures that many perspectives shape the evolution of the taxonomy [5].

18.3   Nursing Interventions Classification (NIC)

The Nursing Interventions Classification (NIC) is a comprehensive, standardized approach that identifies and categorizes interventions nurses utilize in diverse healthcare settings. Developed to promote communication among nurses and interdisciplinary teams, NIC serves as a tool for planning, executing, and evaluating nursing care [2]. This categorization connects nursing diagnoses, as established by NANDA International, with the outcomes specified in the Nursing Outcomes categorization (NOC) [2, 3, 5].

The NIC establishes a comprehensive framework for nursing practice by guaranteeing that interventions are grounded in evidence and widely comprehensible. It facilitates the uninterrupted delivery of care across various settings and specialties, allowing nurses to modify interventions to address unique patient requirements. In doing so, NIC ensures the provision of consistent and high-quality care.

18.3.1 Organization of NIC

The NIC taxonomy categorizes nursing interventions into a three-tiered hierarchical framework to enhance clarity and use. NIC encompasses seven domains that include essential aspects of nursing practice. These domains encompass fundamental nursing responsibilities, from physiological requirements to community health. Each domain contains categories that aggregate relevant interventions [2].

NIC delineates more than 550 distinct interventions at the most granular level. Every intervention is distinctly identified, comprehensively defined, and substantiated by related actions. The hierarchy facilitates adaptability and accuracy, allowing nurses to meet specific patient requirements while upholding evidence-based best practices. The organized nature of NIC facilitates its incorporation into electronic health records (EHR), allowing for the standardization and optimization of interventions across healthcare systems [2].

18.3.2 Applications of NIC

NIC is extensively utilized in teaching, clinical practice, and research, solidifying its status as a fundamental component of nursing technique. In education, NIC offers students a standardized framework for comprehending and executing nursing interventions. Nursing curriculum often integrates NIC into case studies, simulations, and clinical skills training. By interacting with NIC early in their schooling, students cultivate a systematic method for formulating care plans, choosing interventions, and assessing outcomes.

In clinical practice, NIC improves patient care by standardizing intervention terminology, enhancing documentation, and facilitating better communication among interdisciplinary teams. Nurses can create personalized treatment plans associated with quantifiable outcomes while promoting quality improvement activities with comprehensive intervention data. NIC interventions assist nurses in customizing treatment to address individual patient requirements, enhancing resource utilization and elevating patient satisfaction.

In research, the Nursing Interventions Classification (NIC) provides a basis for assessing the efficacy of nursing interventions. Researchers employ NIC's standardized terminology to formulate comparison research, evaluate intervention effects, and enhance evidence-based practice. NIC fosters interdisciplinary and geographic collaboration by offering a standardized language for interventions, so assuring that findings are reproducible and generalizable [2].

18.3.3 Integration with NANDA International and Nursing Outcomes Classification

NIC operates in conjunction with NANDA-I nursing diagnoses and NOC outcomes to establish a cohesive framework for nursing care. This triadic link optimizes the nursing process, guaranteeing coherence from diagnosis to intervention and evaluation. Integration further promotes interdisciplinary collaboration. Healthcare professionals, including physicians and physical therapists, can readily comprehend and synchronize with nursing care plans utilizing this standardized methodology. This integration enhances care coordination by promoting a mutual comprehension of objectives and strategies [2, 3, 5].

18.3.4 NIC and Infection Control

NIC is essential in infection prevention by providing evidence-based interventions aimed at reducing risks, managing current infections, and educating both patients and healthcare personnel. The "Infection Control" intervention emphasizes the preservation of aseptic procedures, the instruction of patients and families regarding preventive measures, and the implementation of isolation precautions when warranted. Through the documentation and monitoring of these actions, nurses guarantee that care is consistent, focused, and responsive to patient requirements [2].

18.3.5 NIC and Evidence-Based Practice

NIC endorses evidence-based practice by correlating therapies with contemporary research and clinical protocols. Every intervention in NIC is meticulously validated, minimizing variability in care delivery and guaranteeing compliance with the best practices. By advocating for evidence-based interventions, NIC enables nurses to deliver care that is both effective and cost-efficient. This linkage with research guarantees that NIC remains pertinent and responsive to rising healthcare concerns, such as changing patient demographics and technological progress [2].

NIC also plays a vital part in the execution of clinical routes and procedures. In the realm of infection prevention, NIC interventions are included in hospital-wide protocols to guarantee adherence to standards established by regulatory organizations such as the CDC or the WHO. Nurses are proficient in assessing outcomes meticulously, hence enhancing patient safety continuously [6].

18.3.6 Fundamental Interventions for Nursing Specialties

NIC addresses the specific requirements of diverse nursing specialties via focused interventions. These specialized treatments guarantee that NIC is versatile across many practice domains, equipping nurses with resources to successfully address distinct patient populations while upholding a uniform methodology. This adaptability also benefits nursing students focusing on specialized disciplines, as they acquire interventions that directly correspond with their prospective jobs [2, 7].

18.3.7 The Prospects of NIC

As healthcare progresses, NIC adjusts to new trends and technologies. The integration with health information technology, especially electronic health records, improves care coordination and data analysis. International initiatives to standardize NIC enhance its accessibility across varied healthcare systems, guaranteeing its relevance in multiple cultural and clinical environments. Furthermore, NIC addresses current difficulties, such as telehealth and pandemic response, by creating innovative solutions designed for contemporary healthcare delivery [8].

NIC's involvement in tackling socioeconomic determinants of health represents an additional domain of expansion. Interventions that account for socioeconomic variables, access to care, and community engagement are progressively incorporated into NIC's taxonomy. This progression integrates nursing care with overarching public health objectives, ensuring that interventions effectively address health inequities [2].

18.4   Nursing Outcomes Classification (NOC)

The NOC correlates anticipated results with diagnoses and actions. The amalgamation of NANDA-I with NIC and NOC facilitates a cohesive workflow from diagnosis to intervention and assessment. This alignment facilitates comprehensive and evidence-based patient care, guaranteeing that nursing practices are both efficient and responsible [3]. The Nursing Outcomes Classification (NOC) is a cornerstone resource for evaluating nursing care outcomes, providing a standardized language that enables clear communication, effective education, and robust research. Developed to complement the Nursing Interventions Classification (NIC) and NANDA-I diagnoses, NOC offers measurable outcomes that reflect the results of nursing interventions.

NOC serves as a critical tool for improving nursing practice by offering detailed outcome measures for various health conditions. By linking interventions to specific patient outcomes, NOC ensures a results-driven approach to care that is both evidence-based and adaptable to individual patient needs. Its integration into electronic health records and its use across educational, clinical, and research settings demonstrate its versatility and importance in modern nursing [3].

18.4.1 Clinical Utilizations

The systematic organization of NOC provides nurses with a robust framework to evaluate patient progress and assess the effectiveness of interventions. Outcomes are clearly defined with specific indicators and measurement scales, allowing for consistent application in practice. This clarity supports seamless integration into electronic health records (EHR), where standardized documentation enhances communication across interdisciplinary teams.

NOC's ability to support decision-making is vital in creating realistic, patient-centered goals. Nurses are equipped to monitor progress effectively and adapt care plans based on measurable indicators. By fostering interdisciplinary collaboration, NOC ensures all healthcare professionals are aligned in their approach to achieving optimal patient outcomes.

In addition to its use in practice, NOC is a valuable resource for policy development. Its standardized metrics provide a foundation for assessing quality measures and identifying areas for improvement within healthcare systems. This adaptability across various contexts underscores NOC's critical role in advancing nursing and healthcare delivery [3].

18.4.1.1 Improving Patient-Centered Care
The taxonomy facilitates a comprehensive approach to patient treatment by encompassing physical, psychological, social, and spiritual aspects. This method guarantees that care is empathetic and customized to specific requirements [3].

18.4.1.2 Documentation and Correspondence Support
Standardized diagnoses enhance communication across healthcare teams, promoting interdisciplinary collaboration. In clinical settings, NOC enhances patient care by providing measurable benchmarks tailored to specific health conditions. When nurses use NOC in electronic health records, they streamline communication among care teams, reduce redundancies, and promote continuity of care. Furthermore, the measurable nature of NOC outcomes enables nurses to demonstrate the impact of their interventions, fostering accountability and continuous improvement in clinical practice. Electronic health records (EHRs) can integrate these diagnoses, enhancing documentation and promoting continuity of care. This standardization improves the precision and efficacy of health records [3] .

18.4.1.3 Enhancing Education and Research
The document functions as a significant asset for educators and academics. The integration of NOC into nursing education ensures that students are equipped with the skills necessary to deliver evidence-based care. By teaching students to establish patient-centered goals, select effective interventions, and evaluate outcomes, NOC prepares them for the complexities of clinical environments. In educational settings, case studies and role-playing exercises simulate real-world scenarios, allowing students to practice applying NOC outcomes to patient care.

Nursing students acquire a comprehensive understanding of diagnostic processes, while researchers can enhance the evidence foundation to further nursing science. The taxonomy offers a comprehensive framework that facilitates the development of nursing courses and enhances clinical research.

NOC's standardized metrics are essential for advancing nursing research. Researchers use NOC to design studies that evaluate the effectiveness of specific nursing interventions, ensuring that findings are consistent and reproducible. For example, a study examining the impact of wound care techniques on healing progress might use NOC outcomes like "Wound Healing Progress" and "Infection Severity" to measure results accurately [3].

18.4.2 Obstacles and Prospective Pathways

Notwithstanding its advantages, the taxonomy has difficulties. For example:

- Evidence Deficiencies: Certain diagnoses lack substantial validation, requiring additional investigation. Rectifying these deficiencies will augment the taxonomy's dependability and applicability.
- Global Standardization: Variations in healthcare systems and practices necessitate continuous collaboration to maintain global relevance. Initiatives to align taxonomy with worldwide standards will enhance its efficacy.

Subsequent versions will probably emphasize improving clinical validation, incorporating technological innovations, and tackling emerging health trends, including pandemics and climate-related health concerns. These advancements will guarantee that the taxonomy continues leading in nursing science [3].

By providing a common language for outcomes, NOC facilitates collaboration among researchers across disciplines and geographic locations. This universality enhances the generalizability of findings and supports the development of global evidence-based practices. NOC also provides a framework for exploring emerging healthcare challenges, such as the impact of telemedicine on patient outcomes.

18.4.3 Outcomes and NOC Taxonomy

Each NOC outcome is meticulously detailed to ensure precision in its application. Outcomes include a title, a clear definition, a list of specific indicators, and a five-point Likert scale measuring the degree of achievement. This systematic approach allows nurses to tailor care plans to the unique needs of each patient.

The organization of NOC taxonomy ensures that all aspects of patient well-being are considered. Nurses can select outcomes that align with clinical goals, ensuring that care remains patient-centered and holistic. By addressing physical, emotional, and social dimensions of health, NOC empowers nurses to provide comprehensive care [3].

18.4.4 NOC and NIC Linkages

The integration of NOC with NIC facilitates seamless care planning and evaluation [9]. This alignment ensures that each intervention is purposeful and measurable. By linking outcomes to interventions, NOC and NIC together create a workflow that supports continuous quality improvement. Nurses can evaluate the effectiveness of interventions in real time, making adjustments to optimize patient outcomes. This integration also fosters interdisciplinary collaboration, as other healthcare professionals can easily understand the rationale behind nursing interventions and their expected outcomes [2, 3].

18.4.5 Core Outcomes for Nursing Specialties

NOC provides core outcome sets designed for specific nursing specialties. These specialty-specific outcomes allow nurses to customize care plans while maintaining a standardized approach. By focusing on relevant metrics, nurses can address the unique challenges of their patient populations [3, 10].

The application of NOC in infection prevention highlights its relevance in addressing one of healthcare's most critical challenges. Outcomes allow nurses to track patient progress, identify potential complications, and adjust care plans as needed. NOC outcomes are closely tied to NIC interventions aimed at reducing infection risks. By linking these interventions to measurable outcomes, nurses can ensure that infection prevention efforts are both effective and evidence-based [11].

The Nursing Outcomes Classification (NOC) is an essential resource for advancing nursing practice, education, and research. By providing a standardized taxonomy of measurable outcomes, NOC empowers nurses to deliver patient-centered care, evaluate intervention effectiveness, and contribute to evidence-based practices. Its integration with NIC and NANDA-I ensures a holistic approach to care, making NOC indispensable in improving patient outcomes and advancing the nursing profession [3].

18.5   Conclusion

The amalgamation of NANDA International (NANDA-I) taxonomy, Nursing Interventions Classification (NIC), and Nursing Outcomes Classification (NOC) frameworks signifies a revolutionary advancement in nursing practice. This triangle offers a systematic approach for examining, diagnosing, intervening, and evaluating patient treatment. By integrating these procedures, the frameworks standardize nursing practice and enhance its scientific basis, guaranteeing that treatment is consistent, evidence-based, and oriented on the patient.

The NANDA-I taxonomy functions as the essential foundation, providing nurses with the resources to precisely identify patient conditions and dangers. Subsequently, NIC offers an extensive array of therapies designed to target diagnoses. Ultimately, NOC guarantees that the outcomes of these treatments are quantifiable and assessable, facilitating ongoing enhancement in care provision.

This integrated architecture significantly contributes to infection prevention. NANDA-I enables nurses to diagnose issues such as "Risk for Infection" or "Impaired Skin Integrity," hence identifying patients in need of specific preventative interventions. NIC provides comprehensive, evidence-based programs including

"Infection Control," "Wound Care," and "Hand Hygiene Education." These actions enable nurses to proactively mitigate infection risks, guaranteeing that patients receive the highest standard of care. Simultaneously, NOC outcomes like "Infection Severity" and "Wound Healing Progress" let nurses to assess and appraise the efficacy of these interventions, yielding quantifiable insights into patient recovery and general health.

Infection prevention is fundamental to patient safety and public health, with the NANDA-I, NIC, and NOC frameworks provide a solid basis for tackling this vital issue. By encouraging interdisciplinary teamwork and enhancing responsibility, these frameworks guarantee that nursing care significantly reduces healthcare-associated infections and improves patient outcomes.

The ongoing evolution of healthcare necessitates the continued integration of NANDA-I, NIC, and NOC in determining the future of nursing. This framework empowers nurses to provide high-quality care and enhances the profession's capacity to adapt to new challenges, including rising infectious diseases, technological improvements, and changing patient demographics. The NANDA-I, NIC, and NOC frameworks illustrate the integration of theory and practice, highlighting the essential contribution of nursing to enhancing global health outcomes.

References

1. Heather T. NANDA international nursing diagnoses: definitions & classification, 2012–2014. Wiley-Blackwell; 2011.
2. Wagner CM, Butcher HK, Clarke MF. Nursing interventions classification (NIC)-E-book: nursing interventions classification (NIC)-E-book. Elsevier Health Sciences; 2023.
3. Moorhead S, Swanson E, Johnson M. Nursing outcomes classification (NOC)-E-book: nursing outcomes classification (NOC)-E-Book. Elsevier Health Sciences; 2023.
4. Rabelo-Silva ER, Monteiro Mantovani V, López Pedraza L, Cardoso PC, Takao Lopes C, Herdman TH. International collaboration and new research evidence on Nanda international terminology. Int J Nurs Knowl. 2021;32(2):103–7.
5. Herdman TH, Kamitsuru S. Nursing diagnoses. Elsevier Health Sciences; 2021.
6. De Cordova PB, Lucero RJ, Hyun S, Quinlan P, Price K, Stone PW. Using the nursing interventions classification as a potential measure of nurse workload. J Nurs Care Qual. 2010;25(1):39–45.
7. Molina-Mula J, Gallo-Estrada J. Impact of nurse-patient relationship on quality of care and patient autonomy in decision-making. Int J Environ Res Public Health. 2020;17(3):835.
8. Maleki Varnosfaderani S, Forouzanfar M. The role of AI in hospitals and clinics: transforming healthcare in the 21st century. Bioengineering. 2024;11(4):337.
9. Prophet C, Dorr G, Gibbs T, Porcella A, editors. Implementation of standardized nursing languages (NIC, NOC) in on-line care planning and documentation, Nursing informatics. IOS Press; 1997.
10. Anderson CA, Keenan G, Jones J. Using bibliometrics to support your selection of a nursing terminology set. Comput Inform Nurs. 2009;27(2):82–90.
11. Lippens B. Use of NANDA, NIC, and NOC in infection control. Int J Nurs Terminol Classif. 2003;14:20.